THE 2022 COMPLETE CALORIE COUNTER

YOUR ESSENTIAL GUIDE TO COUNTING CALORIES FOR WEIGHT LOSS AND HEALTH

DR. H. MAHER

CONTENTS

INTRODUCTION

The best diets, those that work, restrict calories, supply sufficient and high-quality nutrients, banish bad foods, and balance hormones that help lower your blood sugar, improve your glycemic control, and regulate your weight. Diets do this in three main ways:

1. getting you to eat sufficient good foods and/or banish bad ones
2. getting you aware of foods and nutrients you should include in your diet to achieve weight loss, better diabetes control, and prevent complications.
3. changing some of your bad eating habits and the ways you consider highly processed foods and refined carbohydrates

The best diet for losing weight and/or diabetes control is one that is good for all body parts, from your brain to your heart to your pancreas. It is also a diet you can embrace and live with for a long time. In other words, a powerful diet rooted in nature that controls your calorie intake, offers flexible eating patterns, provides healthy choices, banishes unhealthy foods, and doesn't require an extensive (and probably expensive) shopping list or supplements.

Getting the right amount of calories from a variety of healthy foods, including whole foods, minimally processed foods, fruits, vegetables, whole grains, high-quality proteins, healthy fats, constitute the patterns of the healthiest diet. Several studies have established that a balanced caloric consumption from fruits, vegetables, minimally processed foods, and whole grains is associated with a significant decrease in the risk of obesity, diabetes, cardiovascular illnesses, and chronic inflammatory diseases. In addition, counting calories while avoiding highly processed foods and increasing exercise have been found to produce a noticeable effect on weight loss, glycemic control, and inflammation.

To actually achieve and maintain a healthy weight, you should focus on the type of calories you put on your plate. Calories have long been mistakenly considered equal. The same reasoning was applied to carbohydrates, fats, and proteins. And thus, the obesity epidemic was viewed as a result of an increase in caloric consumption of fats. Recent research has established that highly processed foods and refined carbohydrates are the real culprits. Some high-fat-containing foods are very healthy, battle inflammation diabetes, and fight obesity, provided you respect your caloric intake. In contrast, ultra-processed foods, refined carbohydrates, and high glycemic foods are associated with an increased risk of obesity, diabetes, cardiovascular and autoimmune diseases, and chronic inflammatory disorders.

Counting calories doesn't necessarily mean eating less food. Instead, you'll have the tools to make smarter foods choices and cut calories without eating less and feeling hungry. With "The 2022 Calorie Counter", you'll discover how to make healthier food choices, replace some higher calorie foods with better alternatives, avoid high glycemic foods that cause blood sugar spikes, and increase the release of insulin, and ghrelin— the hunger hormone which stimulates your appetite, increases food consumption and promotes fat storage.

This book is based on the USDA (U.S. Department of Agriculture) National Nutrient Database for Standard Reference SR11-SR28, Release 28, which is the primary source of food composition data in the United States. It is designed to help you count carbohydrates and calories accurately and easily. Alphabetical listings make locating your foods easy and quick. Foods are divided into 19 categories:

- Beverages
- Baked Foods
- Beans and Lentils
- Breakfast Cereals
- Dairy and Egg Products
- Fast Foods
- Fats and Oils
- Fish & Seafood
- Fruits & Fruits Products
- Grains and Pasta
- Meats and Poultry
- Nuts and Seeds
- Prepared Meals
- Restaurant Foods
- Snacks
- Soups and Sauces
- Spices and Herbs
- Sweets
- Vegetables & vegetable products

PART I

CALORIES AND THE HEALTHY DIET

1

FOOD, WEIGHT LOSS AND DIABETES

The Healthy Eating

Adhering to a healthy diet is more than restricting your calories, selecting foods you eat, limiting your carbohydrates intake, and avoiding high glycemic index foods; it's also about sticking to the proper lifestyle that promotes effective weight loss, better diabetes management, healthier life, and well-being. Thus, you have to focus simultaneously on your diet and lifestyle to reap all the health benefits of healthy eating.

You can only focus on diet and keep your habits, but you'll not experience optimum health and achieve your goals. The two significant areas in which change is highly advised are physical activity and sleeping habits. Practicing regular physical activity will drive many beneficial effects in improving blood sugar control, insulin sensitivity, and hormones balance. Sleeping well helps your body and brain function correctly, boost your immune system, improve your mental health. By committing to these easy and positive changes, you will expect to achieve a healthy weight, better blood glucose control, positive health outcomes, and prevent diabetes and some chronic disorders.

People who adhere to the healthy eating patterns more closely have consistently lower levels of blood sugar levels, lower blood pressure, increased LDL cholesterol, reduced HDL cholesterol, and reduced triglycerides than those following other diets. It is considered healthier than modern fad diets (e.g., keto diet, low-carb, high-fat diets) because it is centered around restricting calories, reducing carbohydrates intakes, eating whole, unprocessed, or minimally processed foods, and avoiding high glycemic foods and pro-inflammatory agents.

- **Diet, Weight Loss, and Diabetes**

For years, hundreds of diets have been created with a lot of promises in terms of weight loss, inflammation reduction, diabetes reversal. Low-fat diets, low carb high fats diets were thought to be the best approaches to lose weight, control diabetes, and achieve a healthy weight. However, a growing body of evidence shows that these diets often don't work:

- low-fat diets have the tendency to replace fat with easily digested carbohydrates.
- low-carb high-fat diets overlook the importance of carbohydrates and often replace carbohydrates with highly processed fat-containing foods.
- fad diets often overlook the body's fundamental need for a balanced diet

The best diets, those that work, restrict calories, supply sufficient and high-quality nutrients, banish bad foods, and balance hormones that help lower your blood sugar, improve your glycemic control, and regulate your weight. Diets do this in three main ways:

1. getting you to eat sufficient good foods and/or banish bad ones
2. getting you aware of foods and nutrients you should include in your diet to achieve weight loss, better diabetes control, and prevent complications.
3. changing some of your bad eating habits and the ways you consider highly processed foods and refined carbohydrates

The best diet for losing weight and/or diabetes control is one that is good for all body parts, from your brain to your heart to your pancreas. It is also a diet you can embrace and live with for a long time. In other words, a powerful diet rooted in nature that offers a flexible eating pattern, provides healthy choices, banishes unhealthy foods, and doesn't require an extensive (and probably expensive) shopping list or supplements.

A diabetic balanced diet with sufficient and right nutritional elements is critical for battling diabetes, weight gain, and obesity. Both nutritional deficiency and excess are tied with diseases and poor health conditions. Nutritional excess, particularly in highly-processed foods, refined carbohydrates, saturated fats, trans-fatty acids, sugar-sweetened foods, and sodium, can result in severe chronic inflammatory illnesses such as autoimmune disease, cardio-vascular disease, bone disorders, diabetes as well as obesity. In contrast, nutritional deficiencies can lead to impairments of body function, weight loss, fatigue, and conditions associated with vitamin and mineral deficiencies.

One diet that allows that is a Low glycemic type diet. Such a diet—and its many variations—usually include:

- several servings of plant foods (e.g., vegetables, fruits) a day
- whole and minimally processed foods

- daily serving of seeds and nuts
- healthy fats and oils high in omega-3 fatty acids (canola, cod liver oil, fatty fish, flaxseed oil, Walnut oil, sunflower oil, etc.)
- lean protein mainly from fish, poultry, and nuts
- limited amounts of red meat
- limited amounts of sodium
- very limited quantities of refined carbohydrates (e.g., white flour, white, rice, white sugar, brown sugar, honey, corn syrup)
- limited alcoholic drinks
- NO high glycemic index foods
- NO trans fats
- NO highly processed foods

- **Dietary carbohydrates and diabetes**

Increased intake of carbohydrates-containing foods with a higher glycemic index is found to cause a high spike in blood sugar and insulin release, making it harder to control diabetes, increasing the risk of developing diabetes for healthy people, increasing the risk of severe complications, and worsening inflammation. Conversely, eating carbohydrates-containing foods with a low glycemic index is associated with positive health outcomes, including modulating inflammation, regulating immune system responses, and will help you gain close control over your blood sugar.

In addition, many studies have established that the quality of carbohydrates has a significant impact on inflammation, and the occurrence of diabetes complications. Low-quality carbohydrates such as highly processed foods and refined carbs are associated with increased inflammation, both acute and chronic, impaired immune system responses, poor blood glucose control, and increased risk of diabetes complications. Conversely, high-quality foods such as whole foods or minimally processed food with low glycemic index food are linked with better health outcomes, including better control of blood glucose, and reduced acute and chronic inflammation.

- **Dietary fats and diabetes**

Another important nutrient you should consider as part of healthy eating is fat. Eating the right amount of the right type of fat is essential whether you are managing diabetes or aiming to achieve a healthy weight.

In addition, fats are higher in calories per gram compared to proteins or carbohydrates. A gram of dietary fat has nearly 9 calories, while a gram of carbohydrate has roughly 4 calories or protein has about 4 calories. Thus, you should be aware of serving sizes when eating fats.

Eating the right types of fat is also critical for managing type 1 and type 2 diabetes and lowering the risk of developing some chronic diseases such as heart illnesses, strokes, kidneys diseases, and chronic inflammatory diseases.

Several studies have established that replacing trans fats and saturated fats with unsaturated fats (monounsaturated and polyunsaturated) reduces the risk of cardiovascular diseases in high-risk populations, including individuals with diabetes.

In addition, studies also found that replacing trans fats and saturated fat intake with low glycemic carbohydrates (e.g., wholegrain, fiber-rich fruits, fiber-rich vegetables, beans) results in cardiovascular benefits without altering the blood glucose control.

On the other side, a growing body of evidence has revealed how dietary fat intake affects the inflammatory status and focused on the gut microbiome as an important factor explaining the increase of inflammation biomarkers and fat intake. Trans fats are tied with various adverse health effects, worsen inflammation, and trigger some diabetes complications. The consumption of high amounts of saturated fats increases the LDL cholesterol (bad form) promotes and aggravates inflammation.

The American Diabetes Association recommends swapping saturated and trans fats in your diet by healthiest choices such as monounsaturated and polyunsaturated fats.

Healthy fats such as omega-3 fatty acids are associated with decreased inflammation and reduced risk of developing some chronic conditions. Several studies have investigated the role of omega-3 fatty acids in association with metformin to reduce triglyceride levels in diabetic patients with hypertriglyceridemia. Omega-3 fatty acids were found effective in reducing the triglyceride level significantly by 20-65%. Omega-3 fatty acids were also found to improve the effectiveness of statins and thus decrease the risk of cardiovascular diseases among diabetic patients with hypertriglyceridemia.

- **The Essential Role of Vitamin D**

It is established that Vitamin D is essential for normal glucose metabolism and improvement of insulin sensitivity. Therefore, vitamin D supplementation appears to promote glucose-mediated insulin secretion allowing vitamin D to play a beneficial role in glucose metabolism by:

1. regulating insulin secretion and promoting the survival of beta-cells, which results in releasing insulin in a tightly regulated manner to maintain blood glucose levels in the adequate range.
2. regulating the calcium flux within beta-cells, which results

in improving insulin secretion directly because insulin secretion is a calcium-dependent process. Vitamin D stimulates insulin secretion and benefits beta-cell secretory function when calcium levels are adequate.

3. modulating the adaptive and innate immune responses which results in a preventative effect on autoimmune such as type 1 diabetes. Vitamin D modulates the immune system's response and prevents the destruction of insulin-secreting pancreatic beta-cells, which causes the development of type 1 diabetes.

4. reducing substantially systemic inflammation involved in insulin resistance and the development of type 2 diabetes. Recent studies have established that vitamin D plays an essential role in modulating the inflammation system by inhibiting the proliferation of pro-inflammatory cells and regulating the production of inflammatory cytokines.

5. improving insulin sensitivity and enhancing pancreatic beta-cell function.

2

EATING WHOLE AND MINIMALLY PROCESSED FOODS

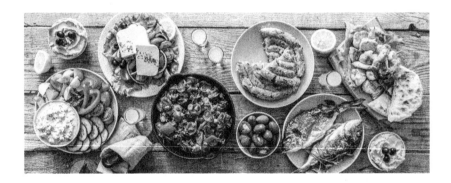

Most Americans don't eat whole foods anymore. They eat processed and highly-processed foods that are generally inferior to unprocessed or minimally processed foods. In fact, highly-processed foods are generally industrially-made and contain many ingredients, including high-fructose corn syrup, trans fats, monosodium glutamate, artificial sweeteners, flavors, colors, and other chemical additives. Highly-processed foods are believed to be a significant contributor to the obesity epidemic in the world, promoting diabetes, chronic inflammation, and the prevalence of autoimmune diseases. Therefore, we must distinguish between healthy processed foods to include in your diet and those to exclude because they are considered unhealthy and pro-inflammatory. For this reason, the next chapter (chapter 10) is fundamental because it contains foods groups based on the NOVA classification system. To adhere to a healthy diet, you must get familiar with the four NOVA foods groups.

Whole food refers to unprocessed or minimally processed food— a nature-made food without added sugars, fat, sodium, flavorings, or other artificial ingredients. It has not been broken down by the man intervention into its components and refined into a new form. Whole Foods are generally close to their natural state, unprocessed, and unrefined. Whole foods have little to no additives or preservatives.

A healthy diet is not a specific diet with strict recommendations. Instead, it refers to an eating plan that primarily restricts calories, and selects whole and minimally processed foods that result in many health benefits, including effective weight loss, better glycemic control, inflammation reduction, diabetes prevention, and hypertension prevention and treatment.

- **The Healthy Eating Main Principles**

The healthy diet is a balanced, easy, long-term, and sustainable diet that counts calories, selects whole, minimally processed foods, and limits animal products. It mainly focuses on plants, including vegetables, fruits, whole grains, legumes, seeds, and nuts, which should make up most of what you eat. You then have to design your eating plan around **unprocessed and minimally processed foods (NOVA group 1 of foods)** and, as much as you can, **avoid those that are processed (NOVA group 2 of foods)** and **absolutely exclude highly-processed (NOVA group 3 of foods)**.

The healthy diet supplies your body with low glycemic unprocessed or minimally processed foods **(NOVA group 1 of foods)**, with little to no unhealthy added constituents.

Carbohydrates, Proteins, and Fats: How do macronutrients fit into the healthy diet?

1. Carbohydrates

The choice of high-quality macronutrients is crucial for the success of the healthy diet.

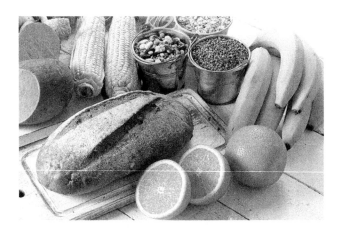

- **Knowing how carbohydrates can work for you or against you**

The healthy eating isn't just about counting calories and eating unprocessed and minimally processed foods; a large part of controlling your blood glucose, and hormones release is strongly impacted by the type of carbohydrates you eat.

Types of Carbohydrates in Your Diet

When you eat carbohydrates, your body breaks them down into glucose, which is absorbed into the bloodstream. As the glucose level rises in your body, the pancreas releases insulin, a peptide hormone responsible for maintaining normal blood glucose levels. Insulin moves glucose from the blood into the cells, where it can be used as an energy source. Dietary carbohydrates can be divided into three major categories:

- sugars: Short-chain carbs found in foods such as fructose, glucose, sucrose, and galactose.
- starches: Long-chain of glucose molecules, which get transformed into glucose during digestion.
- fibers: are divided into soluble and insoluble.

Carbohydrates can also be divided according to their chemical composition into simple and complex carbs:

- complex carbohydrates are formed by sugar molecules that are linked together in complex and long chains. Complex carbs are found in vegetables, fruits, peas, beans, and whole grains and contain natural fiber. These types of food are considered healthy.
- simple carbohydrates are transformed quickly by the body and induce blood sugar spikes. They are found in high amounts in processed foods and refined sugars. The consumption of this type of carbs is associated with medical conditions such as type 2 diabetes, obesity, metabolism problem. Simple carbs foods are also deprived of essential nutrients and vitamins.

Choosing the best carbohydrate-containing foods

The quality of the carbohydrates you eat is crucial in adjusting the level of some hormones that influences inflammation or controls weight gain, including insulin, cortisol, leptin, peptide YY. For instance, low-quality carbs (high glycemic foods) are quickly digested and lead to blood glucose spikes, which may aggravate diabetes, worsen inflammation, cause weight gain, obesity, insulin resistance, and increased cortisol levels. Conversely, the soluble and insoluble fibers in whole foods (low glycemic foods) are known to offset glucose conversion, prevent higher insulin supplies, and avoid irregular blood sugar variations that induce an excess of cortisol and insulin release.

2. Protein

Eating an adequate amount of protein is extremely important for your health because it plays a crucial role in your body's vital processes and metabolisms, such as building and repairing tissues, building muscles, blood, hair, and skin, and producing hormones, enzymes, and other body chemicals.

Unlike carbohydrates and fat, your body does not store protein, and you need to eat the necessary amount to keep the right hormonal balance and a healthy body.

Plus, eating protein reduces levels of ghrelin (the hunger hormone) and stimulates the production of the satiety hormones (PYY and GLP-1)

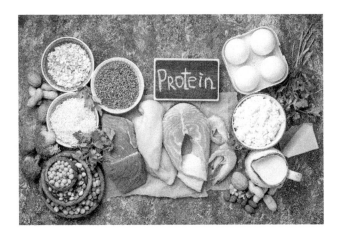

When you eat protein, it's transformed into amino acids, which help your body with various processes such as building muscle and regulating immune function.

However, many studies have established that red meat, processed meats, and highly processed meats promote and aggravate inflammation.

On the adapted whole foods diet, animal protein is consumed very moderately following the degree of food processing. You have to select animal sources of protein from the NOVA food group 1 (unprocessed or minimally processed), which include:

- poultry meat (fresh, chilled, or frozen), whole, steaks, fillets, and other cuts
- fish (fresh, chilled, or frozen), whole, steaks, fillets, and other cuts

You have also to choose vegetable sources of protein from the NOVA food group 1 (unprocessed or minimally processed), which include:

- lentils
- chickpeas
- green peas
- nuts
- seeds
- quinoa
- wild rice
- broccoli
- spinach
- asparagus
- artichokes
- sweet potatoes
- Brussels sprouts

Guidelines for individualized protein intake

The RDA (international Recommended Dietary Allowance) for protein is 0.8 g per kg of body weight, regardless of age. This recommendation is derived as the minimum amount to maintain nitrogen balance; however, it is not optimized for women's needs or physical activity levels.

Based on a recent body of evidence, the protein recommended intake from all sources can be adjusted to 1.4-1.8 grams per kg of your body weight.

The Protein Quality

The optimal source of protein is based on the calculation of the PDCAA (Protein Digestibility Corrected Amino Acid) Score or the DIAA (Digestibility Indispensable Amino Acid) Score. Thus, animal-based foods were identified as a superior source of protein because they offer a complete composition of essential amino acids, with higher bioavailability and digestibility (>90%). Thus, you have to eat a combination of animal proteins and plant proteins, mainly in the NOVA group 1 of foods (unprocessed and minimally processed).

Collagen, an essential ingredient

The most abundant type of protein in your body is collagen. Ligaments, tendons, skin, hair, nails, discs, and bones are collagen. Collagen is rich in amino acids that play an essential role in the building of joint cartilage. It also plays an important role in strengthening and rebuilding the lining of our digestive tract, thus healing gut inflammation and subsequently improving the immune system and helping modulate inflammation.

During the normal aging process, your body begins to experience a decline in the synthesis of collagen proteins. According to studies, this decline in collagen production starts around 30, at a rate of 1% per year. At the age of fifty, the rate jump to up to 3%, causing health issues::

- Muscle stiffness
- Aging joint
- Wrinkles and fine lines
- Lack of tone
- Aging skin
- Healing of wounds slower
- Frequent fatigue.

Consuming more collagen will boost your body's collagen protection. So it is recommended that your daily intake of collagen represent up to 25% of protein.

The beneficial effects include:

• Decreased gut inflammation.

• Improved intestinal health.

• Less articular pain.

• Less hair loss.

• Better skin.

• Increased muscle mass.

Foods rich in collagen

Here are some of the best collagen-rich foods you can add to your diet:

Bone broth

Made by simmering bones, tendons, ligaments, and skin of beef, bone broth is an excellent source of collagen and several essential amino acids. Bone broth is also available in powder, bar, or even capsules, so you can add it to your diet as a supplement.

Spirulina

This seaweed is an excellent source of plant-based amino acids, which are a key component of collagen. Spirulina can be found in dried form at most health food stores.

Codfish

Codfish, like most other types of white fish, is a good source of collagen in addition to selenium, vitamin B6 and phosphorus.

Eggs

Eggs are a good source of collagen, including glycine and proline.

---

3. Fats

After carbohydrates and proteins, it is essential to optimize the choice of your dietary fat.

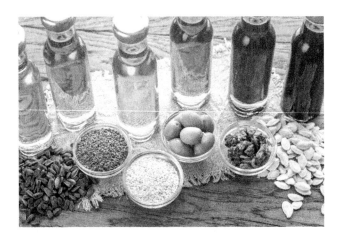

What is fat, and why it is essential for your health?

Dietary fats are found in both animals and vegetables and are essential for your living since they provide your body energy and support cell growth.

Fats also provide some valuable benefits and play essential roles, including:

- helping your body absorb some nutrients such as vitamins A, D, E, and K.
- helping your body produce the necessary hormones.
- regulating inflammation and immunity issues.
- maintaining the health of your cells (skin, hair cells)

How many different fats are there?

There are four major fats in food, based on their chemical structures and physical properties:

- Saturated fat (bad fat; reduce your intake of saturated fat): is a kind of fat in which the fatty acid chain of carbon atoms holds as many hydrogen atoms as possible (saturated with hydrogens). This form of saturated fat is associated with various adverse health effects, including aggravation of inflammation.
- Trans fat (very bad fat; to exclude completely): (trans-unsaturated fatty acids or trans fatty acids) are a form of unsaturated fat associated with various adverse health effects and known to worsen inflammation.
- Monounsaturated fats (healthy fat): are a type of unsaturated fat but have only one double bond. These fats are associated with positive health effects and may replace bad fats. Monounsaturated fats are found in olive oil, avocados, and some nuts
- Polyunsaturated fat (healthy fat): The two major classes of polyunsaturated fats are omega-3 and omega-6 fatty acids. However, many studies have shown that omega-3 and omega-6 have different inflammatory properties. Omega-3 fatty acids have powerful anti-inflammatory effects, while omega-6 tend to promote inflammation.

What is cholesterol?

Cholesterol is a waxy, fat-like substance found in all the cells in your body. Plus, your body needs some cholesterol to produce steroid hormones, vitamin D, and bile acid that helps you digest fats. Contrary to popular belief, your body makes all the cholesterol it needs in the liver. Cholesterol is supplied in small quantities (less than 15%) by plant and animals foods.

More than 85% of the cholesterol in your bloodstream comes from your liver rather than from the food you eat. Dietary cholesterol has little impact on raising blood cholesterol levels, which is valuable information from a diet perspective.

A recent and growing body of evidence has pointed to inflammation as the most important cause of cardiovascular diseases rather than cholesterol. While a high cholesterol level in the blood can be dangerous, maintaining the right balance of cholesterol is essential for your health.

What types of fat should you eat?

Eating an adapted whole foods diet implies selecting fats found naturally in food and not being processed. You have then to choose fat-rich foods belonging to the NOVA group 1 of foods (unprocessed and minimally processed foods).

Examples of healthy sources of fat include:

- butter and ghee (clarified butter)
- cheese
- avocado (the fruit or avocado oil)
- cacao butter and powder
- sardines, anchovies
- salmon
- olives and olive oil
- macadamias and macadamia oil
- almonds and almonds oil

- Brazil nuts and Brazil nuts oil
- hazelnuts and hazelnuts oil
- pecan and pecan oil

What Are Fatty Acids?

Fatty acids are a form of hydrocarbon chains with carboxyl at one end and methyl at the other. The bioloGical activity of fatty acids is determined by the length of their carbon chain and their double bonds' number and position.

While saturated fatty acids do not contain double bonds within the acyl chain, unsaturated fatty acids include at least one double bond.

When two or more double bonds are present in their chain, unsaturated fatty acids are referred to as Dietary polyunsaturated fatty acids (PUFAs) and have been associated with cholesterol-lowering properties. The two families of PUFA are omega-3 and omega-6.

What Are Omega-3 Fatty Acids?

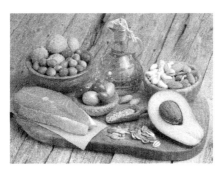

Omega-3 fatty acids are a type of polyunsaturated fats that the body can't produce. Omega-3 fatty acids are essential fats, so you have to get them from your diet.

There are various types of omega-3 fats, which differ by their chemical structure. The three most common types of omega-3 are:

- Eicosapentaenoic acid (EPA)
- Docosahexaenoic acid (DHA)
- Alpha-linolenic acid (ALA)

What Are Omega-6 Fatty Acids?

Like omega-3, omega-6 fatty acids are polyunsaturated fatty acids. omega-6 fatty acids are abundant and account for most polyunsaturated fatty acids in the food supply.

Following different recommendations and guidelines, we recommend a ratio of 4/1 omega-6 to omega-3 or less, which means that for 400 milligrams of omega-6, you have to consume 100 milligrams of omega-3. However, the Western diet has a very high ratio between 10/1 and 50/1.

Why and how is the excess of omega-6 harmful?

A high amount of omega-6 polyunsaturated fatty acids associated with a very high ratio of omega-6/omega-3 is a constant in most Western diets, including the keto diet. That increases the pathogenesis of several diseases, such as cancer, cardiovascular disease, autoimmune and inflammatory diseases. Conversely, high levels of omega-3 associated with a low ratio of omega-6/omega-3 induce health benefits. For example, a ratio omega-6/omega-3 of 4/1 was correlated to a 70% reduction in mortality.

This explains why the notion of the omega-6 / omega-3 ratio is essential in weight loss and health management.

Consuming fatty fish twice a week, eating whole foods, choosing dairy products and meat from grass-fed animals can help you improve your omega-6:omega-3 ratio.

3

EATING LOW GLYCEMIC AND ANTI-INFLAMMATORY FOODS

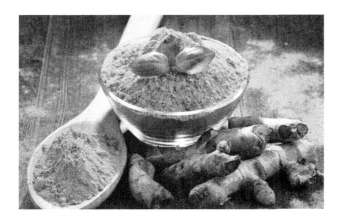

Growing lines of evidence indicate that various dietary polyphenols and flavonoids positively influence blood sugar at different levels, help control and prevent diabetes complications. Antioxidants also play a beneficial and protective role of the pancreatic beta-cells against glucose toxicity in diabetic patients. Thus, consuming polyphenols-rich foods, flavonoids-rich foods, and antioxidants will help you closely control your blood sugar levels, reduce the risk of developing chronic inflammatory diseases and prevent diabetes complications.

- **1. Eating low glycemic index vegetables and fruits**

In the glycemic index diet, you have to eat low glycemic index fruits and vegetables to keep close control of your blood sugar level. In addition, non-starchy vegetables and fruits are good sources of anti-inflammatory nutrients such as polyphenols, antioxidants, and flavonoids which contribute to lowering inflammation and, in turn, reducing the risk of diabetes complications.

The serving sizes for low glycemic index vegetables and fruits are equivalent to:

- 1 cup raw or salad vegetables
- 1/2 cup cooked vegetables
- 3/4 cup (6oz) vegetable juice homemade and unsweetened
- ½ cup of cooked beans, lentils, and peas
- 1 medium piece of fruit
- 1 cup (6 oz) of sliced fruits
- ½ cup (4 oz) of fruit juice

The total vegetable intake (per day) is equivalent to 8-10 servings. You have to vary your meals using the maximal recommended amount as follows:

- "Dark-Green Vegetables" group up to 2 servings
- "Red & Orange Vegetables" group up to 3 servings
- "Beans, Peas, Lentils" group up to 2 servings
- "Starchy Vegetables" group up to 1 serving
- "Other Vegetables" group up to 3 servings

The total fruit intake is equivalent to 2-4 servings per day.

- **2. Increasing your Omega-3 Fatty Acids intake**

Omega-3 fatty acids are a healthy type of polyunsaturated fats associated with beneficial health effects such as

- decreasing inflammation
- improving heart health
- supporting mental health
- decreasing liver fat
- helping in the prevention of many chronic conditions
- promoting bone health

Strategies to increase your weekly intake of omega-3 fatty acids include regularly eating omega-3-rich nuts and seeds—such as chia seed, flaxseed, Hemp seed—, eating fatty fish—such as salmon, sardines, anchovies, mackerel, and herring. The weekly fish intake is equivalent to 10 servings (a serving is equal to 3 to 4 ounces). So target eating 6-8 servings of fatty fish per week.

- **3. Choosing healthy fats**

A healthy diet is rich in omega-3 and lower in omega-6 than most diets. High levels of omega-3 combined with a low (omega-6/omega-3) are associated with many health benefits, including a significant reduction of unnecessary inflammation and diabetes complications. For example, a ratio (omega-6/omega-3) of 4/1 was correlated to a 70% reduction in mortality. So, based on recent studies, you have to keep the ratio (omega-6/omega-3) in the range of 1/1 and 4/1, which is associated with positive health outcomes.

Strategies to achieve an adequate ratio (omega-6/omega-3) include

- consuming fatty fish (e.g., sardines, mackerels, salmon, herring, anchovies) twice a week,
- consuming nuts and seeds (e.g., flax seeds, chia seeds, walnuts) twice a week.

- **4. Increasing olive oil consumption**

Recent studies have established that an extra virgin olive oil-rich diet reduces glucose levels, LDL cholesterol (bad), and triglycerides. And thus, prevents a series of illnesses that are very common among diabetic patients.

The anti-diabetes benefits of Extra Virgin Olive Oil (EVOO) increase with the daily ingested amount. A minimum of extra virgin olive oil of four tablespoons per day is necessary to provide beneficial anti-diabetes and antioxidant effects. When cooking, EVOO is an excellent choice as it has been well established that it helps reduce blood sugar levels, reduce blood pressure, lower bad cholesterol (LDL), and decrease inflammation. The nutritional composition of virgin olive is comprised of mainly

- monounsaturated fatty acids (69.2% for extra virgin olive oil), mainly Oleic acid (omega-9)
- saturated fats (15.4% for extra virgin olive oil) mainly Stearic acid and Palmitic Acid
- polyunsaturated (9.07% for extra virgin olive oil), mainly Linoleic acid (omega-3)
- Polyphenols
- Vitamin E, Carotenoids, and Squalene

Strategies to increase your daily intake of olive oil include

- replacing butter with EVOO,

- using olive oil as finishing oil for your meals,
- replacing the oil you use for cooking,
- roasting, and frying with EVOO.

- **5. Including anti-inflammatory spices in your eating plan**

Over the several last decades, extensive research has revealed that some spices and their active components exhibit tremendous anti-inflammatory benefits. Thus, spices have been found to prevent or decrease the severity of diabetes complications as well as a number of chronic conditions such as arthritis, asthma, multiple sclerosis, cardiovascular diseases, lupus, cancer, and neurodegenerative diseases. The most common spices used for their anti-inflammatory activities are

- turmeric,
- green tea,
- garlic,
- ginger,
- cayenne pepper,
- black pepper,
- black cumin,
- clove,
- cumin,
- ginseng,
- cardamom,
- parsley
- cinnamon,
- rosemary,
- chives,
- basil,
- cilantro

In addition, spices have a unique property to add flavor to any meal without adding fats or salt. Therefore, you should consider integrating herbs as part of your daily diet when cooking.

Some strategies for getting more herbs and spices in your diet include

- using some fresh herbs as the main ingredient (e.g., herb salad, tabbouleh salad),
- replacing some green vegetables in salads with herbs,
- substituting (or reducing) salt in a recipe with spices,
- replacing mayonnaise with basil-olive oil preparation,
- drinking 3–4 cups of green tea daily.

- **6. Drinking more water**

Water is critical for life. Without water, there is no life. All of the organs of our body, such as the heart, brain, lungs, and muscles, contain a significant quantity of water and need water to stay healthy.

Every day we lose water, and we need to replace it through a regular water supply. Otherwise, we can suffer from dehydration, which may alter the normal body's functions.

The recommended water intake for men aged 19+ is 3 liters (13 cups), and for women aged 19+ is 2.2 liters (9 cups) each day.

4

AVOIDING HIGH GLYCEMIC AND INFLAMMATORY FOODS

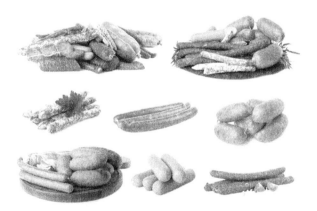

- I. Limiting moderate glycemic index foods and avoiding high glycemic foods

Eating according to the calorie counting principle looks simple because all you need to do is count the calories in all foods you eat and keep the amount of calories ingested at each meal under close control.

Avoiding high glycemic index foods will let you take more control of your glycemic level, avoid insulin spikes, and increased ghrelin secretion. You may follow these simple and complementary guidelines:

- Eat smaller amounts of moderate glycemic index foods (GI value:56 to 69)
- And mostly avoid high glycemic index foods (GI value: 70 and up)

- **2. Excluding Trans-Fats containing Foods**

Trans-fatty acids are mostly industrially manufactured fats produced during the hydrogenation process that adds hydrogen to liquid vegetable oils to transform the liquid to a solid form at room temperature. Trans fats give foods a desirable taste and texture. However, unlike other dietary fats, consuming trans-fatty acids raises the level of your bad cholesterol (LDL), lowers your good cholesterol (HDL) levels, increases your risk of developing severe cardiovascular conditions certain cancers, and aggravates inflammation. Trans fats may be present in several food products, including:

- fried fast foods, including french fries, fried chicken, battered fish, mozzarella sticks, and doughnuts
- margarine
- peanut butter
- baked goods, such as cakes, pies, and cookies made with margarine or vegetable shortening
- vegetable shortening

Strategies to reduce drastically trans fats intake include

- avoiding or reducing intakes of fried fast foods—including french fries, fried chicken, battered fish, mozzarella sticks,

and doughnuts—margarine, peanut butter, frozen pizza,
baked goods made with margarine or vegetable shortening
- eating smaller portion sizes
- consuming trans-fat-containing foods less frequently.

- **3. Eating a little less red meat but enough proteins**

There is little evidence that red meat may contribute to inflammation and alter glycemic control, while some recent studies revealed that unprocessed red meat might be associated with less inflammation and is safe for people with diabetes. However, there is a consensus about the danger of consuming processed red meat such as sausage, bacon, salami, and hot dogs. A 2012 study funded and supported by some health and nutrition government agencies has established the link between processed red meal consumption and increased total mortality. It also revealed that daily unprocessed red meat consumption raised the risk of total mortality by 13%. The study revealed that replacing one serving of red meat per day with other proteins sources such as fish, poultry, and nuts could decrease the risk of mortality by 7-19%.

These findings suggest that you should restrict your red meat intake to reduce inflammation, prevent and delay diabetes complications.

Eating an adequate amount of protein is extremely important for your health because proteins play a crucial role in your body's vital processes and metabolisms, such as building and repairing tissues, building muscles, blood, hair, and skin, regulating some inflammatory response, and producing hormones, enzymes, and other body chemicals. The weekly recommended proteins intake is equivalent to

- 30 servings of animal proteins (mainly lean white meat, and eggs)
- 10 servings of seafood

- 5 servings of nuts and seeds

By restricting red meat intake in the range of 1/5 to 1/4 of animal proteins (e.g., 6 to 7.5 servings of red meat per week), you may experience improvement in your overall health and reduction of some symptoms caused by inflammation.

FOOD PROCESSING CLASSIFICATION: OVERVIEW

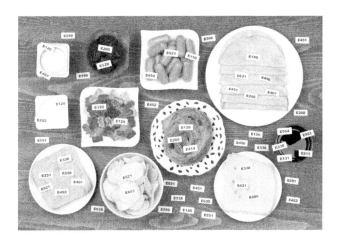

Food processing has been practiced for centuries in form of cooking, dehydrating, fermenting, ultraviolet radiation, and salt preservation. However, modern food processing methods are more sophisticated and complex, and alter considerably foods, by adding many ingredients including trans fats, high-fructose corn syrup, salts, artificial sweeteners, flavors, colors, and other chemical additives. The U.S. Department of Agriculture (USDA) defines processed food as one that has undergone any procedure that alters it from its natural state. Thus, the current definition of processed food is broad, making a diet —like the whole foods diet— that excludes all processed food very hard and challenging to follow.

Therefore, we have to distinguish between healthy processed foods to include in the whole foods diet and those to exclude because considered unhealthy and pro-inflammatory.

Because of the huge heterogeneity among industrially processed foods, researchers have developed frameworks to classify foods based on the category or complexity of processing operations, ranging from minimally to highly processed. The NOVA classification system groups all foods based on the nature, complexity, and outcomes of the industrial processes they undergo. The NOVA classification system is recognized as a legitimate system to classify foods according to their degree of processing by the World Health Organisation (WHO), and the Food and Agriculture Organization (FAO).

NOVA classifies foods and food products into four distinct groups.

- group 1 of the NOVA classification: Unprocessed, natural, or minimally processed foods
- group 2 of the NOVA classification: Processed culinary ingredients
- group 3 of the NOVA classification: Processed foods
- group 4 of the NOVA classification: Ultra-processed foods

However, it can be sometimes challenging to distinguish food that has been minimally processed, processed or highly processed. For example:

1. Plain yogurt belongs to group 1 (minimally processed), but adding food additives such as artificial sweeteners, stabilizers, or preservatives made it ultra-processed (group 4).

2. Freshly made pizzas made from wheat flour, water, salt and yeast, garlic clove, onions, green peppers, black olives, organic mozzarella cheese, raw parmesan cheese, red pepper, belongs to group 3 (processed), but adding food additives such as artificial sweeteners, stabilizers, or changing mozzarella cheese with a non-dairy cheese analog for pizza made it ultra-processed (group 4).

Group 1: Unprocessed or minimally processed foods

Unprocessed foods are obtained directly from plants or animals and include the natural edible food parts of plants and animals.

Minimally processed foods are obtained from unprocessed or natural foods after minimal industrial processing that aims to enhance the edibility and digestibility of food or to increase its shelf life and storability without changing its nutritional content. Food undergoes minor transformations such as removal of non-edible or unwanted parts, crushing, drying, fractioning, grinding, roasting, refrigeration, freezing, vacuum packaging, boiling, pasteurization, non-alcoholic fermentation. The most commonly eaten unprocessed or minimally processed foods are:

- Natural, packaged, cut, chilled, or frozen vegetables
- Natural, packaged, cut, chilled, or frozen fruits
- Natural, packaged, cut, chilled, or frozen salads
- nuts, and other seeds without sugar or salt
- bulk or packaged grains such as wholegrain, brown, parboiled rice, or corn kernel
- fresh and dried herbs and spices (e.g., basil, dill, oregano, pepper, rosemary, thyme, cinnamon, mint, parsley)
- garlic powder

- fresh or pasteurized fruit juices with no added sugar or other ingredients
- fresh or pasteurized vegetable juices with no added sugar or other ingredients
- fresh and dried mushrooms
- cereal grains (e.g. wheat, barley, rye, oats, and sorghum)
- chickpeas, lentils, beans, black beans, peas, chicken beans, and other legumes
- flours made from maize, wheat, corn, or oats, including flours fortified with iron, folic acid, vitamin B (thiamin and niacin)
- flakes, and grits made from maize, wheat, corn, or oats, including flours fortified with iron, folic acid, vitamin B (thiamin and niacin)
- meat (fresh, chilled, or frozen), whole, steaks, fillets, and other cuts
- poultry meat (fresh, chilled, or frozen), whole, steaks, fillets, and other cuts
- fish (fresh, chilled, or frozen), whole, steaks, fillets, and other cuts
- dried or fresh pasta, couscous, and polenta made from water and the grits/flakes/flours described above
- fresh or pasteurized milk
- yogurt unsweetened without added sugar, flavor, or additives
- eggs
- tea
- herbal infusions
- coffee
- dried fruits
- water (tap, spring, and mineral)

Group 2: Processed Culinary Ingredients

The next category of processed foods includes products extracted from unprocessed, minimally processed foods, or directly from nature by pressing, grinding, crushing, milling, drying, or refining.

This group of food referred to as processed culinary ingredients is rather considered as ingredients for cooking various, delicious, and nutritious meals or dishes at home and elsewhere. They are rarely consumed by themselves but used in combination with foods.

The most commonly used processed culinary ingredients foods are:

- oils made from seeds, including sunflower oil, soybean oil, corn oil, cottonseed oil, rapeseed oil, canola oil, grapeseed oil, safflower oil
- oils made from nuts, including almond oil, hazelnut oil, Brazil nut oil, Walnut oil, Macadamia nut oil, and pecan oil.
- oils made from fruits, including olive oil, avocado oil, peach oil, apricot oil, coconut oil
- vegetable oils with added anti-oxidants
- butter
- salted butter
- sugar (white, brown, and other types) obtained from cane or beet
- molasses obtained from cane or beet
- honey (natural)
- lard
- coconut fat
- maple syrup
- cane syrup
- Agave syrup
- salt (refined or raw, mined or from seawater)
- table salt with added drying agents
- potato starch
- corn starch

- starches extracted from other plants
- balsamic vinegar
- Cane vinegar
- Coconut vinegar
- Malt vinegar
- any combination of two items of the NOVA group 2 "processed culinary ingredients"
- any item of the NOVA group 2 "processed culinary ingredients" with added vitamins or minerals, such as iodized salt

---

Group 3: Processed Foods

Processed foods are made by adding salt, oil, fat, sugar, or other ingredients from group 2 to group 1 food. The transformation processes include preservation, cooking, fermentation. These foods usually are made from at least two or three ingredients and can be eaten without further preparation. This group of food includes cheeses, smoked and cured meats, freshly-made bread, salted and sugared nuts, bacon, tinned fruit in syrup, cider, beer, and wine.

Processed foods usually keep an equivalent nutritional value and most nutrients and constituents of the original food. However, when excessive sugar, salt, or saturated oil are added, foods of group 3 become nutritionally unbalanced and may aggravate inflammation.

The most commonly eaten processed foods are::

- legumes canned or bottled preserved in salt (brine) or vinegar, or by pickling
- vegetables canned or bottled preserved in salt (brine) or vinegar, or by pickling
- fruit canned or bottled, packed in syrup
- fruits in sugar syrup (with or without added antioxidants)

- canned fish, such as sardine and tuna, with or without added preservatives
- fish (salted, dried, smoked)
- cured meat (salted, dried, smoked)
- tomato extract concentrates, or pastes, (with salt and/or sugar)
- beef jerky
- freshly-made cheeses
- freshly-made bread made of wheat flour, salt, yeast, and water
- bacon
- nuts (salted or sugared)
- seeds (salted or sugared)
- fermented alcoholic beverages such as alcoholic cider, beer, and wine
- fermented non-alcoholic beverages such as cider

Group 4: Ultra-processed foods

Also commonly referred to as highly processed foods, Ultra-processed foods usually contain substances that you would never add when cooking homemade food. These are foods from group 3 that undergo "heavily" transformation to maintain or improve their taste, texture, safety, freshness, or appearance by the incorporation of substances:

- derived from foods—such as sugar, oils, fats, carbohydrates, and proteins,—or
- derived from food constituents—such as hydrogenated fats and modified starch—, or
- synthesized in laboratories—such as flavor enhancers, preservatives, antioxidants, colors, and other food additives—

Ultra-processed foods are defined as "formulations of several ingredients mostly of exclusive industrial use which, besides sugar, salt, oils, and fats, include food ingredients not used in culinary preparations, in particular, flavor enhancers, preservatives, colors, antioxidants, sweeteners, emulsifiers, and other additives used to provide sensory attributes of natural or minimally processed foods and their culinary preparations or to disguise undesirable sensory attributes of the final product such as odor, appearance, texture, flavor, and taste of foods"

The most commonly eaten ultra-processed foods are:

- Industrialized breads
- packaged breads
- Pre-prepared meals (packaged)
- Pre-prepared fish (packaged)
- Pre-prepared vegetables (packaged)
- pre-prepared pizza and pasta dishes
- pre-prepared pasta dishes
- pre-prepared poultry 'nuggets' and 'sticks'
- pre-prepared fish 'nuggets' and 'sticks'
- Breakfast cereals
- Sausages and other reconstituted meat products
- fatty packaged snacks
- sweet savory or salty packaged snacks
- savory or salty packaged snacks
- biscuits (cookies)
- chocolates
- candies
- gum and jelly products
- sweet fillings
- confectionery products in general
- pasties
- buns and cakes
- industrially-made chips (e.g. potato chips, banana chips, lentil chips)

- soft drinks
- fruit drinks
- fruit juices
- fast foods
- tortilla Chips
- chip Dips
- microwave Popcorn
- pretzels
- salty snacks in general
- ice creams
- frozen desserts
- pre-prepared burgers
- hot dogs
- sausages
- cola, soda, and other carbonated soft drinks
- animal products made from remnants
- energy and sports drinks
- packaged hamburger and hot dog buns
- instant soups
- instant noodles
- canned, packaged sauces
- canned, packaged, or powdered desserts
- canned, packaged, or powdered drink mixes
- canned, packaged, or powdered seasonings
- canned, packaged, powdered desserts, drink mixes, and seasonings
- flavored cheese crackers
- baked products made with ingredients other than those in group 2 (processed culinary ingredients) such as hydrogenated vegetable fat, emulsifiers, flavors, and other food additives.
- breakfast cereals and bars
- dairy drinks, including chocolate milk
- sweetened and/or flavored yogurts, including fruit yogurts
- infant formulas and drinks

- meal replacement shakes or powders
- sweetened juices made from concentrate
- pastries
- cakes and cake mixes
- margarine and spreads
- distilled beverages such as whisky, vodka, gin, rum, tequila.

6

UNDERSTANDING THE FOOD NUTRITION LABELS

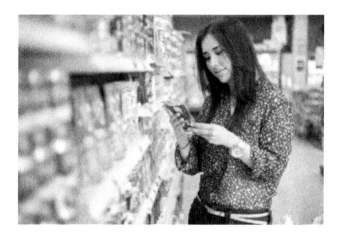

Food labeling regulation is complex, and food labels are filled with a multitude of numbers, percentages, and unusual ingredients making them difficult for consumers to understand. Products nutrition labels are often localized on the front, back, or side of the packaging. Food manufacturers must list on the product label all ingredients in the food to inform consumers what the food contains and to provide support in making healthier choices of processed foods.

Nutrition Facts label

A Nutrition Facts label breaks down the nutritional content of the food to help consumers to make healthier choices and compare between similar products. It includes

- the serving size,
- total fat,
- total carbohydrates,
- dietary fiber,
- protein,
- and vitamins per serving of the food

Example of using nutrition facts label:

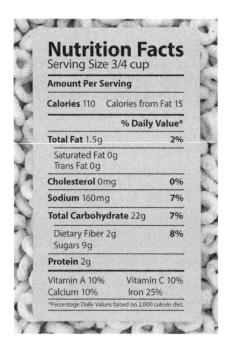

1. The first step is to check the **serving size.** All the values on this label are for a 3/4-cup serving.

2. **calorie** is an important value to many consumers. The label lists the calorie amount for one serving of food (110 calories for 3/4-cup in this example). So if you eat 1.5 cups, the total calorie is 220 calories.

3. **total fat** shows you types of fats in the food, including saturated fat, and trans fat. Avoid foods with trans fat. The total fat per 3/4-cup is 1.5 g

4. **total Carbohydrate** shows you types of carbohydrates in the food, including dietary fiber and sugar.

5. protein shows you the amount of protein in the food,

6. choose foods with lower calories, and that contain little amount of sugar, little amount of sodium, a high amount of fiber, more vitamins, and minerals.

Ingredients list

In addition to the nutrition label, food manufacturers are required to display ingredients label in their products. This is where consumers find all information about the constituents of the food, and can find if this product is suitable for them or not.

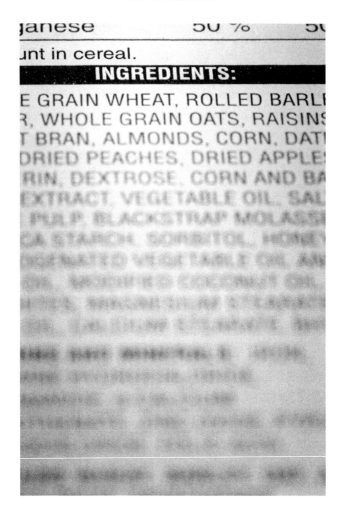

janese   50 %   50

unt in cereal.

INGREDIENTS:

E GRAIN WHEAT, ROLLED BARLE
R, WHOLE GRAIN OATS, RAISINS
T BRAN, ALMONDS, CORN, DATI
DRIED PEACHES, DRIED APPLE
RIN, DEXTROSE, CORN AND BA
EXTRACT, VEGETABLE OIL, SAL
PULP, BLACKSTRAP MOLASSE
CA STARCH, SORBITOL, HONEY

Ingredients are listed in descending order of predominance— ingredients used in the greatest amount are listed first—. Food manufacturers are required to list food additives by their class name (e.g. acidity regulator, antioxidant, color, emulsifier, flavor enhancer, gelling agent, stabilizer, sweetener, thickener), followed by the name of the food additive or the food additive number.

PART II

THE CALORIES COUNTER FOR OVER 12,000 FOODS

ABBREVIATIONS

- dia diameter
- fl oz fluid ounce
- g gram
- kcal kilocalorie (commonly known as calories)
- IU International Units
- lb pound
- mg microgram
- mg milligram
- ml milliliter
- NA not available
- oz ounce
- pkg package
- RE retinol equivalent
- sq square
- tbsp tablespoon
- Tr trace
- tsp teaspoon

BAKED FOODS

Air Filled Fritter Or Fried Puff Without Syrup Puerto Rican Style ☛ 1 turnover= 57 g; Calories = 248.5

Andreas Gluten Free Soft Dinner Roll ☛ 1 roll= 69 g; Calories = 177.3

Apple Strudel ☛ 1 oz= 28.4 g; Calories = 77.8

Archway Home Style Cookies Chocolate Chip Ice Box ☛ 1 serving= 24 g; Calories = 119.3

Archway Home Style Cookies Coconut Macaroon ☛ 1 serving= 22 g; Calories = 101.2

Archway Home Style Cookies Date Filled Oatmeal ☛ 1 serving= 25 g; Calories = 100

Archway Home Style Cookies Dutch Cocoa ☛ 1 serving= 24 g; Calories = 103.4

Archway Home Style Cookies Frosty Lemon ☛ 1 serving= 26 g; Calories = 111.8

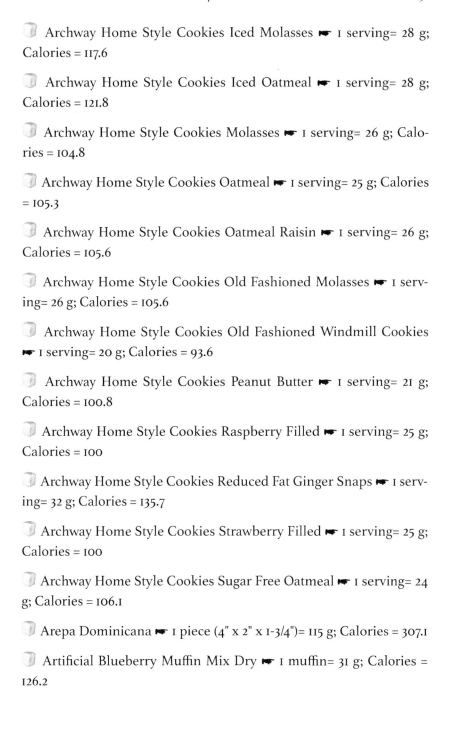

Archway Home Style Cookies Iced Molasses ☛ 1 serving= 28 g; Calories = 117.6

Archway Home Style Cookies Iced Oatmeal ☛ 1 serving= 28 g; Calories = 121.8

Archway Home Style Cookies Molasses ☛ 1 serving= 26 g; Calories = 104.8

Archway Home Style Cookies Oatmeal ☛ 1 serving= 25 g; Calories = 105.3

Archway Home Style Cookies Oatmeal Raisin ☛ 1 serving= 26 g; Calories = 105.6

Archway Home Style Cookies Old Fashioned Molasses ☛ 1 serving= 26 g; Calories = 105.6

Archway Home Style Cookies Old Fashioned Windmill Cookies ☛ 1 serving= 20 g; Calories = 93.6

Archway Home Style Cookies Peanut Butter ☛ 1 serving= 21 g; Calories = 100.8

Archway Home Style Cookies Raspberry Filled ☛ 1 serving= 25 g; Calories = 100

Archway Home Style Cookies Reduced Fat Ginger Snaps ☛ 1 serving= 32 g; Calories = 135.7

Archway Home Style Cookies Strawberry Filled ☛ 1 serving= 25 g; Calories = 100

Archway Home Style Cookies Sugar Free Oatmeal ☛ 1 serving= 24 g; Calories = 106.1

Arepa Dominicana ☛ 1 piece (4" x 2" x 1-3/4")= 115 g; Calories = 307.1

Artificial Blueberry Muffin Mix Dry ☛ 1 muffin= 31 g; Calories = 126.2

Bagel (Oat Bran) ☞ 1 mini bagel (2-1/2 inch dia)= 26 g; Calories = 66.3

Bagel Multigrain ☞ 1 miniature= 26 g; Calories = 65

Bagel Multigrain With Raisins ☞ 1 miniature= 26 g; Calories = 66.3

Bagel Oat Bran ☞ 1 miniature= 26 g; Calories = 65

Bagel Pumpernickel ☞ 1 miniature= 26 g; Calories = 65

Bagel Wheat Bran ☞ 1 miniature= 26 g; Calories = 65

Bagel Wheat With Raisins ☞ 1 miniature= 26 g; Calories = 66.3

Bagel Whole Grain White ☞ 1 miniature= 26 g; Calories = 65

Bagel Whole Wheat ☞ 1 miniature= 26 g; Calories = 65

Bagel Whole Wheat With Raisins ☞ 1 miniature= 26 g; Calories = 66.3

Bagels ☞ 1 bagel= 99 g; Calories = 261.4

Bagels Multigrain ☞ 1 piece bagel= 81 g; Calories = 195.2

Bagels Plain Enriched Without Calcium Propionate (Includes Onion Poppy Sesame) ☞ 1 oz= 28.4 g; Calories = 78.1

Bagels Plain Unenriched With Calcium Propionate (Includes Onion Poppy Sesame) ☞ 1 oz= 28.4 g; Calories = 78.1

Bagels Plain Unenriched Without Calcium Propionate(Includes Onion Poppy Sesame) ☞ 1 oz= 28.4 g; Calories = 78.1

Bagels Wheat ☞ 1 bagel= 98 g; Calories = 245

Bagels Whole Grain White ☞ 1/2 piece bagel 1 serving= 43 g; Calories = 109.7

Baklava ☞ 1 piece (2" x 2" x 1-1/2")= 78 g; Calories = 333.8

Basbousa ☞ 1 piece (about 3 x 2-1/2")= 82 g; Calories = 252.6

Biscuit Baking Powder Or Buttermilk Type Made From Home Recipe ☞ 1 small (1-1/2" dia)= 14 g; Calories = 49.6

Biscuit Baking Powder Or Buttermilk Type Made From Mix ☞ 1 small (1-1/2" dia)= 14 g; Calories = 45.4

Biscuit Cheese ☞ 1 biscuit (2" dia)= 30 g; Calories = 103.8

Biscuit Cinnamon-Raisin ☞ 1 biscuit (3" dia)= 64 g; Calories = 220.8

Biscuit Dough Fried ☞ 1 piece= 43 g; Calories = 150.5

Biscuit Whole Wheat ☞ 1 small (1-1/2" dia)= 14 g; Calories = 43.7

Biscuits Mixed Grain Refrigerated Dough ☞ 1 oz= 28.4 g; Calories = 74.7

Biscuits Plain Or Buttermilk Dry Mix ☞ 1 cup, purchased= 120 g; Calories = 513.6

Biscuits Plain Or Buttermilk Frozen Baked ☞ 1 oz= 28.4 g; Calories = 96

Biscuits Plain Or Buttermilk Prepared From Recipe ☞ 1 oz= 28.4 g; Calories = 100.3

Biscuits Plain Or Buttermilk Refrigerated Dough Higher Fat ☞ 1 biscuit= 58 g; Calories = 178.1

Biscuits Plain Or Buttermilk Refrigerated Dough Higher Fat Baked ☞ 1 biscuit= 51 g; Calories = 165.2

Biscuits Plain Or Buttermilk Refrigerated Dough Lower Fat ☞ 1 serving 1 biscuit= 58 g; Calories = 156.6

Biscuits Plain Or Buttermilk Refrigerated Dough Lower Fat Baked ☞ 1 oz= 28.4 g; Calories = 90.6

Blueberry Pie ☞ 1 oz= 28.4 g; Calories = 65.9

Bread Banana Prepared From Recipe Made With Margarine ☞ 1 oz= 28.4 g; Calories = 92.6

Bread Barley Toasted ☛ 1 small or thin/very thin slice= 22 g; Calories = 66.2

Bread Boston Brown Canned ☛ 1 oz= 28.4 g; Calories = 55.4

Bread Caressed Puerto Rican Style ☛ 1 slice= 25 g; Calories = 68.3

Bread Caressed Toasted Puerto Rican Style ☛ 1 slice= 23 g; Calories = 69

Bread Chapati Or Roti Plain Commercially Prepared ☛ 1 piece= 68 g; Calories = 202

Bread Chapati Or Roti Whole Wheat Commercially Prepared Frozen ☛ 1 piece= 43 g; Calories = 128.6

Bread Cheese ☛ 1 slice= 48 g; Calories = 195.8

Bread Cheese Toasted ☛ 1 small or thin/very thin slice= 22 g; Calories = 98.6

Bread Cinnamon ☛ 1 slice 1 serving= 28 g; Calories = 70.8

Bread Cornbread Dry Mix Enriched (Includes Corn Muffin Mix) ☛ 1 oz= 28.4 g; Calories = 118.7

Bread Cornbread Dry Mix Prepared With 2% Milk 80% Margarine And Eggs ☛ 1 muffin= 51 g; Calories = 168.3

Bread Cornbread Dry Mix Unenriched (Includes Corn Muffin Mix) ☛ 1 oz= 28.4 g; Calories = 118.7

Bread Cornbread Prepared From Recipe Made With Low Fat (2%) Milk ☛ 1 oz= 28.4 g; Calories = 75.5

Bread Cracked-Wheat ☛ 1 oz= 28.4 g; Calories = 73.8

Bread Crumbs Dry Grated Plain ☛ 1 oz= 28.4 g; Calories = 112.2

Bread Crumbs Dry Grated Seasoned ☛ 1 oz= 28.4 g; Calories = 108.8

Bread Cuban Toasted ☛ 1 small or thin/very thin slice= 9 g; Calories = 26.9

Bread Dough Fried ☛ 1 slice or roll= 26 g; Calories = 99.3

Bread Egg ☛ 1 oz= 28.4 g; Calories = 81.5

Bread Egg Challah Toasted ☛ 1 small or thin/very thin slice= 18 g; Calories = 56.7

Bread Egg Toasted ☛ 1 oz= 28.4 g; Calories = 89.5

Bread French Or Vienna Toasted (Includes Sourdough) ☛ 1 oz= 28.4 g; Calories = 90.6

Bread French Or Vienna Whole Wheat ☛ 1 slice 1 serving= 48 g; Calories = 114.7

Bread Fruit ☛ 1 slice= 41 g; Calories = 148.4

Bread Gluten Free Toasted ☛ 1 small or thin/very thin slice= 22 g; Calories = 60.1

Bread Gluten-Free White Made With Potato Extract Rice Starch And Rice Flour ☛ 1 slice= 34 g; Calories = 108.8

Bread Gluten-Free White Made With Rice Flour Corn Starch And/or Tapioca ☛ 1 slice= 35 g; Calories = 86.8

Bread Gluten-Free White Made With Tapioca Starch And Brown Rice Flour ☛ 1 slice= 28 g; Calories = 83.4

Bread Gluten-Free Whole Grain Made With Tapioca Starch And Brown Rice Flour ☛ 1 slice= 25 g; Calories = 77.3

Bread Irish Soda Prepared From Recipe ☛ 1 oz= 28.4 g; Calories = 82.4

Bread Italian ☛ 1 oz= 28.4 g; Calories = 73.6

Bread Italian Grecian Armenian ☛ 1 small or thin/very thin slice= 24 g; Calories = 65

Bread Italian Grecian Armenian Toasted ☞ 1 small or thin/very thin slice= 22 g; Calories = 65.6

Bread Lard Puerto Rican Style ☞ 1 slice= 25 g; Calories = 70

Bread Lard Toasted Puerto Rican Style ☞ 1 slice= 23 g; Calories = 71.5

Bread Made From Home Recipe Or Purchased At A Bakery Ns As To Major Flour ☞ 1 small or thin/very thin slice= 33 g; Calories = 89.1

Bread Made From Home Recipe Or Purchased At A Bakery Toasted Ns As To Major Flour ☞ 1 small or thin/very thin slice= 30 g; Calories = 89.1

Bread Multi-Grain (Includes Whole-Grain) ☞ 1 oz= 28.4 g; Calories = 75.3

Bread Naan Plain Commercially Prepared Refrigerated ☞ 1 piece= 90 g; Calories = 261.9

Bread Naan Whole Wheat Commercially Prepared Refrigerated ☞ 1 piece= 106 g; Calories = 303.2

Bread Native Water Puerto Rican Style ☞ 1 slice= 25 g; Calories = 69.3

Bread Native Water Toasted Puerto Rican Style ☞ 1 slice= 23 g; Calories = 70.2

Bread Nut ☞ 1 slice= 49 g; Calories = 192.1

Bread Oat Bran ☞ 1 oz= 28.4 g; Calories = 67

Bread Oat Bran Toasted ☞ 1 oz= 28.4 g; Calories = 73.6

Bread Oatmeal ☞ 1 oz= 28.4 g; Calories = 76.4

Bread Oatmeal Toasted ☞ 1 oz= 28.4 g; Calories = 82.9

Bread Onion ☞ 1 small or thin/very thin slice= 24 g; Calories = 56.6

Bread Onion Toasted ☛ 1 small or thin/very thin slice= 18 g; Calories = 46.8

Bread Pan Dulce Sweet Yeast Bread ☛ 1 slice (average weight of 1 slice)= 63 g; Calories = 231.2

Bread Paratha Whole Wheat Commercially Prepared Frozen ☛ 1 piece= 79 g; Calories = 257.5

Bread Pita White Unenriched ☛ 1 oz= 28.4 g; Calories = 78.1

Bread Potato ☛ 1 slice= 32 g; Calories = 85.1

Bread Potato Toasted ☛ 1 small or thin/very thin slice= 24 g; Calories = 70.1

Bread Pound Cake Type Pan De Torta Salvadoran ☛ 1 serving= 55 g; Calories = 214.5

Bread Protein (Includes Gluten) ☛ 1 oz= 28.4 g; Calories = 69.6

Bread Protein (Includes Gluten) Toasted ☛ 1 oz= 28.4 g; Calories = 76.7

Bread Pumpernickel ☛ 1 oz= 28.4 g; Calories = 71

Bread Pumpkin ☛ 1 slice= 60 g; Calories = 180

Bread Puri Wheat ☛ 1 puri (approx 4-4/5" dia)= 36 g; Calories = 142.6

Bread Raisin Enriched ☛ 1 oz= 28.4 g; Calories = 77.8

Bread Raisin Enriched Toasted ☛ 1 oz= 28.4 g; Calories = 84.3

Bread Raisin Unenriched ☛ 1 oz= 28.4 g; Calories = 77.8

Bread Reduced-Calorie Oat Bran ☛ 1 oz= 28.4 g; Calories = 57.1

Bread Reduced-Calorie Oat Bran Toasted ☛ 1 oz= 28.4 g; Calories = 67.9

Bread Reduced-Calorie Oatmeal ☛ 1 oz= 28.4 g; Calories = 59.6

Bread Reduced-Calorie Rye ☞ 1 oz= 28.4 g; Calories = 57.7

Bread Reduced-Calorie Wheat ☞ 1 oz= 28.4 g; Calories = 61.6

Bread Reduced-Calorie White ☞ 1 oz= 28.4 g; Calories = 58.8

Bread Rice Bran ☞ 1 oz= 28.4 g; Calories = 69

Bread Rice Bran Toasted ☞ 1 oz= 28.4 g; Calories = 75

Bread Roll Mexican Bollilo ☞ 1 piece= 98 g; Calories = 311.6

Bread Rye Toasted ☞ 1 oz= 28.4 g; Calories = 80.7

Bread Salvadoran Sweet Cheese (Quesadilla Salvadorena) ☞ 1 serving (approximate serving size)= 55 g; Calories = 205.7

Bread Spanish Coffee ☞ 1 piece= 85 g; Calories = 292.4

Bread Sprouted Wheat Toasted ☞ 1 slice= 24 g; Calories = 49.7

Bread Sticks Plain ☞ 1 cup, small pieces= 46 g; Calories = 189.5

Bread Stuffing Bread Dry Mix ☞ 1 oz= 28.4 g; Calories = 109.6

Bread Stuffing Bread Dry Mix Prepared ☞ 1 oz= 28.4 g; Calories = 55.4

Bread Stuffing Cornbread Dry Mix ☞ 1 oz= 28.4 g; Calories = 110.5

Bread Stuffing Cornbread Dry Mix Prepared ☞ 1 oz= 28.4 g; Calories = 50.8

Bread Sweet Potato Toasted ☞ 1 small or thin/very thin slice= 22 g; Calories = 57.9

Bread Vegetable ☞ 1 slice= 44 g; Calories = 114

Bread Vegetable Toasted ☞ 1 slice= 40 g; Calories = 114

Bread Wheat Sprouted ☞ 1 slice 1 serving= 38 g; Calories = 71.4

Bread Wheat Sprouted Toasted ☞ 1 slice 1 serving= 38 g; Calories = 77.9

Bread Wheat Toasted ☞ 1 oz= 28.4 g; Calories = 88.9

Bread White Commercially Prepared Low Sodium No Salt ☞ 1 oz= 28.4 g; Calories = 75.8

Bread White Commercially Prepared Toasted Low Sodium No Salt ☞ 1 oz= 28.4 g; Calories = 83.2

Bread White Made From Home Recipe Or Purchased At A Bakery ☞ 1 small or thin/very thin slice= 33 g; Calories = 89.1

Bread White Made From Home Recipe Or Purchased At A Bakery Toasted ☞ 1 small or thin/very thin slice= 30 g; Calories = 89.1

Bread White Prepared From Recipe Made With Low Fat (2%) Milk ☞ 1 oz= 28.4 g; Calories = 80.9

Bread White Prepared From Recipe Made With Nonfat Dry Milk ☞ 1 oz= 28.4 g; Calories = 77.8

Bread White Wheat ☞ 1 slice= 28 g; Calories = 66.6

Bread White With Whole Wheat Swirl ☞ 1 small or thin/very thin slice= 24 g; Calories = 62.2

Bread White With Whole Wheat Swirl Toasted ☞ 1 small or thin/very thin slice= 22 g; Calories = 65.6

Bread Whole Wheat Made From Home Recipe Or Purchased At Bakery ☞ 1 small or thin/very thin slice= 33 g; Calories = 81.8

Bread Whole Wheat Made From Home Recipe Or Purchased At Bakery Toasted ☞ 1 small or thin/very thin slice= 30 g; Calories = 81.6

Bread Whole Wheat Toasted ☞ 1 small or thin/very thin slice= 22 g; Calories = 60.9

Bread Whole-Wheat Prepared From Recipe ☞ 1 oz= 28.4 g; Calories = 79

Bread Whole-Wheat Prepared From Recipe Toasted ☞ 1 oz= 28.4 g; Calories = 86.6

Bread Zucchini ☞ 1 slice= 40 g; Calories = 120

Breadsticks Nfs ☞ 1 small stick= 28 g; Calories = 95.8

Breadsticks Soft From Fast Food / Restaurant ☞ 1 small stick= 26 g; Calories = 88.9

Breadsticks Soft From Frozen ☞ 1 small stick= 26 g; Calories = 81.1

Breadsticks Soft Nfs ☞ 1 small stick= 28 g; Calories = 95.8

Breadsticks Soft With Parmesan Cheese From Fast Food / Restaurant ☞ 1 small stick= 28 g; Calories = 96.3

Breakfast Tart Low Fat ☞ 1 tart= 52 g; Calories = 193.4

Brioche ☞ 1 piece= 77 g; Calories = 322.6

Butter Croissants ☞ 1 oz= 28.4 g; Calories = 115.3

Cake Angelfood Commercially Prepared ☞ 1 piece (1/12 of 12 oz cake)= 28 g; Calories = 72.2

Cake Angelfood Dry Mix Prepared ☞ 1 piece (1/12 of 10 inch dia)= 50 g; Calories = 128.5

Cake Batter Raw Chocolate ☞ 1 tablespoon= 14 g; Calories = 40.6

Cake Batter Raw Not Chocolate ☞ 1 tablespoon= 15 g; Calories = 42.2

Cake Boston Cream Pie Commercially Prepared ☞ 1 oz= 28.4 g; Calories = 71.6

Cake Cherry Fudge With Chocolate Frosting ☞ 1 oz= 28.4 g; Calories = 75

Cake Cream Without Icing Or Topping ☞ 1 cake (8" dia)= 510 g; Calories = 1887

Cake Dobos Torte ☞ 1 cake (8-1/2" dia)= 1472 g; Calories = 5740.8

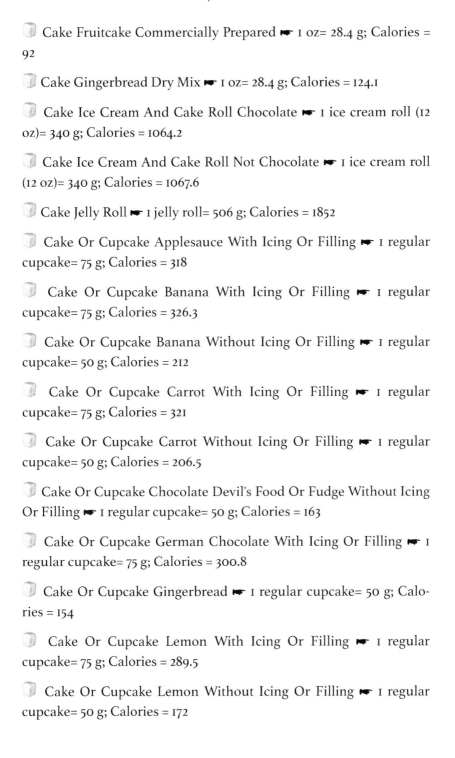

Cake Fruitcake Commercially Prepared ☞ 1 oz= 28.4 g; Calories = 92

Cake Gingerbread Dry Mix ☞ 1 oz= 28.4 g; Calories = 124.1

Cake Ice Cream And Cake Roll Chocolate ☞ 1 ice cream roll (12 oz)= 340 g; Calories = 1064.2

Cake Ice Cream And Cake Roll Not Chocolate ☞ 1 ice cream roll (12 oz)= 340 g; Calories = 1067.6

Cake Jelly Roll ☞ 1 jelly roll= 506 g; Calories = 1852

Cake Or Cupcake Applesauce With Icing Or Filling ☞ 1 regular cupcake= 75 g; Calories = 318

Cake Or Cupcake Banana With Icing Or Filling ☞ 1 regular cupcake= 75 g; Calories = 326.3

Cake Or Cupcake Banana Without Icing Or Filling ☞ 1 regular cupcake= 50 g; Calories = 212

Cake Or Cupcake Carrot With Icing Or Filling ☞ 1 regular cupcake= 75 g; Calories = 321

Cake Or Cupcake Carrot Without Icing Or Filling ☞ 1 regular cupcake= 50 g; Calories = 206.5

Cake Or Cupcake Chocolate Devil's Food Or Fudge Without Icing Or Filling ☞ 1 regular cupcake= 50 g; Calories = 163

Cake Or Cupcake German Chocolate With Icing Or Filling ☞ 1 regular cupcake= 75 g; Calories = 300.8

Cake Or Cupcake Gingerbread ☞ 1 regular cupcake= 50 g; Calories = 154

Cake Or Cupcake Lemon With Icing Or Filling ☞ 1 regular cupcake= 75 g; Calories = 289.5

Cake Or Cupcake Lemon Without Icing Or Filling ☞ 1 regular cupcake= 50 g; Calories = 172

Cake Or Cupcake Marble With Icing Or Filling ☛ 1 regular cupcake= 75 g; Calories = 292.5

Cake Or Cupcake Marble Without Icing Or Filling ☛ 1 regular cupcake= 50 g; Calories = 167.5

Cake Or Cupcake Nut With Icing Or Filling ☛ 1 regular cupcake= 75 g; Calories = 303

Cake Or Cupcake Nut Without Icing Or Filling ☛ 1 regular cupcake= 50 g; Calories = 212.5

Cake Or Cupcake Oatmeal ☛ 1 regular cupcake= 50 g; Calories = 185

Cake Or Cupcake Peanut Butter ☛ 1 regular cupcake= 50 g; Calories = 206.5

Cake Or Cupcake Pumpkin With Icing Or Filling ☛ 1 regular cupcake= 75 g; Calories = 308.3

Cake Or Cupcake Pumpkin Without Icing Or Filling ☛ 1 regular cupcake= 50 g; Calories = 193.5

Cake Or Cupcake Raisin-Nut ☛ 1 regular cupcake= 50 g; Calories = 205.5

Cake Or Cupcake Spice With Icing Or Filling ☛ 1 regular cupcake= 75 g; Calories = 318

Cake Or Cupcake Spice Without Icing Or Filling ☛ 1 regular cupcake= 50 g; Calories = 204

Cake Or Cupcake White Without Icing Or Filling ☛ 1 regular cupcake= 50 g; Calories = 164.5

Cake Or Cupcake Yellow Without Icing Or Filling ☛ 1 regular cupcake= 50 g; Calories = 172

Cake Or Cupcake Zucchini ☛ 1 1-layer cake (8" or 9" dia, 1-1/2" high)= 579 g; Calories = 2530.2

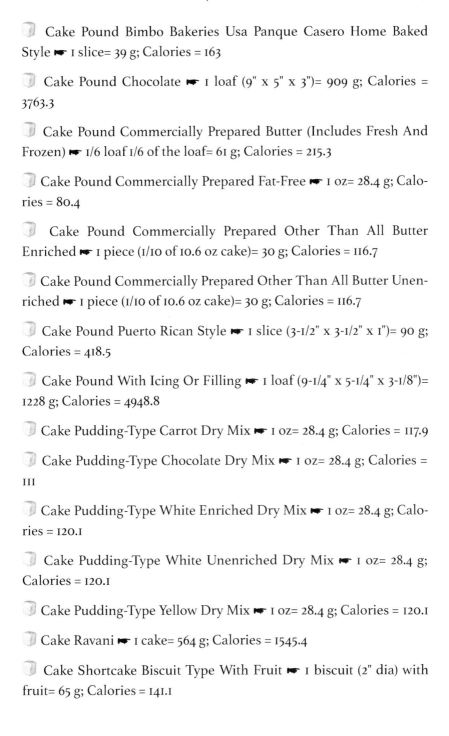

Cake Pound Bimbo Bakeries Usa Panque Casero Home Baked Style ☛ 1 slice= 39 g; Calories = 163

Cake Pound Chocolate ☛ 1 loaf (9" x 5" x 3")= 909 g; Calories = 3763.3

Cake Pound Commercially Prepared Butter (Includes Fresh And Frozen) ☛ 1/6 loaf 1/6 of the loaf= 61 g; Calories = 215.3

Cake Pound Commercially Prepared Fat-Free ☛ 1 oz= 28.4 g; Calories = 80.4

Cake Pound Commercially Prepared Other Than All Butter Enriched ☛ 1 piece (1/10 of 10.6 oz cake)= 30 g; Calories = 116.7

Cake Pound Commercially Prepared Other Than All Butter Unenriched ☛ 1 piece (1/10 of 10.6 oz cake)= 30 g; Calories = 116.7

Cake Pound Puerto Rican Style ☛ 1 slice (3-1/2" x 3-1/2" x 1")= 90 g; Calories = 418.5

Cake Pound With Icing Or Filling ☛ 1 loaf (9-1/4" x 5-1/4" x 3-1/8")= 1228 g; Calories = 4948.8

Cake Pudding-Type Carrot Dry Mix ☛ 1 oz= 28.4 g; Calories = 117.9

Cake Pudding-Type Chocolate Dry Mix ☛ 1 oz= 28.4 g; Calories = 111

Cake Pudding-Type White Enriched Dry Mix ☛ 1 oz= 28.4 g; Calories = 120.1

Cake Pudding-Type White Unenriched Dry Mix ☛ 1 oz= 28.4 g; Calories = 120.1

Cake Pudding-Type Yellow Dry Mix ☛ 1 oz= 28.4 g; Calories = 120.1

Cake Ravani ☛ 1 cake= 564 g; Calories = 1545.4

Cake Shortcake Biscuit Type With Fruit ☛ 1 biscuit (2" dia) with fruit= 65 g; Calories = 141.1

Cake Shortcake Biscuit Type With Whipped Cream And Fruit ☞ 1 biscuit (2" dia) with fruit and whipped cream= 74 g; Calories = 162.1

Cake Shortcake Biscuit-Type Prepared From Recipe ☞ 1 oz= 28.4 g; Calories = 98.3

Cake Shortcake Sponge Type With Fruit ☞ 1 cake (3" dia) with fruit= 102 g; Calories = 251.9

Cake Shortcake Sponge Type With Whipped Cream And Fruit ☞ 1 cake (3" dia) with fruit and whipped cream= 118 g; Calories = 285.6

Cake Shortcake With Whipped Topping And Fruit Diet ☞ 1 individual cake= 94 g; Calories = 204

Cake Snack Cakes Creme-Filled Chocolate With Frosting ☞ 1 oz= 28.4 g; Calories = 113.3

Cake Snack Cakes Creme-Filled Chocolate With Frosting Low-Fat With Added Fiber ☞ 1 cake 1 serving= 27 g; Calories = 110.4

Cake Snack Cakes Creme-Filled Sponge ☞ 1 oz= 28.4 g; Calories = 106.2

Cake Snack Cakes Not Chocolate With Icing Or Filling Low-Fat With Added Fiber ☞ 1 cake 1 serving= 27 g; Calories = 111.2

Cake Sponge Chocolate ☞ 1 tube cake (10" dia, 4" high)= 790 g; Calories = 2796.6

Cake Sponge Commercially Prepared ☞ 1 oz= 28.4 g; Calories = 82.4

Cake Sponge Prepared From Recipe ☞ 1 oz= 28.4 g; Calories = 84.3

Cake Sponge With Icing Or Filling ☞ 1 tube cake (10-1/2" dia, 4-1/4" high)= 1109 g; Calories = 4014.6

Cake Torte ☞ 1 torte= 912 g; Calories = 2581

Cake Tres Leche ☞ 1 cake= 1448 g; Calories = 3866.2

Cake White Dry Mix Special Dietary (Includes Lemon-Flavored) ☛ 1 oz= 28.4 g; Calories = 112.7

Cake White Prepared From Recipe Without Frosting ☛ 1 piece (1/12 of 9 inch dia)= 74 g; Calories = 264.2

Cake Yellow Enriched Dry Mix ☛ 1 serving= 43 g; Calories = 160.8

Cake Yellow Light Dry Mix ☛ 1 oz= 28.4 g; Calories = 114.7

Cake Yellow Prepared From Recipe Without Frosting ☛ 1 piece (1/12 of 8 inch dia)= 68 g; Calories = 245.5

Cake Yellow Unenriched Dry Mix ☛ 1 oz= 28.4 g; Calories = 122.7

Calzone With Cheese Meatless ☛ 1 calzone or stromboli= 424 g; Calories = 1632.4

Calzone With Meat And Cheese ☛ 1 calzone or stromboli= 424 g; Calories = 1475.5

Casabe Cassava Bread ☛ 1 piece (6" dia)= 100 g; Calories = 299

Cheese Croissants ☛ 1 oz= 28.4 g; Calories = 117.6

Cheese Pastry Puffs ☛ 1 puff or cheese straw (5" long)= 6 g; Calories = 15.8

Cheesecake Chocolate ☛ 1 cake or pie (9" dia, approx 1-1/2" high)= 1533 g; Calories = 5733.4

Cheesecake Commercially Prepared ☛ 1 oz= 28.4 g; Calories = 91.2

Cheesecake Prepared From Mix No-Bake Type ☛ 1 oz= 28.4 g; Calories = 77.8

Cheesecake With Fruit ☛ 1 cake or pie (9" dia, approx 1-1/2" high)= 1704 g; Calories = 3561.4

Chocolate Cake ☛ 1 piece (1/12 of 9 inch dia)= 95 g; Calories = 352.5

Chocolate Cake With Frosting ☛ 1 piece (1/12 of a cake)= 138 g; Calories = 536.8

Chocolate Coated Graham Crackers ☛ 3 pieces= 27 g; Calories = 135

Chocolate Coated Marshmallows ☛ 1 oz= 28.4 g; Calories = 119.6

Churros ☛ 1 churro= 26 g; Calories = 125.1

Cinnamon Buns Frosted (Includes Honey Buns) ☛ 1 bun= 65 g; Calories = 293.8

Cinnamon Coffeecake ☛ 1 oz= 28.4 g; Calories = 118.7

Cinnamon Raisin Bagels ☛ 1 mini bagel (2-1/2 inch dia)= 26 g; Calories = 71.2

Cobbler Apple ☛ 1 cup= 217 g; Calories = 423.2

Cobbler Apricot ☛ 1 cup= 217 g; Calories = 408

Cobbler Berry ☛ 1 cup= 217 g; Calories = 499.1

Cobbler Cherry ☛ 1 cup= 217 g; Calories = 421

Cobbler Peach ☛ 1 cup= 217 g; Calories = 431.8

Cobbler Pear ☛ 1 cup= 217 g; Calories = 466.6

Cobbler Pineapple ☛ 1 cup= 217 g; Calories = 414.5

Cobbler Plum ☛ 1 cup= 217 g; Calories = 434

Cobbler Rhubarb ☛ 1 cup= 217 g; Calories = 544.7

Coconut Cream Cake Puerto Rican Style ☛ 1 tablespoon= 15 g; Calories = 47.7

Coconut Custard Pie ☛ 1 oz= 28.4 g; Calories = 73.8

Coffee Cake Crumb Or Quick-Bread Type ☛ 1 cake (9" square)= 692 g; Calories = 2643.4

Coffee Cake Crumb Or Quick-Bread Type Cheese-Filled ☛ 1 cake (8" square)= 568 g; Calories = 2016.4

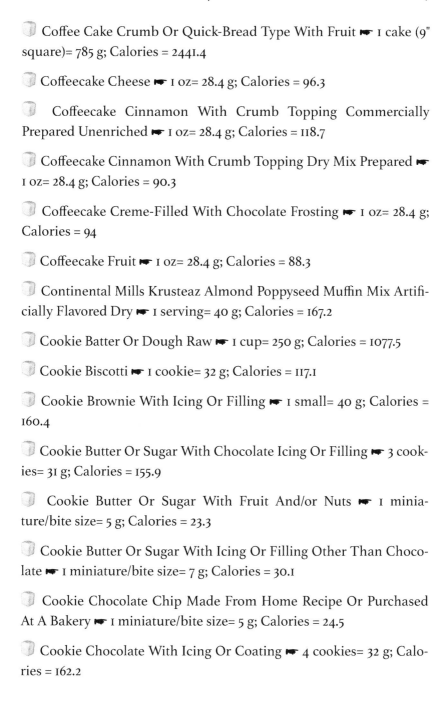

Coffee Cake Crumb Or Quick-Bread Type With Fruit ☛ 1 cake (9" square)= 785 g; Calories = 2441.4

Coffeecake Cheese ☛ 1 oz= 28.4 g; Calories = 96.3

Coffeecake Cinnamon With Crumb Topping Commercially Prepared Unenriched ☛ 1 oz= 28.4 g; Calories = 118.7

Coffeecake Cinnamon With Crumb Topping Dry Mix Prepared ☛ 1 oz= 28.4 g; Calories = 90.3

Coffeecake Creme-Filled With Chocolate Frosting ☛ 1 oz= 28.4 g; Calories = 94

Coffeecake Fruit ☛ 1 oz= 28.4 g; Calories = 88.3

Continental Mills Krusteaz Almond Poppyseed Muffin Mix Artificially Flavored Dry ☛ 1 serving= 40 g; Calories = 167.2

Cookie Batter Or Dough Raw ☛ 1 cup= 250 g; Calories = 1077.5

Cookie Biscotti ☛ 1 cookie= 32 g; Calories = 117.1

Cookie Brownie With Icing Or Filling ☛ 1 small= 40 g; Calories = 160.4

Cookie Butter Or Sugar With Chocolate Icing Or Filling ☛ 3 cookies= 31 g; Calories = 155.9

Cookie Butter Or Sugar With Fruit And/or Nuts ☛ 1 miniature/bite size= 5 g; Calories = 23.3

Cookie Butter Or Sugar With Icing Or Filling Other Than Chocolate ☛ 1 miniature/bite size= 7 g; Calories = 30.1

Cookie Chocolate Chip Made From Home Recipe Or Purchased At A Bakery ☛ 1 miniature/bite size= 5 g; Calories = 24.5

Cookie Chocolate With Icing Or Coating ☛ 4 cookies= 32 g; Calories = 162.2

🍪 Cookie Graham Cracker With Chocolate And Marshmallow ☞ 1 suddenly s'mores cookie= 19 g; Calories = 88.4

🍪 Cookie Oatmeal With Chocolate Chips ☞ 1 miniature/bite size= 5 g; Calories = 22.9

🍪 Cookie Peanut Butter With Chocolate ☞ 1 miniature/bite size= 5 g; Calories = 23.8

🍪 Cookie Shortbread With Icing Or Filling ☞ 1 miniature/bite size= 7 g; Calories = 36.1

🍪 Cookie Vanilla With Caramel Coconut And Chocolate Coating ☞ 2 cookies= 29 g; Calories = 141.8

🍪 Cookie With Peanut Butter Filling Chocolate-Coated ☞ 2 cookies= 25 g; Calories = 140.5

🍪 Cookies Animal Crackers (Includes Arrowroot Tea Biscuits) ☞ 1 oz= 28.4 g; Calories = 126.7

🍪 Cookies Animal With Frosting Or Icing ☞ 8 cookies 1 serving= 31 g; Calories = 157.8

🍪 Cookies Brownies Commercially Prepared ☞ 1 oz= 28.4 g; Calories = 115

🍪 Cookies Brownies Commercially Prepared Reduced Fat With Added Fiber ☞ 1 brownie 1 serving= 36 g; Calories = 124.2

🍪 Cookies Brownies Dry Mix Regular ☞ 1 oz= 28.4 g; Calories = 123.3

🍪 Cookies Brownies Dry Mix Sugar Free ☞ 1 oz= 28.4 g; Calories = 121

🍪 Cookies Brownies Prepared From Recipe ☞ 1 oz= 28.4 g; Calories = 132.3

🍪 Cookies Butter Commercially Prepared Enriched ☞ 1 oz= 28.4 g; Calories = 132.6

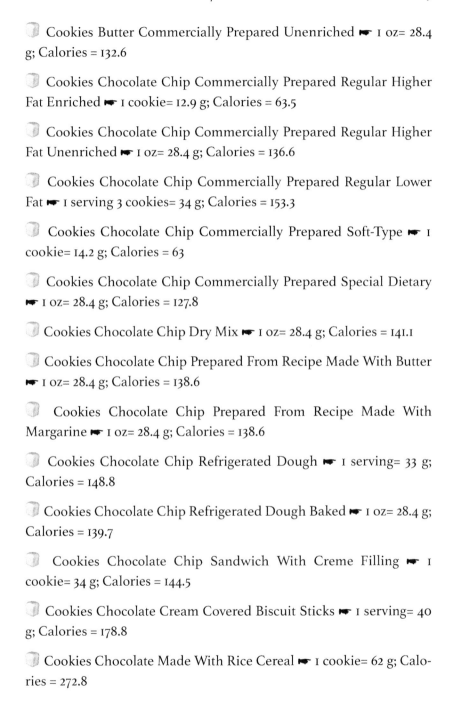

Cookies Butter Commercially Prepared Unenriched ☛ 1 oz= 28.4 g; Calories = 132.6

Cookies Chocolate Chip Commercially Prepared Regular Higher Fat Enriched ☛ 1 cookie= 12.9 g; Calories = 63.5

Cookies Chocolate Chip Commercially Prepared Regular Higher Fat Unenriched ☛ 1 oz= 28.4 g; Calories = 136.6

Cookies Chocolate Chip Commercially Prepared Regular Lower Fat ☛ 1 serving 3 cookies= 34 g; Calories = 153.3

Cookies Chocolate Chip Commercially Prepared Soft-Type ☛ 1 cookie= 14.2 g; Calories = 63

Cookies Chocolate Chip Commercially Prepared Special Dietary ☛ 1 oz= 28.4 g; Calories = 127.8

Cookies Chocolate Chip Dry Mix ☛ 1 oz= 28.4 g; Calories = 141.1

Cookies Chocolate Chip Prepared From Recipe Made With Butter ☛ 1 oz= 28.4 g; Calories = 138.6

Cookies Chocolate Chip Prepared From Recipe Made With Margarine ☛ 1 oz= 28.4 g; Calories = 138.6

Cookies Chocolate Chip Refrigerated Dough ☛ 1 serving= 33 g; Calories = 148.8

Cookies Chocolate Chip Refrigerated Dough Baked ☛ 1 oz= 28.4 g; Calories = 139.7

Cookies Chocolate Chip Sandwich With Creme Filling ☛ 1 cookie= 34 g; Calories = 144.5

Cookies Chocolate Cream Covered Biscuit Sticks ☛ 1 serving= 40 g; Calories = 178.8

Cookies Chocolate Made With Rice Cereal ☛ 1 cookie= 62 g; Calories = 272.8

Cookies Chocolate Sandwich With Creme Filling Reduced Fat ☛ 1 serving= 34 g; Calories = 148.2

Cookies Chocolate Sandwich With Creme Filling Regular ☛ 3 cookie= 36 g; Calories = 167

Cookies Chocolate Sandwich With Creme Filling Regular Chocolate-Coated ☛ 1 oz= 28.4 g; Calories = 136.6

Cookies Chocolate Sandwich With Creme Filling Special Dietary ☛ 1 oz= 28.4 g; Calories = 130.9

Cookies Chocolate Sandwich With Extra Creme Filling ☛ 1 oz= 28.4 g; Calories = 141.1

Cookies Chocolate Wafers ☛ 1 oz= 28.4 g; Calories = 123

Cookies Coconut Macaroon ☛ 2 cookie 1 serving= 36 g; Calories = 165.6

Cookies Fudge Cake-Type (Includes Trolley Cakes) ☛ 1 oz= 28.4 g; Calories = 99.1

Cookies Gluten-Free Chocolate Sandwich With Creme Filling ☛ 3 cookies= 44 g; Calories = 208.6

Cookies Gluten-Free Chocolate Wafer ☛ 3 cookies= 23 g; Calories = 124.4

Cookies Gluten-Free Lemon Wafer ☛ 3 cookies= 30 g; Calories = 154.5

Cookies Gluten-Free Vanilla Sandwich With Creme Filling ☛ 3 cookies= 44 g; Calories = 216.9

Cookies Graham Crackers Plain Or Honey Lowfat ☛ 1 serving= 35 g; Calories = 135.1

Cookies Ladyfingers Without Lemon Juice And Rind ☛ 1 oz= 28.4 g; Calories = 103.1

Cookies Marie Biscuit ☛ 5 cookie= 28 g; Calories = 113.7

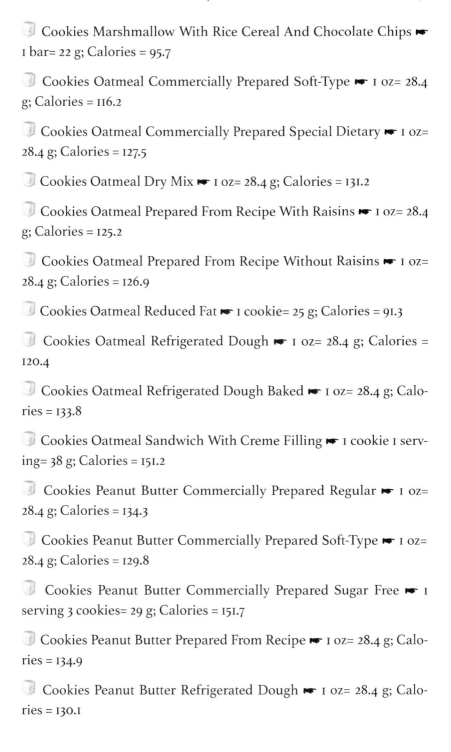

Cookies Marshmallow With Rice Cereal And Chocolate Chips ☞ 1 bar= 22 g; Calories = 95.7

Cookies Oatmeal Commercially Prepared Soft-Type ☞ 1 oz= 28.4 g; Calories = 116.2

Cookies Oatmeal Commercially Prepared Special Dietary ☞ 1 oz= 28.4 g; Calories = 127.5

Cookies Oatmeal Dry Mix ☞ 1 oz= 28.4 g; Calories = 131.2

Cookies Oatmeal Prepared From Recipe With Raisins ☞ 1 oz= 28.4 g; Calories = 125.2

Cookies Oatmeal Prepared From Recipe Without Raisins ☞ 1 oz= 28.4 g; Calories = 126.9

Cookies Oatmeal Reduced Fat ☞ 1 cookie= 25 g; Calories = 91.3

Cookies Oatmeal Refrigerated Dough ☞ 1 oz= 28.4 g; Calories = 120.4

Cookies Oatmeal Refrigerated Dough Baked ☞ 1 oz= 28.4 g; Calories = 133.8

Cookies Oatmeal Sandwich With Creme Filling ☞ 1 cookie 1 serving= 38 g; Calories = 151.2

Cookies Peanut Butter Commercially Prepared Regular ☞ 1 oz= 28.4 g; Calories = 134.3

Cookies Peanut Butter Commercially Prepared Soft-Type ☞ 1 oz= 28.4 g; Calories = 129.8

Cookies Peanut Butter Commercially Prepared Sugar Free ☞ 1 serving 3 cookies= 29 g; Calories = 151.7

Cookies Peanut Butter Prepared From Recipe ☞ 1 oz= 28.4 g; Calories = 134.9

Cookies Peanut Butter Refrigerated Dough ☞ 1 oz= 28.4 g; Calories = 130.1

Cookies Peanut Butter Refrigerated Dough Baked ☞ 1 oz= 28.4 g; Calories = 142.9

Cookies Peanut Butter Sandwich Regular ☞ 1 oz= 28.4 g; Calories = 135.8

Cookies Peanut Butter Sandwich Special Dietary ☞ 1 oz= 28.4 g; Calories = 151.9

Cookies Raisin Soft-Type ☞ 1 oz= 28.4 g; Calories = 113.9

Cookies Shortbread Commercially Prepared Pecan ☞ 1 oz= 28.4 g; Calories = 153.9

Cookies Shortbread Commercially Prepared Plain ☞ 1 oz= 28.4 g; Calories = 146

Cookies Shortbread Reduced Fat ☞ 1 cookie= 11.8 g; Calories = 53.2

Cookies Sugar Commercially Prepared Regular (Includes Vanilla) ☞ 1 oz= 28.4 g; Calories = 131.8

Cookies Sugar Refrigerated Dough ☞ 1 serving= 33 g; Calories = 143.9

Cookies Sugar Refrigerated Dough Baked ☞ 1 oz= 28.4 g; Calories = 138.9

Cookies Sugar Wafer Chocolate-Covered ☞ 3 cookie= 29 g; Calories = 152.5

Cookies Sugar Wafer With Creme Filling Sugar Free ☞ 1 oz= 28.4 g; Calories = 150.8

Cookies Sugar Wafers With Creme Filling Regular ☞ 3 cookies= 36 g; Calories = 180.7

Cookies Vanilla Sandwich With Creme Filling ☞ 1 oz= 28.4 g; Calories = 137.2

Cookies Vanilla Sandwich With Creme Filling Reduced Fat ☞ 1 serving cookie= 48 g; Calories = 203

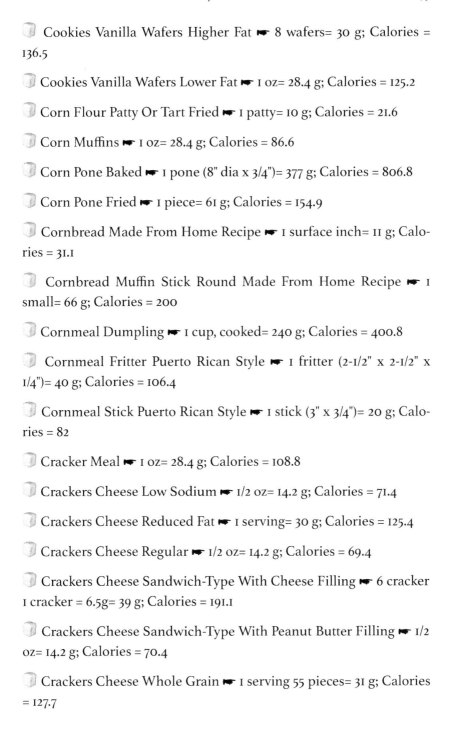

Cookies Vanilla Wafers Higher Fat ☛ 8 wafers= 30 g; Calories = 136.5

Cookies Vanilla Wafers Lower Fat ☛ 1 oz= 28.4 g; Calories = 125.2

Corn Flour Patty Or Tart Fried ☛ 1 patty= 10 g; Calories = 21.6

Corn Muffins ☛ 1 oz= 28.4 g; Calories = 86.6

Corn Pone Baked ☛ 1 pone (8" dia x 3/4")= 377 g; Calories = 806.8

Corn Pone Fried ☛ 1 piece= 61 g; Calories = 154.9

Cornbread Made From Home Recipe ☛ 1 surface inch= 11 g; Calories = 31.1

Cornbread Muffin Stick Round Made From Home Recipe ☛ 1 small= 66 g; Calories = 200

Cornmeal Dumpling ☛ 1 cup, cooked= 240 g; Calories = 400.8

Cornmeal Fritter Puerto Rican Style ☛ 1 fritter (2-1/2" x 2-1/2" x 1/4")= 40 g; Calories = 106.4

Cornmeal Stick Puerto Rican Style ☛ 1 stick (3" x 3/4")= 20 g; Calories = 82

Cracker Meal ☛ 1 oz= 28.4 g; Calories = 108.8

Crackers Cheese Low Sodium ☛ 1/2 oz= 14.2 g; Calories = 71.4

Crackers Cheese Reduced Fat ☛ 1 serving= 30 g; Calories = 125.4

Crackers Cheese Regular ☛ 1/2 oz= 14.2 g; Calories = 69.4

Crackers Cheese Sandwich-Type With Cheese Filling ☛ 6 cracker 1 cracker = 6.5g= 39 g; Calories = 191.1

Crackers Cheese Sandwich-Type With Peanut Butter Filling ☛ 1/2 oz= 14.2 g; Calories = 70.4

Crackers Cheese Whole Grain ☛ 1 serving 55 pieces= 31 g; Calories = 127.7

Crackers Cream Gamesa Sabrosas ☛ 11 crackers (1 nlea serving)= 31 g; Calories = 150

Crackers Cream La Moderna Rikis Cream Crackers ☛ 10 crackers (1 nlea serving)= 32 g; Calories = 148.5

Crackers Flavored Fish-Shaped ☛ 10 goldfish= 5.2 g; Calories = 24.1

Crackers Gluten-Free Multi-Seeded And Multigrain ☛ 3 crackers= 6.1 g; Calories = 27.6

Crackers Gluten-Free Multigrain And Vegetable Made With Corn Starch And White Rice Flour ☛ 3 crackers= 10.7 g; Calories = 48.8

Crackers Matzo Egg And Onion ☛ 1/2 oz= 14.2 g; Calories = 55.5

Crackers Matzo Whole-Wheat ☛ 1/2 oz= 14.2 g; Calories = 49.8

Crackers Melba Toast Plain Without Salt ☛ 1/2 oz= 14.2 g; Calories = 55.4

Crackers Milk ☛ 1/2 oz= 14.2 g; Calories = 63.3

Crackers Multigrain ☛ 4 crackers= 14 g; Calories = 67.5

Crackers Rusk Toast ☛ 1/2 oz= 14.2 g; Calories = 57.8

Crackers Rye Sandwich-Type With Cheese Filling ☛ 1/2 oz= 14.2 g; Calories = 68.3

Crackers Rye Wafers Plain ☛ 1/2 oz= 14.2 g; Calories = 47.4

Crackers Rye Wafers Seasoned ☛ 1/2 oz= 14.2 g; Calories = 54.1

Crackers Saltines (Includes Oyster Soda Soup) ☛ 5 crackers= 14.9 g; Calories = 62.3

Crackers Saltines Fat-Free Low-Sodium ☛ 3 saltines= 15 g; Calories = 59

Crackers Saltines Low Salt (Includes Oyster Soda Soup) ☛ 1/2 oz= 14.2 g; Calories = 59.8

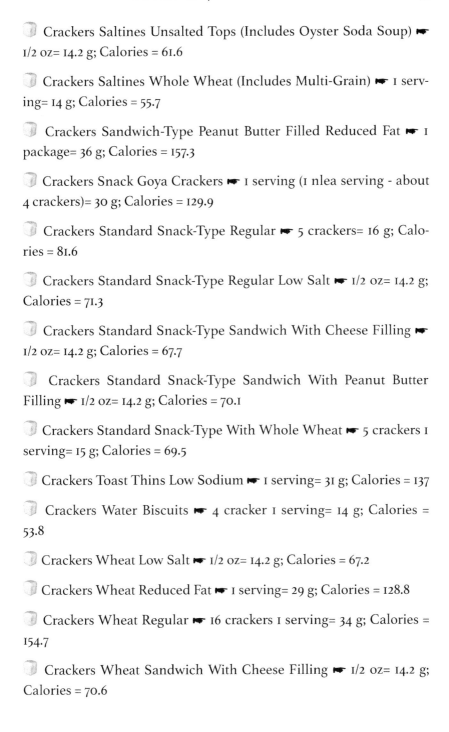

Crackers Saltines Unsalted Tops (Includes Oyster Soda Soup) ☛ 1/2 oz= 14.2 g; Calories = 61.6

Crackers Saltines Whole Wheat (Includes Multi-Grain) ☛ 1 serving= 14 g; Calories = 55.7

Crackers Sandwich-Type Peanut Butter Filled Reduced Fat ☛ 1 package= 36 g; Calories = 157.3

Crackers Snack Goya Crackers ☛ 1 serving (1 nlea serving - about 4 crackers)= 30 g; Calories = 129.9

Crackers Standard Snack-Type Regular ☛ 5 crackers= 16 g; Calories = 81.6

Crackers Standard Snack-Type Regular Low Salt ☛ 1/2 oz= 14.2 g; Calories = 71.3

Crackers Standard Snack-Type Sandwich With Cheese Filling ☛ 1/2 oz= 14.2 g; Calories = 67.7

Crackers Standard Snack-Type Sandwich With Peanut Butter Filling ☛ 1/2 oz= 14.2 g; Calories = 70.1

Crackers Standard Snack-Type With Whole Wheat ☛ 5 crackers 1 serving= 15 g; Calories = 69.5

Crackers Toast Thins Low Sodium ☛ 1 serving= 31 g; Calories = 137

Crackers Water Biscuits ☛ 4 cracker 1 serving= 14 g; Calories = 53.8

Crackers Wheat Low Salt ☛ 1/2 oz= 14.2 g; Calories = 67.2

Crackers Wheat Reduced Fat ☛ 1 serving= 29 g; Calories = 128.8

Crackers Wheat Regular ☛ 16 crackers 1 serving= 34 g; Calories = 154.7

Crackers Wheat Sandwich With Cheese Filling ☛ 1/2 oz= 14.2 g; Calories = 70.6

Crackers Wheat Sandwich With Peanut Butter Filling ☛ 1/2 oz= 14.2 g; Calories = 70.3

Crackers Whole Grain Sandwich-Type With Peanut Butter Filling ☛ 6 cracker 1 serving= 43 g; Calories = 200

Crackers Whole-Wheat ☛ 1 serving= 28 g; Calories = 119.6

Crackers Whole-Wheat Low Salt ☛ 1/2 oz= 14.2 g; Calories = 62.9

Crackers Whole-Wheat Reduced Fat ☛ 1 serving= 29 g; Calories = 120.6

Cream Puff Eclair Custard Or Cream Filled Iced ☛ 4 oz= 113 g; Calories = 377.4

Cream Puff Eclair Custard Or Cream Filled Iced Reduced Fat ☛ 1 eclair, frozen= 60 g; Calories = 142.2

Cream Puff Eclair Custard Or Cream Filled Not Iced ☛ 1 eclair (5" x 2" x 1-3/4")= 90 g; Calories = 234

Cream Puff Eclair Custard Or Cream Filled Ns As To Icing ☛ 1 eclair (5" x 2" x 1-3/4")= 102 g; Calories = 281.5

Cream Puff Shell Prepared From Recipe ☛ 1 oz= 28.4 g; Calories = 102.2

Crisp Apple Apple Dessert ☛ 1 cup= 246 g; Calories = 386.2

Crisp Blueberry ☛ 1 cup= 246 g; Calories = 629.8

Crisp Cherry ☛ 1 cup= 246 g; Calories = 647

Crisp Peach ☛ 1 cup= 246 g; Calories = 524

Crisp Rhubarb ☛ 1 cup= 246 g; Calories = 553.5

Croissants Apple ☛ 1 oz= 28.4 g; Calories = 72.1

Croutons Seasoned ☛ 1/2 oz= 14.2 g; Calories = 66

Crumpet ☛ 1 small (2-1/2" dia)= 20 g; Calories = 38.6

Crumpet Toasted ☛ 1 small (2-1/2" dia)= 18 g; Calories = 39.1

Crunchmaster Multi-Grain Crisps Snack Crackers Gluten-Free ☛ 3 crackers= 3.9 g; Calories = 17.8

Danish Pastry Cheese ☛ 1 oz= 28.4 g; Calories = 106.2

Danish Pastry Cinnamon Enriched ☛ 1 oz= 28.4 g; Calories = 114.5

Danish Pastry Cinnamon Unenriched ☛ 1 oz= 28.4 g; Calories = 114.5

Danish Pastry Fruit Enriched (Includes Apple Cinnamon Raisin Lemon Raspberry Strawberry) ☛ 1 oz= 28.4 g; Calories = 105.4

Danish Pastry Fruit Unenriched (Includes Apple Cinnamon Raisin Strawberry) ☛ 1 oz= 28.4 g; Calories = 105.4

Danish Pastry Lemon Unenriched ☛ 1 oz= 28.4 g; Calories = 105.4

Danish Pastry Raspberry Unenriched ☛ 1 oz= 28.4 g; Calories = 105.4

Dessert Pizza ☛ 1 piece= 108 g; Calories = 225.7

Doughnut Cake Type Chocolate Covered Dipped In Peanuts ☛ 1 doughnut (3-1/4" dia)= 53 g; Calories = 221.5

Doughnut Chocolate Cream-Filled ☛ 1 doughnut= 65 g; Calories = 230.1

Doughnut Chocolate Raised Or Yeast ☛ 1 doughnut (approx 3" dia)= 50 g; Calories = 206

Doughnut Chocolate Raised Or Yeast With Chocolate Icing ☛ 1 doughnut (approx 3" dia)= 71 g; Calories = 287.6

Doughnut Custard-Filled With Icing ☛ 1 doughnut= 70 g; Calories = 252.7

Doughnut Raised Or Yeast Chocolate Covered ☛ 1 doughnut (approx 3" dia)= 71 g; Calories = 287.6

🍩 Doughnuts Cake-Type Chocolate Sugared Or Glazed ☞ 1 oz= 28.4 g; Calories = 118.4

🍩 Doughnuts Cake-Type Plain (Includes Unsugared Old-Fashioned) ☞ 1 donut= 40 g; Calories = 173.6

🍩 Doughnuts Cake-Type Plain Chocolate-Coated Or Frosted ☞ 1 oz= 28.4 g; Calories = 128.4

🍩 Doughnuts Cake-Type Plain Sugared Or Glazed ☞ 1 oz= 28.4 g; Calories = 121

🍩 Doughnuts French Crullers Glazed ☞ 1 oz= 28.4 g; Calories = 117

🍩 Doughnuts Yeast-Leavened Glazed Enriched (Includes Honey Buns) ☞ 1 oz= 28.4 g; Calories = 119.6

🍩 Doughnuts Yeast-Leavened Glazed Unenriched (Includes Honey Buns) ☞ 1 oz= 28.4 g; Calories = 114.5

🍩 Doughnuts Yeast-Leavened With Creme Filling ☞ 1 oz= 28.4 g; Calories = 102.5

🍩 Doughnuts Yeast-Leavened With Jelly Filling ☞ 1 oz= 28.4 g; Calories = 96.6

🍩 Dumpling Plain ☞ 1 small= 18 g; Calories = 22.3

🍩 Dutch Apple Pie ☞ 1/8 pie 1 pie (1/8 of 9 inch pie)= 131 g; Calories = 379.9

🍩 Egg Bagel ☞ 1 oz= 28.4 g; Calories = 79

🍩 Empanada Mexican Turnover Pumpkin ☞ 1 cup= 132 g; Calories = 380.2

🍩 Empanada Mexican Turnover Fruit-Filled ☞ 1 cup= 142 g; Calories = 448.7

🍩 English Muffins ☞ 1 oz= 28.4 g; Calories = 63.3

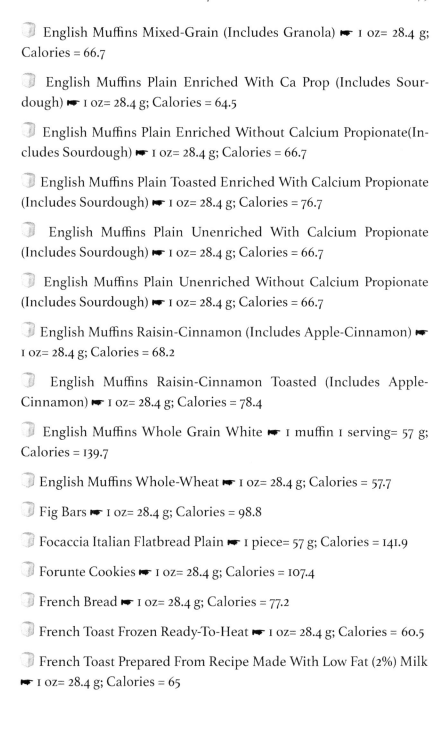

English Muffins Mixed-Grain (Includes Granola) ☞ 1 oz= 28.4 g; Calories = 66.7

English Muffins Plain Enriched With Ca Prop (Includes Sourdough) ☞ 1 oz= 28.4 g; Calories = 64.5

English Muffins Plain Enriched Without Calcium Propionate(Includes Sourdough) ☞ 1 oz= 28.4 g; Calories = 66.7

English Muffins Plain Toasted Enriched With Calcium Propionate (Includes Sourdough) ☞ 1 oz= 28.4 g; Calories = 76.7

English Muffins Plain Unenriched With Calcium Propionate (Includes Sourdough) ☞ 1 oz= 28.4 g; Calories = 66.7

English Muffins Plain Unenriched Without Calcium Propionate (Includes Sourdough) ☞ 1 oz= 28.4 g; Calories = 66.7

English Muffins Raisin-Cinnamon (Includes Apple-Cinnamon) ☞ 1 oz= 28.4 g; Calories = 68.2

English Muffins Raisin-Cinnamon Toasted (Includes Apple-Cinnamon) ☞ 1 oz= 28.4 g; Calories = 78.4

English Muffins Whole Grain White ☞ 1 muffin 1 serving= 57 g; Calories = 139.7

English Muffins Whole-Wheat ☞ 1 oz= 28.4 g; Calories = 57.7

Fig Bars ☞ 1 oz= 28.4 g; Calories = 98.8

Focaccia Italian Flatbread Plain ☞ 1 piece= 57 g; Calories = 141.9

Forunte Cookies ☞ 1 oz= 28.4 g; Calories = 107.4

French Bread ☞ 1 oz= 28.4 g; Calories = 77.2

French Toast Frozen Ready-To-Heat ☞ 1 oz= 28.4 g; Calories = 60.5

French Toast Prepared From Recipe Made With Low Fat (2%) Milk ☞ 1 oz= 28.4 g; Calories = 65

Fritter Apple ☞ 1 fritter (2-1/2" long x 1-5/8" wide)= 17 g; Calories = 64.8

Fritter Banana ☞ 1 fritter (2" long)= 34 g; Calories = 116.3

Fritter Berry ☞ 1 fritter (1-1/4" dia)= 24 g; Calories = 82.1

Funnel Cake With Sugar ☞ 1 cake (6" dia)= 90 g; Calories = 314.1

Funnel Cake With Sugar And Fruit ☞ 1 cake (6" dia)= 135 g; Calories = 509

Garlic Bread From Fast Food / Restaurant ☞ 1 small slice= 37 g; Calories = 129.1

Garlic Bread Frozen ☞ 1 slice presliced= 43 g; Calories = 150.5

Garlic Bread Nfs ☞ 1 small slice= 39 g; Calories = 136.1

Garlic Bread With Melted Cheese From Fast Food / Restaurant ☞ 1 small slice= 44 g; Calories = 148.7

Garlic Bread With Melted Cheese From Frozen ☞ 1 small slice= 44 g; Calories = 150.9

Garlic Bread With Parmesan Cheese From Fast Food / Restaurant ☞ 1 small slice= 39 g; Calories = 136.9

Garlic Bread With Parmesan Cheese From Frozen ☞ 1 small slice= 39 g; Calories = 136.9

George Weston Bakeries Brownberry Sage And Onion Stuffing Mix Dry ☞ 1 serving= 67 g; Calories = 261.3

George Weston Bakeries Thomas English Muffins ☞ 1 serving= 57 g; Calories = 132.2

Gingerbread Cake ☞ 1 oz= 28.4 g; Calories = 101.1

Gingersnaps ☞ 1 oz= 28.4 g; Calories = 118.1

Glutino Gluten Free Cookies Chocolate Vanilla Creme ☞ 3 cookies= 44 g; Calories = 208.6

Glutino Gluten Free Cookies Vanilla Creme ☛ 3 cookies= 45 g; Calories = 219.2

Glutino Gluten Free Wafers Lemon Flavored ☛ 3 cookies= 30 g; Calories = 154.5

Glutino Gluten Free Wafers Milk Chocolate ☛ 3 cookies= 23 g; Calories = 124.4

Heinz Weight Watcher Chocolate Eclair Frozen ☛ 1 eclair, frozen= 59 g; Calories = 142.2

Hush Puppies Prepared From Recipe ☛ 1 oz= 28.4 g; Calories = 95.7

Ice Cream Cones Cake Or Wafer-Type ☛ 1 oz= 28.4 g; Calories = 118.4

Ice Cream Cones Sugar Rolled-Type ☛ 1 oz= 28.4 g; Calories = 114.2

Injera Ethiopian Bread ☛ 1 cup, pieces= 68 g; Calories = 59.8

Interstate Brands Corp Wonder Hamburger Rolls ☛ 1 serving= 43 g; Calories = 117.4

Johnnycake ☛ 1 piece= 49 g; Calories = 134.8

Keebler Keebler Chocolate Graham Selects ☛ 1 serving= 31 g; Calories = 144.2

Keikitos (Muffins) Latino Bakery Item ☛ 1 piece= 42 g; Calories = 196.1

Kraft Foods Shake N Bake Original Recipe Coating For Pork Dry ☛ 1 serving= 28 g; Calories = 105.6

Kraft Stove Top Stuffing Mix Chicken Flavor ☛ 1 nlea serving (makes 1/2 cup prepared)= 28 g; Calories = 106.7

Ladyfingers ☛ 1 oz= 28.4 g; Calories = 103.7

Leavening Agents Baking Powder Double-Acting Sodium Aluminum Sulfate ☞ 1 tsp= 4.6 g; Calories = 2.4

Leavening Agents Baking Powder Double-Acting Straight Phosphate ☞ 1 tsp= 4.6 g; Calories = 2.3

Leavening Agents Baking Powder Low-Sodium ☞ 1 tsp= 5 g; Calories = 4.9

Leavening Agents Baking Soda ☞ 1 tsp= 4.6 g; Calories = 0

Leavening Agents Cream Of Tartar ☞ 1 tsp= 3 g; Calories = 7.7

Leavening Agents Yeast Bakers Active Dry ☞ 1 tsp= 4 g; Calories = 13

Leavening Agents Yeast Bakers Compressed ☞ 1 cake (0.6 oz)= 17 g; Calories = 17.9

Martha White Foods Martha Whites Buttermilk Biscuit Mix Dry ☞ 1 serving= 41 g; Calories = 159.1

Martha White Foods Martha Whites Chewy Fudge Brownie Mix Dry ☞ 1 serving= 28 g; Calories = 114

Marys Gone Crackers Original Crackers Organic Gluten Free ☞ 3 crackers= 7.4 g; Calories = 33

Matzo Egg Crackers ☞ 1/2 oz= 14.2 g; Calories = 55.5

Mckee Baking Little Debbie Nutty Bars Wafers With Peanut Butter Chocolate Covered ☞ 1 serving= 57 g; Calories = 312.4

Melba Toast ☞ 1/2 oz= 14.2 g; Calories = 55.4

Mission Foods Mission Flour Tortillas Soft Taco 8 Inch ☞ 1 serving= 51 g; Calories = 146.4

Mixed Fruit Tart Filled With Custard Or Cream Cheese ☞ 1 tart (9" dia)= 1265 g; Calories = 2188.5

Molasses Cookies ☞ 1 oz= 28.4 g; Calories = 122.1

Muffin Blueberry Commercially Prepared Low-Fat 🖝 1 muffin small= 71 g; Calories = 181.1

Muffin English Cheese 🖝 1 muffin= 58 g; Calories = 136.9

Muffin English Oat Bran With Raisins 🖝 1 muffin= 58 g; Calories = 157.8

Muffin English Wheat Bran With Raisins 🖝 1 muffin= 58 g; Calories = 134

Muffin English Wheat Or Cracked Wheat With Raisins 🖝 1 muffin= 58 g; Calories = 133.4

Muffin English Whole Wheat With Raisins 🖝 1 muffin= 58 g; Calories = 133.4

Muffin English With Fruit Other Than Raisins 🖝 1 muffin= 58 g; Calories = 140.9

Muffin English With Raisins 🖝 1 muffin= 58 g; Calories = 135.7

Muffin Whole Grain 🖝 1 miniature= 25 g; Calories = 90

Muffins Blueberry Commercially Prepared (Includes Mini-Muffins) 🖝 1 oz= 28.4 g; Calories = 106.5

Muffins Blueberry Dry Mix 🖝 1 serving= 43 g; Calories = 126

Muffins Blueberry Prepared From Recipe Made With Low Fat (2%) Milk 🖝 1 oz= 28.4 g; Calories = 80.9

Muffins Blueberry Toaster-Type 🖝 1 oz= 28.4 g; Calories = 88.9

Muffins Blueberry Toaster-Type Toasted 🖝 1 oz= 28.4 g; Calories = 94.6

Muffins Corn Dry Mix Prepared 🖝 1 oz= 28.4 g; Calories = 91.2

Muffins Corn Prepared From Recipe Made With Low Fat (2%) Milk 🖝 1 oz= 28.4 g; Calories = 89.7

Muffins Corn Toaster-Type 🖝 1 oz= 28.4 g; Calories = 98.3

Muffins Oat Bran 🐾 1 oz= 28.4 g; Calories = 76.7

Muffins Plain Prepared From Recipe Made With Low Fat (2%) Milk 🐾 1 oz= 28.4 g; Calories = 84.1

Muffins Wheat Bran Dry Mix 🐾 1 oz= 28.4 g; Calories = 112.5

Muffins Wheat Bran Toaster-Type With Raisins Toasted 🐾 1 oz= 28.4 g; Calories = 88.9

Multi-Grain Toast 🐾 1 oz= 28.4 g; Calories = 81.8

Naan Indian Flatbread 🐾 1 piece (1/4 of 10" dia)= 44 g; Calories = 136.8

Nabisco Nabisco Grahams Crackers 🐾 1 serving= 28 g; Calories = 118.7

Nabisco Nabisco Oreo Crunchies Cookie Crumb Topping 🐾 1 serving= 11 g; Calories = 52.4

Nabisco Nabisco Ritz Crackers 🐾 1 cracker= 3.3 g; Calories = 16.2

Nabisco Nabisco Snackwells Fat Free Devils Food Cookie Cakes 🐾 1 serving= 16 g; Calories = 48.8

Oatmeal Cookies 🐾 1 oz= 28.4 g; Calories = 127.8

Pan Dulce La Ricura Salpora De Arroz Con Azucar Cookie-Like Contains Wheat Flour And Rice Flour 🐾 1 piece (1 serving)= 42 g; Calories = 186.9

Pan Dulce With Raisins And Icing 🐾 1 roll= 93 g; Calories = 342.2

Pancakes Blueberry Prepared From Recipe 🐾 1 oz= 28.4 g; Calories = 63

Pancakes Buckwheat Dry Mix Incomplete 🐾 1 oz= 28.4 g; Calories = 96.6

Pancakes Buttermilk Prepared From Recipe 🐾 1 oz= 28.4 g; Calories = 64.5

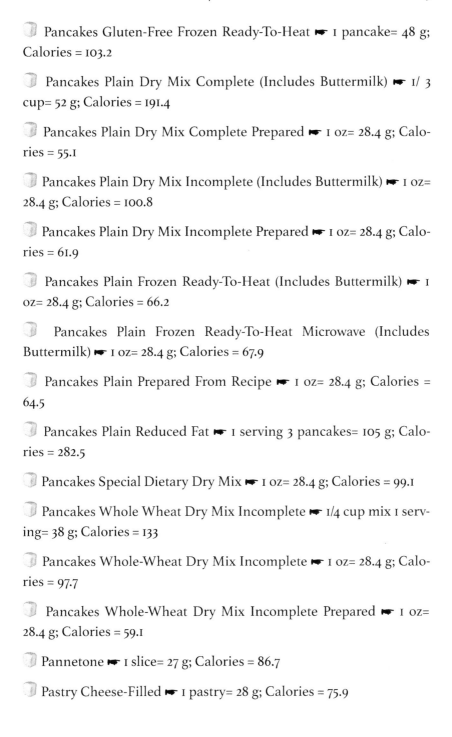

Pancakes Gluten-Free Frozen Ready-To-Heat ☞ 1 pancake= 48 g; Calories = 103.2

Pancakes Plain Dry Mix Complete (Includes Buttermilk) ☞ 1/ 3 cup= 52 g; Calories = 191.4

Pancakes Plain Dry Mix Complete Prepared ☞ 1 oz= 28.4 g; Calories = 55.1

Pancakes Plain Dry Mix Incomplete (Includes Buttermilk) ☞ 1 oz= 28.4 g; Calories = 100.8

Pancakes Plain Dry Mix Incomplete Prepared ☞ 1 oz= 28.4 g; Calories = 61.9

Pancakes Plain Frozen Ready-To-Heat (Includes Buttermilk) ☞ 1 oz= 28.4 g; Calories = 66.2

Pancakes Plain Frozen Ready-To-Heat Microwave (Includes Buttermilk) ☞ 1 oz= 28.4 g; Calories = 67.9

Pancakes Plain Prepared From Recipe ☞ 1 oz= 28.4 g; Calories = 64.5

Pancakes Plain Reduced Fat ☞ 1 serving 3 pancakes= 105 g; Calories = 282.5

Pancakes Special Dietary Dry Mix ☞ 1 oz= 28.4 g; Calories = 99.1

Pancakes Whole Wheat Dry Mix Incomplete ☞ 1/4 cup mix 1 serving= 38 g; Calories = 133

Pancakes Whole-Wheat Dry Mix Incomplete ☞ 1 oz= 28.4 g; Calories = 97.7

Pancakes Whole-Wheat Dry Mix Incomplete Prepared ☞ 1 oz= 28.4 g; Calories = 59.1

Pannetone ☞ 1 slice= 27 g; Calories = 86.7

Pastry Cheese-Filled ☞ 1 pastry= 28 g; Calories = 75.9

Pastry Chinese Made With Rice Flour ☛ 1 oz= 28 g; Calories = 68

Pastry Cookie Type Fried ☛ 1 pastry= 46 g; Calories = 179.4

Pastry Fruit-Filled ☛ 1 pastry= 78 g; Calories = 264.4

Pastry Italian With Cheese ☛ 1 pastry= 85 g; Calories = 234.6

Pastry Made With Bean Or Lotus Seed Paste Filling Baked ☛ 1 small square moon cake= 51 g; Calories = 169.8

Pastry Made With Bean Paste And Salted Egg Yolk Filling Baked ☛ 1 large square moon cake= 204 g; Calories = 679.3

Pastry Pastelitos De Guava (Guava Pastries) ☛ 1 piece= 86 g; Calories = 325.9

Pastry Puff Custard Or Cream Filled Iced Or Not Iced ☛ 1 cream horn= 57 g; Calories = 233.1

Pepperidge Farm Goldfish Baked Snack Crackers Cheddar ☛ 10 goldfish= 5.2 g; Calories = 23.8

Pepperidge Farm Goldfish Baked Snack Crackers Explosive Pizza ☛ 10 goldfish= 5.3 g; Calories = 24.3

Pepperidge Farm Goldfish Baked Snack Crackers Original ☛ 10 goldfish= 5.2 g; Calories = 24.3

Pepperidge Farm Goldfish Baked Snack Crackers Parmesan ☛ 10 goldfish= 5.3 g; Calories = 24.3

Pepperidge Farm Goldfish Baked Snack Crackers Pizza ☛ 10 goldfish= 5.1 g; Calories = 23.9

Phyllo Dough ☛ 1 oz= 28.4 g; Calories = 84.9

Pie Apple Commercially Prepared Enriched Flour ☛ 1 oz= 28.4 g; Calories = 67.3

Pie Apple Commercially Prepared Unenriched Flour ☛ 1 oz= 28.4 g; Calories = 67.3

Pie Apple Diet ☞ 1 individual serving= 85 g; Calories = 193

Pie Apple One Crust ☞ 1 pie (9" dia)= 1203 g; Calories = 2911.3

Pie Apple Prepared From Recipe ☞ 1 oz= 28.4 g; Calories = 75.3

Pie Apple-Sour Cream ☞ 1 pie (9" dia)= 1274 g; Calories = 2611.7

Pie Apricot Two Crust ☞ 1 pie (9" dia)= 1203 g; Calories = 3344.3

Pie Banana Cream Individual Size Or Tart ☞ 1 tart= 117 g; Calories = 277.3

Pie Banana Cream Prepared From Mix No-Bake Type ☞ 1 oz= 28.4 g; Calories = 71.3

Pie Banana Cream Prepared From Recipe ☞ 1 oz= 28.4 g; Calories = 76.4

Pie Berry Not Blackberry Blueberry Boysenberry Huckleberry Raspberry Or Strawberry Individual Size Or Tart ☞ 1 tart= 117 g; Calories = 362.7

Pie Berry Not Blackberry Blueberry Boysenberry Huckleberry Raspberry Or Strawberry; One Crust ☞ 1 pie (9" dia)= 1096 g; Calories = 2729

Pie Berry Not Blackberry Blueberry Boysenberry Huckleberry Raspberry Or Strawberry; Two Crust ☞ 1 pie (9" dia)= 1203 g; Calories = 3476.7

Pie Black Bottom ☞ 1 pie (9" dia)= 792 g; Calories = 2439.4

Pie Blackberry Individual Size Or Tart ☞ 1 tart= 117 g; Calories = 332.3

Pie Blackberry Two Crust ☞ 1 pie (10" dia)= 1521 g; Calories = 3985

Pie Blueberry Individual Size Or Tart ☞ 1 tart= 117 g; Calories = 335.8

Pie Blueberry One Crust ☞ 1 pie (9" dia)= 1096 g; Calories = 2334.5

Pie Blueberry Prepared From Recipe ☛ 1 oz= 28.4 g; Calories = 69.6

Pie Buttermilk ☛ 1 pie (9" dia)= 1154 g; Calories = 4385.2

Pie Cherry Commercially Prepared ☛ 1 oz= 28.4 g; Calories = 73.8

Pie Cherry Made With Cream Cheese And Sour Cream ☛ 1 pie (9" dia)= 1274 g; Calories = 3605.4

Pie Cherry One Crust ☛ 1 pie (9" dia)= 1096 g; Calories = 2498.9

Pie Cherry Prepared From Recipe ☛ 1 oz= 28.4 g; Calories = 76.7

Pie Chess ☛ 1 pie (9" dia)= 714 g; Calories = 2920.3

Pie Chiffon Chocolate ☛ 1 pie (9" dia)= 792 g; Calories = 2574

Pie Chiffon Not Chocolate ☛ 1 pie (9" dia)= 792 g; Calories = 2296.8

Pie Chocolate Cream Individual Size Or Tart ☛ 1 tart= 117 g; Calories = 338.1

Pie Chocolate Creme Commercially Prepared ☛ 1 serving .167 pie= 120 g; Calories = 423.6

Pie Chocolate Mousse Prepared From Mix No-Bake Type ☛ 1 oz= 28.4 g; Calories = 73.8

Pie Chocolate-Marshmallow ☛ 1 pie (8" dia)= 819 g; Calories = 3194.1

Pie Coconut Cream Individual Size Or Tart ☛ 1 tart= 117 g; Calories = 263.3

Pie Coconut Cream Prepared From Mix No-Bake Type ☛ 1 oz= 28.4 g; Calories = 78.4

Pie Coconut Creme Commercially Prepared ☛ 1 oz= 28.4 g; Calories = 84.6

Pie Crust Cookie-Type Chocolate Ready Crust ☛ 1 crust= 182 g; Calories = 880.9

Pie Crust Cookie-Type Graham Cracker Ready Crust ☛ 1 oz= 28.4 g; Calories = 142.3

Pie Crust Cookie-Type Prepared From Recipe Graham Cracker Chilled ☛ 1 piece (1/8 of 9 inch crust)= 30 g; Calories = 145.2

Pie Crust Cookie-Type Prepared From Recipe Vanilla Wafer Chilled ☛ 1 cup= 129 g; Calories = 685

Pie Crust Deep Dish Frozen Baked Made With Enriched Flour ☛ 1 pie crust (average weight)= 202 g; Calories = 1052.4

Pie Crust Deep Dish Frozen Unbaked Made With Enriched Flour ☛ 1 pie crust (average weight)= 225 g; Calories = 1053

Pie Crust Refrigerated Regular Baked ☛ 1 pie crust= 198 g; Calories = 1001.9

Pie Crust Refrigerated Regular Unbaked ☛ 1 pie crust (average weight)= 229 g; Calories = 1019.1

Pie Crust Standard-Type Dry Mix ☛ 1 oz= 28.4 g; Calories = 147.1

Pie Crust Standard-Type Dry Mix Prepared Baked ☛ 1 piece (1/8 of 9 inch crust)= 20 g; Calories = 100.2

Pie Crust Standard-Type Frozen Ready-To-Bake Enriched ☛ 1 piece (1/8 of 9 inch crust)= 18 g; Calories = 82.3

Pie Crust Standard-Type Frozen Ready-To-Bake Enriched Baked ☛ 1 pie crust (average weight of 1 baked crust)= 154 g; Calories = 782.3

Pie Crust Standard-Type Frozen Ready-To-Bake Unenriched ☛ 1 crust, single 9 inch= 142 g; Calories = 648.9

Pie Crust Standard-Type Prepared From Recipe Baked ☛ 1 piece (1/8 of 9 inch crust)= 23 g; Calories = 121.2

Pie Crust Standard-Type Prepared From Recipe Unbaked ☛ 1 piece (1/8 of 9 inch crust)= 24 g; Calories = 112.6

Pie Custard Individual Size Or Tart ☛ 1 tart= 117 g; Calories = 201.2

Pie Egg Custard Commercially Prepared ☛ 1 oz= 28.4 g; Calories = 59.6

Pie Fried Pies Cherry ☛ 1 oz= 28.4 g; Calories = 89.7

Pie Fried Pies Fruit ☛ 1 oz= 28.4 g; Calories = 89.7

Pie Fried Pies Lemon ☛ 1 oz= 28.4 g; Calories = 89.7

Pie Lemon Cream ☛ 1 pie (9" dia)= 1154 g; Calories = 3081.2

Pie Lemon Cream Individual Size Or Tart ☛ 1 tart= 117 g; Calories = 331.1

Pie Lemon Meringue Commercially Prepared ☛ 1 oz= 28.4 g; Calories = 76.1

Pie Lemon Meringue Prepared From Recipe ☛ 1 oz= 28.4 g; Calories = 80.9

Pie Lemon Not Cream Or Meringue ☛ 1 pie (9" dia)= 791 g; Calories = 3037.4

Pie Lemon Not Cream Or Meringue Individual Size Or Tart ☛ 1 tart= 117 g; Calories = 462.2

Pie Mince Individual Size Or Tart ☛ 1 tart= 117 g; Calories = 358

Pie Mince Prepared From Recipe ☛ 1 oz= 28.4 g; Calories = 82.1

Pie Oatmeal ☛ 1 pie (9" dia)= 915 g; Calories = 3568.5

Pie Peach ☛ 1 oz= 28.4 g; Calories = 63.6

Pie Peach Individual Size Or Tart ☛ 1 tart= 117 g; Calories = 342.8

Pie Peach One Crust ☛ 1 pie (9" dia)= 1203 g; Calories = 2791

Pie Peanut Butter Cream ☛ 1 pie (9" dia)= 1154 g; Calories = 3381.2

Pie Pear Individual Size Or Tart ☛ 1 tart= 117 g; Calories = 339.3

Pie Pear Two Crust ☛ 1 pie (9" dia)= 1203 g; Calories = 3212

Pie Pecan Commercially Prepared ☛ 1 oz= 28.4 g; Calories = 115.6

Pie Pecan Prepared From Recipe ☛ 1 oz= 28.4 g; Calories = 117

Pie Pineapple Cream ☛ 1 pie (9" dia)= 1154 g; Calories = 2319.5

Pie Pineapple Two Crust ☛ 1 pie (9" dia)= 1203 g; Calories = 3163.9

Pie Plum Two Crust ☛ 1 pie (9" dia)= 1203 g; Calories = 3512.8

Pie Prune One Crust ☛ 1 pie (9" dia)= 1203 g; Calories = 3621

Pie Pudding Chocolate With Chocolate Coating Individual Size ☛ 1 individual pie= 142 g; Calories = 552.4

Pie Pudding Flavors Other Than Chocolate ☛ 1 pie (8" dia)= 885 g; Calories = 1982.4

Pie Pudding Flavors Other Than Chocolate Individual Size Or Tart ☛ 1 small tart= 117 g; Calories = 390.8

Pie Pudding Flavors Other Than Chocolate With Chocolate Coating Individual Size ☛ 1 individual pie= 142 g; Calories = 545.3

Pie Pumpkin Commercially Prepared ☛ 1 oz= 28.4 g; Calories = 69

Pie Pumpkin Prepared From Recipe ☛ 1 oz= 28.4 g; Calories = 57.9

Pie Raisin Individual Size Or Tart ☛ 1 tart= 117 g; Calories = 339.3

Pie Raisin Two Crust ☛ 1 pie (9" dia)= 1203 g; Calories = 3019.5

Pie Raspberry Cream ☛ 1 pie (9" dia)= 1154 g; Calories = 2284.9

Pie Raspberry One Crust ☛ 1 pie (9" dia)= 1096 g; Calories = 2630.4

Pie Raspberry Two Crust ☛ 1 pie (9" dia)= 1203 g; Calories = 3380.4

Pie Rhubarb Individual Size Or Tart ☛ 1 tart= 117 g; Calories = 372.1

Pie Rhubarb One Crust ☛ 1 pie (9" dia)= 1096 g; Calories = 2685.2

Pie Rhubarb Two Crust ☛ 1 pie (9" dia)= 1203 g; Calories = 3560.9

Pie Shoo-Fly ☛ 1 pie (9" dia)= 915 g; Calories = 3239.1

Pie Sour Cream Raisin ☛ 1 pie (9" dia)= 1154 g; Calories = 4085.2

Pie Squash ☛ 1 pie (9" dia)= 1235 g; Calories = 2334.2

Pie Strawberry Cream ☛ 1 pie (10" dia)= 1449 g; Calories = 2956

Pie Strawberry Cream Individual Size Or Tart ☛ 1 tart= 117 g; Calories = 280.8

Pie Strawberry Individual Size Or Tart ☛ 1 tart= 117 g; Calories = 310.1

Pie Strawberry One Crust ☛ 1 pie (9" dia)= 1343 g; Calories = 3088.9

Pie Strawberry-Rhubarb Two Crust ☛ 1 pie (10" dia)= 1521 g; Calories = 4274

Pie Sweet Potato ☛ 1 pie (10" dia)= 1530 g; Calories = 3978

Pie Tofu With Fruit ☛ 1 pie (9" dia)= 1154 g; Calories = 2411.9

Pie Toll House Chocolate Chip ☛ 1 pie (9" dia)= 915 g; Calories = 4895.3

Pie Vanilla Cream Prepared From Recipe ☛ 1 oz= 28.4 g; Calories = 79

Pie Yogurt Frozen ☛ 1 pie (9" dia)= 1154 g; Calories = 2850.4

Pillsbury Buttermilk Biscuits Artificial Flavor Refrigerated Dough ☛ 1 biscuit= 64 g; Calories = 151

Pillsbury Chocolate Chip Cookies Refrigerated Dough ☛ 1 serving 2 cookies= 38 g; Calories = 171

Pillsbury Cinnamon Rolls With Icing Refrigerated Dough ☛ 1 serving 1 roll with icing= 44 g; Calories = 145.2

Pillsbury Crusty French Loaf Refrigerated Dough ☛ 1 serving= 52 g; Calories = 126.4

Pillsbury Golden Layer Buttermilk Biscuits Artificial Flavor Refrigerated Dough ☛ 1 serving= 34 g; Calories = 104.4

Pillsbury Grands Buttermilk Biscuits Refrigerated Dough ☞ 1 biscuit= 34 g; Calories = 99.6

Pita Bread ☞ 1 pita, large (6-1/2 inch dia)= 60 g; Calories = 165

Pizza Cheese And Vegetables Gluten-Free Thick Crust ☞ 1 piece, nfs= 149 g; Calories = 339.7

Pizza Cheese And Vegetables Gluten-Free Thin Crust ☞ 1 piece, nfs= 133 g; Calories = 296.6

Pizza Cheese And Vegetables Whole Wheat Thick Crust ☞ 1 piece, nfs= 149 g; Calories = 353.1

Pizza Cheese And Vegetables Whole Wheat Thin Crust ☞ 1 piece, nfs= 133 g; Calories = 307.2

Pizza Cheese From School Lunch Medium Crust ☞ 1 piece, nfs= 147 g; Calories = 367.5

Pizza Cheese Gluten-Free Thick Crust ☞ 1 piece, nfs= 132 g; Calories = 344.5

Pizza Cheese Gluten-Free Thin Crust ☞ 1 piece, nfs= 119 g; Calories = 314.2

Pizza Cheese Whole Wheat Thick Crust ☞ 1 piece, nfs= 132 g; Calories = 359

Pizza Cheese Whole Wheat Thin Crust ☞ 1 piece, nfs= 119 g; Calories = 324.9

Pizza Cheese With Fruit Medium Crust ☞ 1 piece, nfs= 137 g; Calories = 327.4

Pizza Cheese With Fruit Thick Crust ☞ 1 piece, nfs= 150 g; Calories = 369

Pizza Cheese With Fruit Thin Crust ☞ 1 piece, nfs= 104 g; Calories = 270.4

Pizza Cheese With Vegetables From Frozen Thick Crust ☞ I piece, nfs= 143 g; Calories = 350.4

Pizza Cheese With Vegetables From Frozen Thin Crust ☞ I piece, nfs= 109 g; Calories = 261.6

Pizza Cheese With Vegetables From Restaurant Or Fast Food Medium Crust ☞ I piece, nfs= 133 g; Calories = 321.9

Pizza Cheese With Vegetables From Restaurant Or Fast Food Thick Crust ☞ I piece, nfs= 149 g; Calories = 365.1

Pizza Cheese With Vegetables From Restaurant Or Fast Food Thin Crust ☞ I piece, nfs= 100 g; Calories = 265

Pizza Extra Cheese Thick Crust ☞ I piece, nfs= 141 g; Calories = 383.5

Pizza Extra Cheese Thin Crust ☞ I piece, nfs= 92 g; Calories = 277.8

Pizza No Cheese Thick Crust ☞ I piece, nfs= 124 g; Calories = 362.1

Pizza No Cheese Thin Crust ☞ I piece, nfs= 75 g; Calories = 207

Pizza Rolls ☞ I cup= 119 g; Calories = 410.6

Pizza With Beans And Vegetables Thick Crust ☞ I piece, nfs= 173 g; Calories = 389.3

Pizza With Beans And Vegetables Thin Crust ☞ I piece, nfs= 129 g; Calories = 291.5

Pizza With Cheese And Extra Vegetables Medium Crust ☞ I piece, nfs= 152 g; Calories = 334.4

Pizza With Cheese And Extra Vegetables Thick Crust ☞ I piece, nfs= 155 g; Calories = 372

Pizza With Cheese And Extra Vegetables Thin Crust ☞ I piece, nfs= 120 g; Calories = 279.6

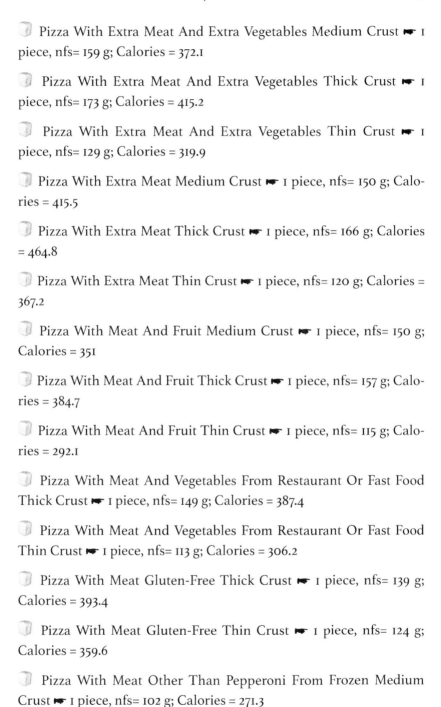

Pizza With Extra Meat And Extra Vegetables Medium Crust ☛ 1 piece, nfs= 159 g; Calories = 372.1

Pizza With Extra Meat And Extra Vegetables Thick Crust ☛ 1 piece, nfs= 173 g; Calories = 415.2

Pizza With Extra Meat And Extra Vegetables Thin Crust ☛ 1 piece, nfs= 129 g; Calories = 319.9

Pizza With Extra Meat Medium Crust ☛ 1 piece, nfs= 150 g; Calories = 415.5

Pizza With Extra Meat Thick Crust ☛ 1 piece, nfs= 166 g; Calories = 464.8

Pizza With Extra Meat Thin Crust ☛ 1 piece, nfs= 120 g; Calories = 367.2

Pizza With Meat And Fruit Medium Crust ☛ 1 piece, nfs= 150 g; Calories = 351

Pizza With Meat And Fruit Thick Crust ☛ 1 piece, nfs= 157 g; Calories = 384.7

Pizza With Meat And Fruit Thin Crust ☛ 1 piece, nfs= 115 g; Calories = 292.1

Pizza With Meat And Vegetables From Restaurant Or Fast Food Thick Crust ☛ 1 piece, nfs= 149 g; Calories = 387.4

Pizza With Meat And Vegetables From Restaurant Or Fast Food Thin Crust ☛ 1 piece, nfs= 113 g; Calories = 306.2

Pizza With Meat Gluten-Free Thick Crust ☛ 1 piece, nfs= 139 g; Calories = 393.4

Pizza With Meat Gluten-Free Thin Crust ☛ 1 piece, nfs= 124 g; Calories = 359.6

Pizza With Meat Other Than Pepperoni From Frozen Medium Crust ☛ 1 piece, nfs= 102 g; Calories = 271.3

Pizza With Meat Other Than Pepperoni From Frozen Thick Crust 1 piece, nfs= 144 g; Calories = 380.2

Pizza With Meat Other Than Pepperoni From Frozen Thin Crust 1 piece, nfs= 97 g; Calories = 260.9

Pizza With Meat Other Than Pepperoni From School Lunch Medium Crust 1 piece, nfs= 147 g; Calories = 373.4

Pizza With Meat Other Than Pepperoni Stuffed Crust 1 piece, nfs= 164 g; Calories = 460.8

Pizza With Meat Whole Wheat Thick Crust 1 piece, nfs= 139 g; Calories = 405.9

Pizza With Meat Whole Wheat Thin Crust 1 piece, nfs= 124 g; Calories = 368.3

Pizza With Pepperoni From Frozen Medium Crust 1 piece, nfs= 102 g; Calories = 276.4

Pizza With Pepperoni From Frozen Thick Crust 1 piece, nfs= 144 g; Calories = 385.9

Pizza With Pepperoni From Frozen Thin Crust 1 piece, nfs= 97 g; Calories = 265.8

Pizza With Pepperoni From School Lunch Medium Crust 1 piece, nfs= 147 g; Calories = 376.3

Pizza With Pepperoni Stuffed Crust 1 piece, nfs= 164 g; Calories = 485.4

Plain Buttermilk Biscuits 1 oz= 28.4 g; Calories = 95.1

Plain Croutons 1/2 oz= 14.2 g; Calories = 57.8

Plain Graham Crackers 1 oz= 28.4 g; Calories = 122.1

Plain Matzo Crackers 1/2 oz= 14.2 g; Calories = 56.1

Popover 1 popover= 31 g; Calories = 82.2

Popovers Dry Mix Enriched ☛ 1 oz= 28.4 g; Calories = 105.4

Popovers Dry Mix Unenriched ☛ 1 oz= 28.4 g; Calories = 105.4

Puff Pastry ☛ 1 oz= 28.4 g; Calories = 156.5

Puff Pastry Frozen Ready-To-Bake Baked ☛ 1 oz= 28.4 g; Calories = 158.5

Pumpernickel Melba Rye Toast ☛ 1/2 oz= 14.2 g; Calories = 55.2

Roll Cheese ☛ 1 roll= 41 g; Calories = 129.2

Roll Sweet Frosted ☛ 1 small= 54 g; Calories = 216

Roll Sweet With Fruit Frosted ☛ 1 small= 54 g; Calories = 204.7

Rolls Dinner Egg ☛ 1 oz= 28.4 g; Calories = 87.2

Rolls Dinner Oat Bran ☛ 1 oz= 28.4 g; Calories = 67

Rolls Dinner Plain Commercially Prepared (Includes Brown-And-Serve) ☛ 1 roll (1 oz)= 28 g; Calories = 86.8

Rolls Dinner Plain Prepared From Recipe Made With Low Fat (2%) Milk ☛ 1 oz= 28.4 g; Calories = 89.7

Rolls Dinner Rye ☛ 1 large (approx 3-1/2 inch to 4 inch dia)= 43 g; Calories = 123

Rolls Dinner Sweet ☛ 1 roll= 30 g; Calories = 96.3

Rolls Dinner Wheat ☛ 1 roll (1 oz)= 28 g; Calories = 76.4

Rolls Dinner Whole-Wheat ☛ 1 roll (1 oz)= 28 g; Calories = 74.5

Rolls French ☛ 1 oz= 28.4 g; Calories = 78.7

Rolls Gluten-Free White Made With Brown Rice Flour Tapioca Starch And Potato Starch ☛ 1 roll= 36 g; Calories = 111.6

🍞 Rolls Gluten-Free White Made With Brown Rice Flour Tapioca Starch And Sorghum Flour 🐮 1 roll= 69 g; Calories = 177.3

🍞 Rolls Gluten-Free White Made With Rice Flour Rice Starch And Corn Starch 🐮 1 roll= 78 g; Calories = 186.4

🍞 Rolls Gluten-Free Whole Grain Made With Tapioca Starch And Brown Rice Flour 🐮 1 roll= 44 g; Calories = 144.8

🍞 Rolls Hamburger Or Hot Dog Wheat/cracked Wheat 🐮 1 roll= 51 g; Calories = 137.2

🍞 Rolls Hamburger Or Hot Dog Whole Wheat 🐮 1 roll= 56 g; Calories = 150.6

🍞 Rolls Hamburger Or Hotdog Mixed-Grain 🐮 1 oz= 28.4 g; Calories = 74.7

🍞 Rolls Hamburger Or Hotdog Plain 🐮 1 roll 1 serving= 44 g; Calories = 122.8

🍞 Rolls Hamburger Whole Grain White Calcium-Fortified 🐮 1 piece roll= 43 g; Calories = 109.7

🍞 Rolls Hard (Includes Kaiser) 🐮 1 oz= 28.4 g; Calories = 83.2

🍞 Rolls Pumpernickel 🐮 1 medium (2-1/2 inch dia)= 36 g; Calories = 99.4

🍞 Rudis Gluten-Free Bakery Original Sandwich Bread 🐮 1 slice= 34 g; Calories = 108.8

🍞 Rye Bread 🐮 1 oz= 28.4 g; Calories = 73.6

🍞 Rye Crispbread 🐮 1/2 oz= 14.2 g; Calories = 52

🍞 Sage Valley Gluten Free Vanilla Sandwich Cookies 🐮 3 cookies= 44 g; Calories = 219.6

🍞 Schar Gluten-Free Classic White Rolls 🐮 1 roll= 78 g; Calories = 186.4

Scone 🐄 1 scone= 42 g; Calories = 148.3

Scone With Fruit 🐄 1 scone= 42 g; Calories = 147.8

Sopaipilla With Syrup Or Honey 🐄 1 sopaipilla (1 1/2" x 1 1/2")= 12 g; Calories = 43.2

Sopaipilla Without Syrup Or Honey 🐄 1 sopaipilla (1 1/2" x 1 1/2")= 10 g; Calories = 36.6

Spoonbread 🐄 1 cup= 187 g; Calories = 306.7

Strudel Berry 🐄 1 piece (approx 2" - 2-1/2" square)= 64 g; Calories = 159.4

Strudel Cheese 🐄 1 piece (approx 2" - 2-1/2" square)= 64 g; Calories = 195.2

Strudel Cheese And Fruit 🐄 1 piece (approx 2" - 2-1/2" square)= 64 g; Calories = 140.8

Strudel Cherry 🐄 1 piece (approx 2" - 2-1/2" square)= 64 g; Calories = 179.2

Strudel Peach 🐄 1 piece (approx 2" - 2-1/2" square)= 64 g; Calories = 130.6

Strudel Pineapple 🐄 1 piece (approx 2" - 2-1/2" square)= 64 g; Calories = 159.4

Sweet Bread Dough Filled With Bean Paste Meatless Steamed 🐄 1 manapua= 103 g; Calories = 273

Sweet Rolls Cheese 🐄 1 oz= 28.4 g; Calories = 102.2

Sweet Rolls Cinnamon Commercially Prepared With Raisins 🐄 1 oz= 28.4 g; Calories = 105.6

Sweet Rolls Cinnamon Refrigerated Dough With Frosting 🐄 1 oz= 28.4 g; Calories = 94.6

Sweet Rolls Cinnamon Refrigerated Dough With Frosting Baked
☞ 1 oz= 28.4 g; Calories = 102.8

Taco Shells Baked ☞ 1 shell= 12.9 g; Calories = 61.4

Taco Shells Baked Without Added Salt ☞ 1 oz= 28.4 g; Calories =
132.9

Tamale Sweet ☞ 1 tamale= 34 g; Calories = 87.4

Tamale Sweet With Fruit ☞ 1 tamale= 49 g; Calories = 98

Tiramisu ☞ 1 piece= 174 g; Calories = 616

Toasted Bagels ☞ 1 mini bagel (2-1/2 inch dia)= 24 g; Calories = 68.9

Toasted Cinnamon Raisin Bagels ☞ 1 mini bagel (2-1/2 inch dia)=
24 g; Calories = 70.6

Toasted White Bread ☞ 1 oz= 28.4 g; Calories = 82.4

Toasted Whole Wheat Bread ☞ 1 oz= 28.4 g; Calories = 86.9

Toaster Pastries Brown-Sugar-Cinnamon ☞ 1 oz= 28.4 g; Calories =
105.1

Toaster Pastries Fruit (Includes Apple Blueberry Cherry Strawberry) ☞ 1 oz= 28.4 g; Calories = 110.2

Toaster Pastries Fruit Frosted (Include Apples Blueberry Cherry
Strawberry) ☞ 1 piece= 53 g; Calories = 204.1

Toaster Pastries Fruit Toasted (Include Apple Blueberry Cherry
Strawberry) ☞ 1 pastry= 51 g; Calories = 208.6

Topping From Cheese Pizza ☞ topping from 1 piece= 40 g; Calories = 91.2

Topping From Meat And Vegetable Pizza ☞ topping from 1 piece=
51 g; Calories = 155.6

Topping From Meat Pizza ☞ topping from 1 piece= 41 g; Calories =
134.5

Topping From Vegetable Pizza ☛ topping from 1 piece= 49 g; Calories = 120.5

Tortillas Ready-To-Bake Or -Fry Corn ☛ 1 oz= 28.4 g; Calories = 61.9

Tortillas Ready-To-Bake Or -Fry Corn Without Added Salt ☛ 1 oz= 28.4 g; Calories = 63

Tortillas Ready-To-Bake Or -Fry Flour Refrigerated ☛ 1 tortilla= 48 g; Calories = 146.9

Tortillas Ready-To-Bake Or -Fry Flour Shelf Stable ☛ 1 tortilla= 49 g; Calories = 145.5

Tortillas Ready-To-Bake Or -Fry Flour Without Added Calcium ☛ 1 oz= 28.4 g; Calories = 92.3

Tortillas Ready-To-Bake Or -Fry Whole Wheat ☛ 1 tortilla 1 serving= 41 g; Calories = 127.1

Tostada Shells Corn ☛ 1 piece= 12.3 g; Calories = 58.3

Turnover Guava ☛ 1 turnover= 78 g; Calories = 239.5

Turnover Or Dumpling Apple ☛ 1 turnover= 82 g; Calories = 285.4

Turnover Or Dumpling Berry ☛ 1 turnover= 78 g; Calories = 275.3

Turnover Or Dumpling Cherry ☛ 1 turnover= 78 g; Calories = 238.7

Turnover Or Dumpling Lemon ☛ 1 turnover= 78 g; Calories = 234.8

Turnover Or Dumpling Peach ☛ 1 turnover= 78 g; Calories = 261.3

Turnover Pumpkin ☛ 1 turnover= 78 g; Calories = 195.8

Udis Gluten Free Classic French Dinner Rolls ☛ 1 roll= 36 g; Calories = 111.6

Udis Gluten Free Soft & Delicious White Sandwich Bread ☞ 1 slice= 28 g; Calories = 83.4

Udis Gluten Free Soft & Hearty Whole Grain Bread ☞ 1 slice= 25 g; Calories = 77.3

Udis Gluten Free Whole Grain Dinner Rolls ☞ 1 roll= 44 g; Calories = 144.8

Upside-Down Pineapple Cake ☞ 1 oz= 28.4 g; Calories = 90.6

Vans Gluten Free Totally Original Pancakes ☞ 1 pancake= 48 g; Calories = 103.2

Vans Gluten Free Totally Original Waffles ☞ 1 waffle= 47 g; Calories = 116.6

Vans The Perfect 10 Crispy Six Whole Grain + Four Seed Baked Crackers Gluten Free ☞ 3 crackers= 8.4 g; Calories = 39.6

Waffle Buttermilk Frozen Ready-To-Heat Microwaved ☞ 1 waffle= 35 g; Calories = 101.2

Waffle Buttermilk Frozen Ready-To-Heat Toasted ☞ 1 oz= 28 g; Calories = 86.5

Waffle Plain Frozen Ready-To-Heat Microwave ☞ 1 waffle, round (4 inchdia)= 32 g; Calories = 95.4

Waffles Buttermilk Frozen Ready-To-Heat ☞ 1 waffle, square= 39 g; Calories = 106.5

Waffles Chocolate Chip Frozen Ready-To-Heat ☞ 2 waffles= 70 g; Calories = 207.9

Waffles Gluten-Free Frozen Ready-To-Heat ☞ 1 waffle= 45 g; Calories = 118.4

Waffles Plain Frozen Ready -To-Heat Toasted ☞ 1 oz= 28.4 g; Calories = 88.6

Waffles Plain Frozen Ready-To-Heat ☞ 1 oz= 28.4 g; Calories = 80.9

Waffles Plain Prepared From Recipe ☛ 1 oz= 28.4 g; Calories = 82.6

Waffles Whole Wheat Lowfat Frozen Ready-To-Heat ☛ 1 serving 2 waffles= 70 g; Calories = 179.9

Wheat Bread ☛ 1 oz= 28.4 g; Calories = 77.8

Wheat Flour Fritter Without Syrup ☛ 1 fritter= 22 g; Calories = 105.2

Wheat Melba Toast Crackers ☛ 1/2 oz= 14.2 g; Calories = 53.1

White Bread ☛ 1 slice= 29 g; Calories = 77.1

White Cake With Coconut Frosting ☛ 1 oz= 28.4 g; Calories = 101.1

White Pizza Cheese Thick Crust ☛ 1 piece, nfs= 141 g; Calories = 407.5

White Pizza Cheese Thin Crust ☛ 1 piece, nfs= 92 g; Calories = 270.5

White Pizza Cheese With Meat And Vegetables Thick Crust ☛ 1 piece, nfs= 155 g; Calories = 432.5

White Pizza Cheese With Meat And Vegetables Thin Crust ☛ 1 piece, nfs= 118 g; Calories = 331.6

White Pizza Cheese With Meat Thick Crust ☛ 1 piece, nfs= 154 g; Calories = 472.8

White Pizza Cheese With Meat Thin Crust ☛ 1 piece, nfs= 100 g; Calories = 314

White Pizza Cheese With Vegetables Thick Crust ☛ 1 piece, nfs= 155 g; Calories = 390.6

White Pizza Cheese With Vegetables Thin Crust ☛ 1 piece, nfs= 106 g; Calories = 262.9

Whole Wheat Bread ☛ 1 slice= 32 g; Calories = 80.6

Whole Wheat Pita ☞ 1 pita, large (6-1/2 inch dia)= 64 g; Calories = 167.7

Wonton Wrappers (Includes Egg Roll Wrappers) ☞ 1 oz= 28.4 g; Calories = 82.6

Yam Buns; Puerto Rican Style ☞ 1 cup= 153 g; Calories = 462.1

Yellow Cake With Chocolate Frosting ☞ 1 piece (1/12 of a cake)= 144 g; Calories = 545.8

Yellow Cake With Vanilla Frosting ☞ 1 serving= 67 g; Calories = 262

9

BEANS AND LENTILS

Adzuki Beans ☛ 1 cup, diced= 130 g; Calories = 294.4

Bacon Bits Meatless ☛ 1 cup= 262 g; Calories = 33.3

Baked Beans ☛ 1 cup= 253 g; Calories = 392.2

Bean Cake ☛ 1 cup= 165 g; Calories = 130.6

Beans Adzuki Mature Seed Cooked Boiled With Salt ☛ 1 cup= 155 g; Calories = 294.4

Beans Adzuki Mature Seeds Canned Sweetened ☛ 1 cup= 126 g; Calories = 701.5

Beans Adzuki Mature Seeds Raw ☛ 1 cup= 253 g; Calories = 648.1

Beans And Franks ☛ 1 slice, thin= 14 g; Calories = 357.4

Beans And Tomatoes Fat Added In Cooking ☛ 1 cup= 144 g; Calories = 341.2

Beans And Tomatoes Fat Not Added In Cooking ☛ 1 fillet= 85 g; Calories = 244.4

Beans And Tomatoes Ns As To Fat Added In Cooking ☛ 1 tbsp= 15 g; Calories = 341.2

Beans Baked Canned No Salt Added ☛ 1 cup= 225 g; Calories = 265.7

Beans Baked Canned With Franks ☛ 1 cup= 256 g; Calories = 367.8

Beans Baked Canned With Pork ☛ 1 cup= 180 g; Calories = 268.2

Beans Baked Canned With Pork And Sweet Sauce ☛ 1 tbsp= 16 g; Calories = 261.5

Beans Baked Canned With Pork And Tomato Sauce ☛ 1 cup= 140 g; Calories = 231.2

Beans Black Mature Seeds Canned Low Sodium ☛ 1 cup= 240 g; Calories = 218.4

Beans Black Mature Seeds Cooked Boiled With Salt ☛ 1 cup= 168 g; Calories = 227

Beans Black Mature Seeds Raw ☛ 1 cup, sliced= 140 g; Calories = 661.5

Beans Black Turtle Mature Seeds Canned ☛ 1 slice= 56 g; Calories = 218.4

Beans Black Turtle Mature Seeds Cooked Boiled With Salt ☛ 1 tbsp= 7 g; Calories = 240.5

Beans Canned Drained Ns As To Type And As To Fat Added In Cooking ☛ 1 cup= 192 g; Calories = 340.2

Beans Canned Drained Ns As To Type Fat Added In Cooking ☛ 1 cup= 198 g; Calories = 340.2

Beans Canned Drained Ns As To Type Fat Not Added In Cooking ☛ 1 cup= 182 g; Calories = 246.6

Beans Chili Barbecue Ranch Style Cooked ☛ 1 cup= 180 g; Calories = 245.4

Beans Cranberry (Roman) Mature Seeds Cooked Boiled With Salt ☞ 1 cup= 166 g; Calories = 240.7

Beans Cranberry (Roman) Mature Seeds Raw ☞ 1 cup= 196 g; Calories = 653.3

Beans Dry Cooked Ns As To Type And As To Fat Added In Cooking ☞ 1 cup= 177 g; Calories = 354.6

Beans Dry Cooked Ns As To Type Fat Added In Cooking ☞ 1 cup= 180 g; Calories = 354.6

Beans Dry Cooked Ns As To Type Fat Not Added In Cooking ☞ 1 cup= 197 g; Calories = 255.6

Beans Dry Cooked With Ground Beef ☞ 1 cup= 196 g; Calories = 540

Beans Dry Cooked With Pork ☞ 1 oz= 28.4 g; Calories = 336.4

Beans French Mature Seeds Cooked Boiled With Salt ☞ 1 cup= 147 g; Calories = 228.3

Beans French Mature Seeds Cooked Boiled Without Salt ☞ 1 cup= 146 g; Calories = 228.3

Beans French Mature Seeds Raw ☞ 1 cup= 144 g; Calories = 631.1

Beans Great Northern Mature Seeds Canned ☞ 1 cup= 146 g; Calories = 298.7

Beans Great Northern Mature Seeds Canned Low Sodium ☞ 1 cup= 60 g; Calories = 298.7

Beans Great Northern Mature Seeds Cooked Boiled With Salt ☞ 1 cup= 205 g; Calories = 208.9

Beans Great Northern Mature Seeds Raw ☞ 1 cup= 168 g; Calories = 620.4

Beans Kidney All Types Mature Seeds Cooked Boiled With Salt ☞ 1 cup= 238 g; Calories = 224.8

Beans Kidney All Types Mature Seeds Raw ☛ 1 cup= 144 g; Calories = 612.7

Beans Kidney California Red Mature Seeds Cooked Boiled With Salt ☛ 1 cup= 172 g; Calories = 219.5

Beans Kidney California Red Mature Seeds Raw ☛ 1 cup= 93 g; Calories = 607.2

Beans Kidney Red Mature Seeds Canned Drained Solids ☛ 1 tbsp= 17 g; Calories = 329.8

Beans Kidney Red Mature Seeds Canned Drained Solids Rinsed In Tap Water ☛ 1 cup= 175 g; Calories = 191.2

Beans Kidney Red Mature Seeds Canned Solids And Liquid Low Sodium ☛ 1 cup, stirred= 88 g; Calories = 207.4

Beans Kidney Red Mature Seeds Cooked Boiled With Salt ☛ 1 cup= 122 g; Calories = 224.8

Beans Kidney Red Mature Seeds Raw ☛ 1 cup= 243 g; Calories = 620.1

Beans Kidney Royal Red Mature Seeds Cooked Boiled With Salt ☛ 1 oz= 28.4 g; Calories = 217.7

Beans Kidney Royal Red Mature Seeds Raw ☛ 1/2 cup= 126 g; Calories = 605.4

Beans Liquid From Stewed Kidney Beans ☛ 1 piece (2-1/2 inch x 2-3/4 inch x 1 inch)= 120 g; Calories = 112.8

Beans Navy Mature Seeds Cooked Boiled With Salt ☛ 1 piece= 17 g; Calories = 254.8

Beans Navy Mature Seeds Raw ☛ 1 oz= 28.4 g; Calories = 701

Beans Pink Mature Seeds Cooked Boiled With Salt ☛ 1 cup= 122 g; Calories = 251.8

Beans Pink Mature Seeds Cooked Boiled Without Salt ☛ 1 cup= 172 g; Calories = 251.8

Beans Pink Mature Seeds Raw ☛ 1 tablespoon= 15 g; Calories = 720.3

Beans Pinto Canned Drained Solids ☛ 1 patty (approx 2-1/4 inch dia)= 17 g; Calories = 315.8

Beans Pinto Mature Seeds Canned Drained Solids Rinsed In Tap Water ☛ 1 cup= 243 g; Calories = 197.7

Beans Pinto Mature Seeds Canned Solids And Liquids ☛ 2 tbsp= 31 g; Calories = 196.8

Beans Pinto Mature Seeds Canned Solids And Liquids Low Sodium ☛ 2 tablespoon= 36 g; Calories = 196.8

Beans Pinto Mature Seeds Cooked Boiled With Salt ☛ 2 tbsp= 32 g; Calories = 244.5

Beans Pinto Mature Seeds Raw ☛ 2 tbsp= 32 g; Calories = 669.7

Beans Small White Mature Seeds Cooked Boiled With Salt ☛ 1 slice= 84 g; Calories = 254.2

Beans Small White Mature Seeds Raw ☛ 1 slice= 84 g; Calories = 722.4

Beans White Mature Seeds Canned ☛ 1 slice= 84 g; Calories = 298.7

Beans White Mature Seeds Cooked Boiled With Salt ☛ 1 slice= 84 g; Calories = 248.8

Beans White Mature Seeds Raw ☛ 1 cup= 231 g; Calories = 672.7

Beans Yellow Mature Seeds Cooked Boiled With Salt ☛ 1 cup= 233 g; Calories = 254.9

Beans Yellow Mature Seeds Raw ☛ 1/5 package= 79 g; Calories = 676.2

Black Bean Salad ☞ 2 tbsp= 32 g; Calories = 251.8

Black Beans ☞ 2 tbsp= 32 g; Calories = 227

Black Beans Cuban Style ☞ 1 tbsp= 16 g; Calories = 294.3

Black Brown Or Bayo Beans Canned Drained Fat Added In Cooking Ns As To Type Of Fat ☞ 1 cup= 168 g; Calories = 336.6

Black Brown Or Bayo Beans Canned Drained Fat Not Added In Cooking ☞ 1 tbsp= 14.2 g; Calories = 241.2

Black Brown Or Bayo Beans Canned Drained Low Sodium Fat Added In Cooking ☞ 1 tbsp= 15 g; Calories = 336.6

Black Brown Or Bayo Beans Canned Drained Low Sodium Fat Not Added In Cooking ☞ 1/2 cup= 126 g; Calories = 241.2

Black Brown Or Bayo Beans Canned Drained Low Sodium Ns As To Fat Added In Cooking ☞ 1/2 cup= 124 g; Calories = 336.6

Black Brown Or Bayo Beans Canned Drained Made With Animal Fat Or Meat Drippings ☞ 1 cup= 172 g; Calories = 325.8

Black Brown Or Bayo Beans Canned Drained Made With Margarine ☞ 1 cup= 197 g; Calories = 293.4

Black Brown Or Bayo Beans Canned Drained Made With Oil ☞ 1 cup= 230 g; Calories = 336.6

Black Brown Or Bayo Beans Canned Drained Ns As To Fat Added In Cooking ☞ 1 cup= 296 g; Calories = 336.6

Black Brown Or Bayo Beans Dry Cooked Fat Added In Cooking Ns As To Type Of Fat ☞ 1 slice= 14 g; Calories = 331.2

Black Brown Or Bayo Beans Dry Cooked Fat Not Added In Cooking ☞ 1 cup= 253 g; Calories = 235.8

Black Brown Or Bayo Beans Dry Cooked Made With Animal Fat Or Meat Drippings ☞ 1 cup= 249 g; Calories = 320.4

Black Brown Or Bayo Beans Dry Cooked Made With Margarine ☛ 1 cup= 246 g; Calories = 289.8

Black Brown Or Bayo Beans Dry Cooked Made With Oil ☛ 1 cup= 194 g; Calories = 334.8

Black Brown Or Bayo Beans Dry Cooked Ns As To Fat Added In Cooking ☛ 1 cup= 172 g; Calories = 331.2

Black Turtle Beans ☛ 1 cup= 177 g; Calories = 240.5

Black-Eyed Peas (Cowpeas) ☛ 1 cup= 260 g; Calories = 198.4

Boiled Lupin Beans ☛ 1 cup= 184 g; Calories = 197.5

Boiled Red Kidney Beans ☛ 1 cup= 177 g; Calories = 217.7

Boiled Soybeans (Edamame) ☛ 1 cup= 177 g; Calories = 295.8

Broad Beans (Fava) ☛ 1 cup= 256 g; Calories = 187

Broadbeans (Fava Beans) Mature Seeds Canned ☛ 1 cup= 184 g; Calories = 181.8

Broadbeans (Fava Beans) Mature Seeds Cooked Boiled With Salt ☛ 1 cup= 177 g; Calories = 187

Broadbeans (Fava Beans) Mature Seeds Raw ☛ 1 cup= 184 g; Calories = 511.5

California Red Kidney Beans ☛ 1 cup= 208 g; Calories = 219.5

Canned Baked Beans ☛ 1 cup= 182 g; Calories = 238.8

Canned Baked Beans With Beef ☛ 1 cup= 262 g; Calories = 321.9

Canned Chili With Beans ☛ 1 cup= 210 g; Calories = 263.7

Canned Cranberry Beans ☛ 1 cup= 215 g; Calories = 215.8

Canned Kidney Beans ☛ 1 cup= 179 g; Calories = 215

Canned Mature (White) Lima Beans ☛ 1 cup= 196 g; Calories = 190.4

Canned Navy Beans ☛ 1 cup= 177 g; Calories = 296.1

Canned Red Kidney Beans ☛ 1 cup= 170 g; Calories = 207.4

Canned Refried Beans ☛ 1 cup= 256 g; Calories = 200.9

Carob Flour ☛ 1 cup= 103 g; Calories = 228.7

Chicken Meatless ☛ 1 cup= 200 g; Calories = 376.3

Chicken Meatless Breaded Fried ☛ 1 cup= 164 g; Calories = 304.2

Chickpea Flour (Besan) ☛ 1 cup= 167 g; Calories = 356

Chickpeas (Garbanzo Beans Bengal Gram) Mature Seeds Canned Drained Rinsed In Tap Water ☛ 1 cup= 171 g; Calories = 350.5

Chickpeas (Garbanzo Beans Bengal Gram) Mature Seeds Canned Drained Solids ☛ 1 cup= 240 g; Calories = 351.7

Chickpeas (Garbanzo Beans Bengal Gram) Mature Seeds Canned Solids And Liquids ☛ 1 cup= 240 g; Calories = 211.2

Chickpeas (Garbanzo Beans Bengal Gram) Mature Seeds Canned Solids And Liquids Low Sodium ☛ 1/5 package= 79 g; Calories = 211.2

Chickpeas (Garbanzo Beans Bengal Gram) Mature Seeds Cooked Boiled With Salt ☛ 1/5 package= 79 g; Calories = 269

Chickpeas (Garbanzo Beans Bengal Gram) Mature Seeds Raw ☛ 1/5 package= 91 g; Calories = 756

Chickpeas (Garbanzo Beans) (Cooked) ☛ 1 cup= 243 g; Calories = 269

Chickpeas Canned Drained Fat Added In Cooking Ns As To Type Of Fat ☛ 1 cup= 243 g; Calories = 356.4

Chickpeas Canned Drained Fat Not Added In Cooking ☛ 1 cup= 243 g; Calories = 262.8

Chickpeas Canned Drained Low Sodium Fat Added In Cooking ☛ 1 cup= 243 g; Calories = 358.2

Chickpeas Canned Drained Low Sodium Fat Not Added In Cooking ☞ 1 cup= 243 g; Calories = 264.6

Chickpeas Canned Drained Low Sodium Ns As To Fat Added In Cooking ☞ 1 cup= 243 g; Calories = 358.2

Chickpeas Canned Drained Made With Oil ☞ 1 cup= 243 g; Calories = 356.4

Chickpeas Canned Drained Ns As To Fat Added In Cooking ☞ 1 cup= 243 g; Calories = 356.4

Chickpeas Dry Cooked Fat Added In Cooking Ns As To Type Of Fat ☞ 1 cup= 243 g; Calories = 392.4

Chickpeas Dry Cooked Fat Not Added In Cooking ☞ 1 cup= 243 g; Calories = 293.4

Chickpeas Dry Cooked Made With Animal Fat Or Meat Drippings ☞ 1/2 cup= 122 g; Calories = 381.6

Chickpeas Dry Cooked Made With Margarine ☞ 1 cup= 243 g; Calories = 347.4

Chickpeas Dry Cooked Made With Oil ☞ 1 cup= 243 g; Calories = 392.4

Chickpeas Dry Cooked Ns As To Fat Added In Cooking ☞ 1 container= 170 g; Calories = 392.4

Chickpeas Stewed With Pig's Feet Puerto Rican Style ☞ 1 container= 170 g; Calories = 305

Chili With Beans Without Meat ☞ 1 container= 170 g; Calories = 106.3

Cooked Blackeyed Peas ☞ 1 container= 170 g; Calories = 160.1

Cooked Catjang Beans ☞ 1/5 package= 79 g; Calories = 200.1

Cooked Green Soybeans ☞ 1/5 package= 91 g; Calories = 253.8

Cooked Large White Beans ☛ 3 oz= 85 g; Calories = 248.8

Cooked Red Kidney Beans ☛ 1/5 package= 91 g; Calories = 224.8

Cooked Small White Beans ☛ 2 oz= 56 g; Calories = 254.2

Cowpeas Catjang Mature Seeds Cooked Boiled With Salt ☛ 2 oz= 56 g; Calories = 200.1

Cowpeas Catjang Mature Seeds Raw ☛ 1 cup= 230 g; Calories = 572.8

Cowpeas Common (Blackeyes Crowder Southern) Mature Seeds Canned Plain ☛ 1 cup= 177 g; Calories = 184.8

Cowpeas Common (Blackeyes Crowder Southern) Mature Seeds Canned With Pork ☛ 1 cup= 262 g; Calories = 199.2

Cowpeas Common (Blackeyes Crowder Southern) Mature Seeds Cooked Boiled With Salt ☛ 1 cup= 177 g; Calories = 198.4

Cowpeas Common (Blackeyes Crowder Southern) Mature Seeds Raw ☛ 1 cup= 177 g; Calories = 561.1

Cowpeas Dry Cooked Fat Added In Cooking ☛ 1 cup= 182 g; Calories = 309.6

Cowpeas Dry Cooked Fat Not Added In Cooking ☛ 1 cup= 169 g; Calories = 207

Cowpeas Dry Cooked Ns As To Fat Added In Cooking ☛ 1 cup= 171 g; Calories = 309.6

Cowpeas Dry Cooked With Pork ☛ 1 cup= 169 g; Calories = 309.7

Cranberry Beans (Roman Beans) ☛ 1 cup= 170 g; Calories = 240.7

Dry-Roasted Soybeans ☛ 1 cup= 164 g; Calories = 417.6

Edamame ☛ 1 can drained= 253 g; Calories = 187.6

Extra Firm Fortified Tofu ☛ 1 can drained, rinsed= 254 g; Calories = 78.2

Falafel ☛ 1 cup= 188 g; Calories = 56.6

Fava Beans (Raw) ☛ 1 cup= 182 g; Calories = 110.9

Fava Beans Canned Drained Fat Added In Cooking ☛ 1 cup= 166 g; Calories = 293.4

Fava Beans Dry Cooked Fat Added In Cooking ☛ 1 cup= 177 g; Calories = 300.6

Fava Beans Dry Cooked Fat Not Added In Cooking ☛ 1 cup= 147 g; Calories = 196.2

Fava Beans Dry Cooked Ns As To Fat Added In Cooking ☛ 1 cup= 144 g; Calories = 300.6

Firm Tofu ☛ 1 cup= 143 g; Calories = 181.4

Firm Tofu (With Calcium And Magnesium) ☛ 1 cup= 178 g; Calories = 98.3

Fortified Chocolate Soy Milk ☛ 1 cup= 188 g; Calories = 153.1

Fortified Silken Tofu ☛ 1 cup= 241 g; Calories = 39.1

Frankfurter Meatless ☛ 1 cup= 202 g; Calories = 326.2

Fried Chickpeas With Bacon Puerto Rican Style ☛ 1 cup= 207 g; Calories = 370.8

Frijoles Rojos Volteados (Refried Beans Red Canned) ☛ 1 cup= 202 g; Calories = 335.5

Great Northern Beans ☛ 1 cup= 140 g; Calories = 208.9

Green Or Yellow Split Peas Dry Cooked Fat Added In Cooking Ns As To Type Of Fat ☛ 1 cup= 207 g; Calories = 300.6

Green Or Yellow Split Peas Dry Cooked Fat Not Added In Cooking ☛ 1 cup in shell, edible yield= 63 g; Calories = 210.6

Green Or Yellow Split Peas Dry Cooked Made With Animal Fat Or Meat Drippings ☛ 1 cup, chopped= 144 g; Calories = 291.6

Green Or Yellow Split Peas Dry Cooked Made With Margarine ☞
1 oz= 28.4 g; Calories = 262.8

Green Or Yellow Split Peas Dry Cooked Made With Oil ☞ 1 cup=
146 g; Calories = 300.6

Green Or Yellow Split Peas Dry Cooked Ns As To Fat Added In
Cooking ☞ 1 cup= 143 g; Calories = 300.6

Green Soybeans ☞ 2 tbsp= 32 g; Calories = 376.3

House Foods Premium Firm Tofu ☞ 2 tbsp= 32 g; Calories = 47.6

House Foods Premium Soft Tofu ☞ 1 cup= 60 g; Calories = 33

Hummus (Commercial) ☞ 1 cup= 88 g; Calories = 35.6

Hummus (Homemade) ☞ 1 link= 25 g; Calories = 26.6

Hyacinth Beans Mature Seeds Cooked Boiled With Salt ☞ 1 cup=
186 g; Calories = 227

Hyacinth Beans Mature Seeds Cooked Boiled Without Salt ☞ 1
cup= 172 g; Calories = 227

Hyacinth Beans Mature Seeds Raw ☞ 1 cup= 166 g; Calories = 722.4

Kidney Beans ☞ 1 cup, stirred= 84 g; Calories = 224.8

Lentils (Cooked) ☞ 1 cup, stirred= 85 g; Calories = 229.7

Lentils Dry Cooked Fat Added In Cooking Ns As To Type Of Fat
☞ 1 cup= 105 g; Calories = 297

Lentils Dry Cooked Fat Not Added In Cooking ☞ 1 oz= 28.4 g;
Calories = 207

Lentils Dry Cooked Made With Animal Fat Or Meat Drippings ☞
1 tbsp= 16 g; Calories = 286.2

Lentils Dry Cooked Made With Margarine ☞ 1 tbsp= 18 g; Calories
= 257.4

Lentils Dry Cooked Made With Oil ☛ 1 tbsp= 18 g; Calories = 297

Lentils Dry Cooked Ns As To Fat Added In Cooking ☛ 1 block= 11 g; Calories = 297

Lentils Mature Seeds Cooked Boiled With Salt ☛ 1 cup= 167 g; Calories = 225.7

Lentils Pink Or Red Raw ☛ 1 cup= 171 g; Calories = 687.4

Lentils Raw ☛ 1 cup= 182 g; Calories = 675.8

Lima Beans ☛ 1 cup= 192 g; Calories = 216.2

Lima Beans Dry Cooked Fat Added In Cooking Ns As To Type Of Fat ☛ 1 can drained solids= 266 g; Calories = 298.8

Lima Beans Dry Cooked Fat Not Added In Cooking ☛ 1 can drained solids= 277 g; Calories = 205.2

Lima Beans Dry Cooked Made With Animal Fat Or Meat Drippings ☛ 1 pattie= 70 g; Calories = 289.8

Lima Beans Dry Cooked Made With Margarine ☛ 1 cup= 92 g; Calories = 259.2

Lima Beans Dry Cooked Made With Oil ☛ 1 tbsp= 15 g; Calories = 298.8

Lima Beans Dry Cooked Ns As To Fat Added In Cooking ☛ 1/5 block= 91 g; Calories = 298.8

Lima Beans Large Mature Seeds Cooked Boiled With Salt ☛ 1/4 block= 122 g; Calories = 216.2

Lima Beans Large Mature Seeds Raw ☛ 1 slice= 84 g; Calories = 601.6

Lima Beans Thin Seeded (Baby) Mature Seeds Cooked Boiled With Salt ☛ 1 cup= 243 g; Calories = 229.3

Lima Beans Thin Seeded (Baby) Mature Seeds Cooked Boiled Without Salt ☞ 2 tbsp= 32 g; Calories = 229.3

Lima Beans Thin Seeded (Baby) Mature Seeds Raw ☞ 1 cup= 243 g; Calories = 676.7

Loaf Lentil ☞ 1 cup= 242 g; Calories = 33.8

Luncheon Slices Meatless ☞ 1/5 package= 79 g; Calories = 26.5

Lupin Beans (Cooked) ☞ 1 cup= 238 g; Calories = 192.6

Lupins Mature Seeds Raw ☞ 1 cup= 172 g; Calories = 667.8

Meat Extender ☞ 1 cup= 172 g; Calories = 273.7

Meat Substitute Cereal- And Vegetable Protein-Based Fried ☞ 1 oz= 28.4 g; Calories = 487.6

Meatballs Meatless ☞ 1 oz= 28.4 g; Calories = 283.7

Miso ☞ 1 piece= 17 g; Calories = 33.7

Mori-Nu Tofu Silken Extra Firm ☞ 1 piece= 13 g; Calories = 46.2

Mori-Nu Tofu Silken Firm ☞ 1 block= 11 g; Calories = 52.1

Mori-Nu Tofu Silken Lite Extra Firm ☞ 1 cup= 171 g; Calories = 31.9

Mori-Nu Tofu Silken Lite Firm ☞ 1 cup= 254 g; Calories = 31.1

Mori-Nu Tofu Silken Soft ☞ 1 cup= 266 g; Calories = 46.2

Mothbeans Mature Seeds Cooked Boiled With Salt ☞ 1 cup= 259 g; Calories = 207.1

Mothbeans Mature Seeds Cooked Boiled Without Salt ☞ 1 cup= 253 g; Calories = 207.1

Mothbeans Mature Seeds Raw ☞ 1 cup= 184 g; Calories = 672.3

Mung Beans (Cooked) ☞ 1 cup= 185 g; Calories = 212.1

Mung Beans Canned Drained Ns As To Fat Added In Cooking ☛ 1 cup= 240 g; Calories = 286.2

Mung Beans Dry Cooked Fat Added In Cooking ☛ 1 cup= 195 g; Calories = 277.2

Mung Beans Dry Cooked Fat Not Added In Cooking ☛ 1 cup= 183 g; Calories = 187.2

Mung Beans Dry Cooked Ns As To Fat Added In Cooking ☛ 1 cup= 177 g; Calories = 277.2

Mung Beans Mature Seeds Cooked Boiled With Salt ☛ 1 cup= 262 g; Calories = 212.1

Mung Beans Mature Seeds Raw ☛ 1 cup= 184 g; Calories = 718.3

Mungo Beans (Cooked) ☛ 1 cup= 177 g; Calories = 189

Mungo Beans Mature Seeds Cooked Boiled With Salt ☛ 1 cup= 256 g; Calories = 189

Mungo Beans Mature Seeds Raw ☛ 1 cup= 184 g; Calories = 705.9

Natto ☛ 1 cup= 177 g; Calories = 369.3

Navy Beans ☛ 1 cup= 169 g; Calories = 254.8

Noodles Chinese Cellophane Or Long Rice (Mung Beans) Dehydrated ☛ 1 cup= 193 g; Calories = 491.4

Okara ☛ 1 cup= 171 g; Calories = 92.7

Peanut Butter (Chunk Style) ☛ 1 cup= 202 g; Calories = 188.5

Peanut Butter (Smooth) ☛ 1 cup= 179 g; Calories = 188.2

Peanut Butter Chunk Style With Salt ☛ 1 cup= 262 g; Calories = 188.5

Peanut Butter Chunky Vitamin And Mineral Fortified ☛ 1 cup= 150 g; Calories = 189.8

Peanut Butter Reduced Sodium ☛ 1 cup= 240 g; Calories = 94.4

Peanut Butter Smooth Reduced Fat ☛ 1 cup= 256 g; Calories = 187.2

Peanut Butter Smooth Style With Salt ☛ 1 cup= 167 g; Calories = 191.4

Peanut Butter Smooth Vitamin And Mineral Fortified ☛ 1 cup= 171 g; Calories = 189.1

Peanut Butter With Omega-3 Creamy ☛ 1 cup= 210 g; Calories = 97.3

Peanut Flour Defatted ☛ 1 cup= 194 g; Calories = 196.2

Peanut Flour Low Fat ☛ 1 cup= 243 g; Calories = 256.8

Peanut Spread Reduced Sugar ☛ 1 cup= 243 g; Calories = 201.5

Peanuts All Types Cooked Boiled With Salt ☛ 1 cup= 243 g; Calories = 200.3

Peanuts All Types Dry-Roasted With Salt ☛ 1 cup= 243 g; Calories = 166.7

Peanuts All Types Oil-Roasted With Salt ☛ 1 cup= 243 g; Calories = 862.6

Peanuts All Types Oil-Roasted Without Salt ☛ 1 cup= 243 g; Calories = 862.6

Peanuts Spanish Oil-Roasted With Salt ☛ 1 cup= 243 g; Calories = 851.1

Peanuts Spanish Oil-Roasted Without Salt ☛ 1 cup= 243 g; Calories = 851.1

Peanuts Spanish Raw ☛ 1 cup= 243 g; Calories = 832.2

Peanuts Valencia Oil-Roasted With Salt ☛ 1 cup= 243 g; Calories = 848.2

Peanuts Valencia Oil-Roasted Without Salt ☛ I cup= 243 g; Calories = 848.2

Peanuts Valencia Raw ☛ I cup= 243 g; Calories = 832.2

Peanuts Virginia Oil-Roasted With Salt ☛ I cup= 243 g; Calories = 826.5

Peanuts Virginia Oil-Roasted Without Salt ☛ I container= 227 g; Calories = 826.5

Peanuts Virginia Raw ☛ I container= 170 g; Calories = 822

Peas Dry Cooked With Pork ☛ I container= 227 g; Calories = 332.9

Peas Green Split Mature Seeds Raw ☛ I container= 170 g; Calories = 717.1

Peas Split Mature Seeds Cooked Boiled With Salt ☛ I container= 170 g; Calories = 227.4

Pigeon Peas (Red Gram) Mature Seeds Cooked Boiled With Salt ☛ I container= 170 g; Calories = 203.3

Pigeon Peas (Red Gram) Mature Seeds Cooked Boiled Without Salt ☛ I tbsp= 15 g; Calories = 203.3

Pigeon Peas (Red Gram) Mature Seeds Raw ☛ I tbsp= 15 g; Calories = 703.2

Pink Beans Canned Drained Fat Added In Cooking ☛ 3 oz= 85 g; Calories = 360

Pink Beans Canned Drained Fat Not Added In Cooking ☛ 3 oz= 85 g; Calories = 266.4

Pink Beans Dry Cooked Fat Added In Cooking ☛ 1/5 package= 79 g; Calories = 365.4

Pink Beans Dry Cooked Fat Not Added In Cooking ☛ 1/5 package= 79 g; Calories = 266.4

Pink Beans Dry Cooked Ns As To Fat Added In Cooking ☛ 1 cup= 172 g; Calories = 365.4

Pinto Beans (Cooked) ☛ 1 cup= 240 g; Calories = 244.5

Pinto Calico Or Red Mexican Beans Canned Drained Fat Added In Cooking Ns As To Type Of Fat ☛ 1 cup= 185 g; Calories = 340.2

Pinto Calico Or Red Mexican Beans Canned Drained Fat Not Added In Cooking ☛ 1 cup= 177 g; Calories = 246.6

Pinto Calico Or Red Mexican Beans Canned Drained Low Sodium Fat Added In Cooking ☛ 1 cup= 177 g; Calories = 336.4

Pinto Calico Or Red Mexican Beans Canned Drained Low Sodium Fat Not Added In Cooking ☛ 1 cup= 177 g; Calories = 237

Pinto Calico Or Red Mexican Beans Canned Drained Low Sodium Ns As To Fat Added In Cooking ☛ 1 cup cup rinsed solids= 158 g; Calories = 336.4

Pinto Calico Or Red Mexican Beans Canned Drained Made With Animal Fat Or Meat Drippings ☛ 1 cup= 177 g; Calories = 329.4

Pinto Calico Or Red Mexican Beans Canned Drained Made With Margarine ☛ 1 cup= 256 g; Calories = 298.8

Pinto Calico Or Red Mexican Beans Canned Drained Made With Oil ☛ 1 cup= 179 g; Calories = 340.2

Pinto Calico Or Red Mexican Beans Canned Drained Ns As To Fat Added In Cooking ☛ 1 cup= 240 g; Calories = 340.2

Pinto Calico Or Red Mexican Beans Dry Cooked Fat Added In Cooking Ns As To Type Of Fat ☛ 1 cup= 177 g; Calories = 354.6

Pinto Calico Or Red Mexican Beans Dry Cooked Fat Not Added In Cooking ☛ 1 cup= 179 g; Calories = 255.6

Pinto Calico Or Red Mexican Beans Dry Cooked Made With Animal Fat Or Meat Drippings ☛ 1 cup= 240 g; Calories = 343.8

Pinto Calico Or Red Mexican Beans Dry Cooked Made With Margarine ☛ 1 cup= 171 g; Calories = 309.6

Pinto Calico Or Red Mexican Beans Dry Cooked Made With Oil ☛ 1 cup= 171 g; Calories = 354.6

Pinto Calico Or Red Mexican Beans Dry Cooked Ns As To Fat Added In Cooking ☛ 1 cup= 194 g; Calories = 354.6

Raw Peanuts ☛ 1 cup= 198 g; Calories = 161

Red Kidney Beans Canned Drained Fat Added In Cooking Ns As To Type Of Fat ☛ 1 cup= 202 g; Calories = 338.4

Red Kidney Beans Canned Drained Fat Not Added In Cooking ☛ 1 cup= 180 g; Calories = 243

Red Kidney Beans Canned Drained Low Sodium Fat Added In Cooking ☛ 1 cup= 196 g; Calories = 338.4

Red Kidney Beans Canned Drained Low Sodium Fat Not Added In Cooking ☛ 1 cup,= 144 g; Calories = 243

Red Kidney Beans Canned Drained Low Sodium Ns As To Fat Added In Cooking ☛ 1 cup= 180 g; Calories = 338.4

Red Kidney Beans Canned Drained Made With Oil ☛ 1 cup= 180 g; Calories = 338.4

Red Kidney Beans Dry Cooked Fat Added In Cooking Ns As To Type Of Fat ☛ 1 cup= 180 g; Calories = 324

Red Kidney Beans Dry Cooked Fat Not Added In Cooking ☛ 1 cup= 180 g; Calories = 226.8

Red Kidney Beans Dry Cooked Made With Animal Fat Or Meat Drippings ☛ 1 cup= 180 g; Calories = 313.2

Red Kidney Beans Dry Cooked Made With Margarine ☛ 1 cup= 180 g; Calories = 282.6

Red Kidney Beans Dry Cooked Made With Oil ☛ 1 cup= 180 g;

Calories = 324

Red Kidney Beans Dry Cooked Ns As To Fat Added In Cooking ☛ 1 cup= 180 g; Calories = 324

Refried Beans Canned Fat-Free ☛ 1 cup= 180 g; Calories = 182.5

Refried Beans Canned Traditional Reduced Sodium ☛ 1 cup= 180 g; Calories = 211.8

Refried Beans Canned Traditional Style (Includes USDA Commodity) ☛ 1 cup= 180 g; Calories = 214.2

Refried Beans Fat Added In Cooking Ns As To Type Of Fat ☛ 1 cup= 180 g; Calories = 364.3

Refried Beans Made With Animal Fat Or Meat Drippings ☛ 1 cup= 180 g; Calories = 354.2

Refried Beans Made With Margarine ☛ 1 cup= 180 g; Calories = 326.4

Refried Beans Made With Oil ☛ 1 cup= 180 g; Calories = 364.3

Refried Beans Ns As To Fat Added In Cooking ☛ 1 cup, nfs= 180 g; Calories = 364.3

Refried Beans With Cheese ☛ 1 cup= 180 g; Calories = 270.7

Refried Beans With Meat ☛ 1 cup= 180 g; Calories = 293.5

Sandwich Spread Meatless ☛ 1 cup= 180 g; Calories = 22.4

Sausage Meatless ☛ 1 cup= 180 g; Calories = 63.8

Silk (Soy Milk) ☛ 1 cup= 180 g; Calories = 99.6

Silk Banana-Strawberry Soy Yogurt ☛ 1 cup= 180 g; Calories = 149.6

Silk Black Cherry Soy Yogurt ☛ 1 cup= 180 g; Calories = 149.6

Silk Blueberry Soy Yogurt ☛ 1 cup= 180 g; Calories = 149.6

- Silk Chai Soy Milk ☛ 1 cup= 180 g; Calories = 128.8

- Silk Chocolate Soy Milk ☛ 1 cup= 180 g; Calories = 140.9

- Silk Coffee Soy Milk ☛ 1 cup= 180 g; Calories = 150.7

- Silk French Vanilla Creamer ☛ 1 cup= 180 g; Calories = 20

- Silk Hazelnut Creamer ☛ 1 cup= 180 g; Calories = 20

- Silk Key Lime Soy Yogurt ☛ 1 cup= 180 g; Calories = 149.6

- Silk Light Chocolate Soy Milk ☛ 1 cup= 180 g; Calories = 119.1

- Silk Light Plain Soy Milk ☛ 1 cup= 180 g; Calories = 70.5

- Silk Light Vanilla Soy Milk ☛ 1 cup= 180 g; Calories = 80.2

- Silk Mocha Soy Milk ☛ 1 cup= 180 g; Calories = 140.9

- Silk Nog Soy Milk ☛ 1 cup= 180 g; Calories = 90.3

- Silk Original Creamer ☛ 1 cup= 180 g; Calories = 15

- Silk Peach Soy Yogurt ☛ 1 cup= 180 g; Calories = 159.8

- Silk Plain Soy Yogurt ☛ 1 cup= 180 g; Calories = 149.8

- Silk Plus Fiber Soy Milk ☛ 1 cup= 180 g; Calories = 99.6

- Silk Plus For Bone Health Soy Milk ☛ 1 cup= 180 g; Calories = 99.6

- Silk Plus Omega-3 Dha Soy Milk ☛ 1 cup= 180 g; Calories = 109.4

- Silk Raspberry Soy Yogurt ☛ 1 cup= 180 g; Calories = 149.6

- Silk Strawberry Soy Yogurt ☛ 1 cup= 180 g; Calories = 159.8

- Silk Vanilla Soy Milk ☛ 1 cup= 180 g; Calories = 99.6

- Silk Vanilla Soy Yogurt (Family Size) ☛ 1 cup= 180 g; Calories = 179.3

- Silk Vanilla Soy Yogurt (Single Serving Size) ☛ 1 cup= 180 g; Calories = 149.6

Silk Very Vanilla Soy Milk ☞ 1 cup= 180 g; Calories = 128.8

Soft Tofu ☞ 1 cup= 180 g; Calories = 73.2

Soy Flour Defatted ☞ 1 cup= 180 g; Calories = 343.4

Soy Flour Full-Fat Raw ☞ 1 cup= 180 g; Calories = 364.6

Soy Flour Full-Fat Roasted ☞ 1 cup= 180 g; Calories = 373.2

Soy Flour Low-Fat ☞ 1 cup= 180 g; Calories = 327.4

Soy Meal Defatted Raw ☞ 1 cup= 180 g; Calories = 411.1

Soy Milk ☞ 1 cup= 180 g; Calories = 80.2

Soy Milk (All Flavors) Enhanced ☞ 1 cup= 180 g; Calories = 109.4

Soy Milk (All Flavors) Lowfat With Added Calcium Vitamins A And D ☞ 1 cup= 180 g; Calories = 104.5

Soy Milk (All Flavors) Nonfat With Added Calcium Vitamins A And D ☞ 1 cup= 180 g; Calories = 68

Soy Milk Chocolate And Other Flavors Light With Added Calcium Vitamins A And D ☞ 1 cup= 180 g; Calories = 114.2

Soy Milk Chocolate Nonfat With Added Calcium Vitamins A And D ☞ 1 cup= 180 g; Calories = 106.9

Soy Milk Chocolate Unfortified ☞ 1 cup= 180 g; Calories = 153.1

Soy Milk Original And Vanilla Light Unsweetened With Added Calcium Vitamins A And D ☞ 1 cup= 178 g; Calories = 82.6

Soy Milk Original And Vanilla Light With Added Calcium Vitamins A And D ☞ 1 cup= 178 g; Calories = 72.9

Soy Milk Original And Vanilla With Added Calcium Vitamins A And D ☞ 1 cup= 173 g; Calories = 104.5

Soy Protein Concentrate Produced By Acid Wash ☞ 1 cup= 180 g; Calories = 93.2

Soy Protein Concentrate Produced By Alcohol Extraction ☞ 1 cup= 180 g; Calories = 93.2

Soy Protein Isolate Potassium Type ☞ 1 cup= 180 g; Calories = 91.2

Soy Protein Powder (Isolate) ☞ 1 cup= 180 g; Calories = 95.1

Soy Sauce ☞ 1 cup= 180 g; Calories = 8.5

Soy Sauce Made From Hydrolyzed Vegetable Protein ☞ 1 cup= 180 g; Calories = 10.8

Soy Sauce Made From Soy And Wheat (Shoyu) Low Sodium ☞ 1 cup= 180 g; Calories = 8.1

Soy Sauce Reduced Sodium Made From Hydrolyzed Vegetable Protein ☞ 1 cup= 180 g; Calories = 13.5

Soybean Curd Breaded Fried ☞ 1 cup= 180 g; Calories = 43.5

Soybean Curd Cheese ☞ 1 cup= 180 g; Calories = 339.8

Soybeans Dry Cooked Fat Added In Cooking ☞ 1 cup= 180 g; Calories = 401.4

Soybeans Dry Cooked Fat Not Added In Cooking ☞ 1 cup= 180 g; Calories = 307.8

Soybeans Dry Cooked Ns As To Fat Added In Cooking ☞ 1 cup= 180 g; Calories = 401.4

Soybeans Mature Seeds Cooked Boiled With Salt ☞ 1 cup= 180 g; Calories = 295.8

Soybeans Mature Seeds Raw ☞ 1 cup= 180 g; Calories = 829.6

Soybeans Mature Seeds Roasted No Salt Added ☞ 1 cup= 180 g; Calories = 806.7

Soybeans Mature Seeds Roasted Salted ☞ 1 cup= 180 g; Calories = 806.7

Soyburger Meatless With Cheese On Bun ☞ 1 cup= 180 g; Calories = 291.2

Split Peas ☞ 1 cup= 180 g; Calories = 231.3

Stewed Beans With Pork Tomatoes And Chili Peppers Mexican Style ☞ 1 cup= 180 g; Calories = 329.1

Stewed Chickpeas Puerto Rican Style ☞ 1 cup= 180 g; Calories = 231.4

Stewed Chickpeas With Potatoes Puerto Rican Style ☞ 1 cup= 180 g; Calories = 416

Stewed Chickpeas With Spanish Sausages Puerto Rican Style ☞ 1 cup= 180 g; Calories = 530

Stewed Pink Beans With Pig's Feet Puerto Rican Style ☞ 1 cup= 180 g; Calories = 288.9

Stewed Pink Beans With White Potatoes And Ham Puerto Rican Style ☞ 1 cup= 180 g; Calories = 219.3

Stewed Red Beans Puerto Rican Style ☞ 1 cup= 180 g; Calories = 210

Stewed Red Beans With Pig's Feet And Potatoes Puerto Rican Style ☞ 1 cup= 242 g; Calories = 332.2

Stewed Red Beans With Pig's Feet Puerto Rican Style ☞ 1 cup= 242 g; Calories = 286.8

Stinky Tofu ☞ 1 cup= 242 g; Calories = 12.8

Swiss Steak With Gravy Meatless ☞ 1 cup= 231 g; Calories = 165.6

Tamari ☞ 1 cup= 253 g; Calories = 10.8

Tempeh ☞ 1 cup= 253 g; Calories = 318.7

Tofu Dried-Frozen (Koyadofu) ☞ 1 cup= 253 g; Calories = 81.1

Tofu Dried-Frozen (Koyadofu) Prepared With Calcium Sulfate ☛ 1 cup= 253 g; Calories = 79.9

Tofu Extra Firm Prepared With Nigari ☛ 1 cup= 253 g; Calories = 75.5

Tofu Fried ☛ 1 cup= 253 g; Calories = 76.7

Tofu Fried Prepared With Calcium Sulfate ☛ 1 cup= 259 g; Calories = 35.1

Tofu Hard Prepared With Nigari ☛ 1 cup= 266 g; Calories = 176.9

Tofu Prepared With Calcium ☛ 1 cup= 178 g; Calories = 94.2

Tofu Salted And Fermented (Fuyu) Prepared With Calcium Sulfate ☛ 1 cake= 32 g; Calories = 12.8

Tofu Yogurt ☛ 1 cup= 242 g; Calories = 246.3

Unsalted Peanut Butter (Smooth) ☛ 1 cup= 250 g; Calories = 191.4

Unsweetened Soy Milk ☛ 1 cup= 255 g; Calories = 80.2

Vanilla Soy Milk ☛ 1 cup, with bone (yield after bone removed)= 202 g; Calories = 131.2

Vegetarian Chili Made With Meat Substitute ☛ 1 cup, with bone (yield after bone removed)= 202 g; Calories = 271.8

Vegetarian Fillets ☛ 1 cup, with bone (yield after bone removed)= 220 g; Calories = 246.5

Vegetarian Meatloaf Or Patties ☛ 1 cup= 270 g; Calories = 110.3

Vegetarian Pot Pie ☛ 1 cup= 253 g; Calories = 508.5

Vegetarian Stew ☛ 1 cup= 180 g; Calories = 76.6

Vegetarian Stroganoff ☛ 1 cup= 180 g; Calories = 773.6

Veggie Burgers ☛ 1 cup= 180 g; Calories = 123.9

Vermicelli Made From Soy ☛ 1 cup= 180 g; Calories = 463.4

Vitasoy Usa Azumaya Extra Firm Tofu ☞ 1 cup= 180 g; Calories = 69.5

Vitasoy Usa Azumaya Firm Tofu ☞ 1 cup= 180 g; Calories = 63.2

Vitasoy Usa Azumaya Silken Tofu ☞ 1 cup= 180 g; Calories = 39.1

Vitasoy Usa Nasoya Lite Firm Tofu ☞ 1 cup= 180 g; Calories = 42.7

Vitasoy Usa Organic Nasoya Extra Firm Tofu ☞ 1 cup= 180 g; Calories = 77.4

Vitasoy Usa Organic Nasoya Firm Tofu ☞ 1 cup= 180 g; Calories = 66.4

Vitasoy Usa Organic Nasoya Silken Tofu ☞ 1 cup= 180 g; Calories = 42.8

Vitasoy Usa Organic Nasoya Soft Tofu ☞ 1 cup= 180 g; Calories = 55.3

Vitasoy Usa Organic Nasoya Sprouted Tofu Plus Super Firm ☞ 1 cup= 180 g; Calories = 97.8

Vitasoy Usa Organic Nasoya Super Firm Cubed Tofu ☞ 1 cup= 180 g; Calories = 93.2

Vitasoy Usa Organic Nasoya Tofu Plus Firm ☞ 1 cup= 180 g; Calories = 62.9

Vitasoy Usa Vitasoy Light Vanilla Soy Milk ☞ 1 cup= 180 g; Calories = 72.9

Vitasoy Usa Vitasoy Organic Classic Original Soy Milk ☞ 1 cup= 180 g; Calories = 114.2

Vitasoy Usa Vitasoy Organic Creamy Original Soy Milk ☞ 1 cup= 180 g; Calories = 106.9

White Beans Canned Drained Fat Added In Cooking Ns As To Type Of Fat ☞ 1 cup= 180 g; Calories = 392.4

White Beans Canned Drained Fat Not Added In Cooking ☛ 1 cup= 180 g; Calories = 302.4

White Beans Canned Drained Low Sodium Fat Added In Cooking ☛ 1 cup= 180 g; Calories = 392.4

White Beans Canned Drained Low Sodium Fat Not Added In Cooking ☛ 1 cup= 180 g; Calories = 302.4

White Beans Canned Drained Low Sodium Ns As To Fat Added In Cooking ☛ 1 cup= 197 g; Calories = 392.4

White Beans Canned Drained Made With Oil ☛ 1 cup= 179 g; Calories = 392.4

White Beans Dry Cooked Fat Added In Cooking Ns As To Type Of Fat ☛ 1 cup= 180 g; Calories = 343.8

White Beans Dry Cooked Fat Not Added In Cooking ☛ 1 cup= 180 g; Calories = 248.4

White Beans Dry Cooked Made With Animal Fat Or Meat Drippings ☛ 1 cup= 180 g; Calories = 333

White Beans Dry Cooked Made With Margarine ☛ 1 cup= 180 g; Calories = 300.6

White Beans Dry Cooked Made With Oil ☛ 1 cup= 180 g; Calories = 343.8

White Beans Dry Cooked Ns As To Fat Added In Cooking ☛ 1 cup= 180 g; Calories = 343.8

Winged Beans Mature Seeds Cooked Boiled With Salt ☛ 1 slice (3/4" thick)= 47 g; Calories = 252.8

Winged Beans Mature Seeds Cooked Boiled Without Salt ☛ 1 cup= 260 g; Calories = 252.8

Winged Beans Mature Seeds Raw ☛ 1 cup= 260 g; Calories = 744.4

Yardlong Beans Mature Seeds Cooked Boiled With Salt ☛ 1 cup, with bone (yield after bone removed)= 202 g; Calories = 201.8

Yardlong Beans Mature Seeds Cooked Boiled Without Salt ☛ 1 cup= 250 g; Calories = 201.8

Yardlong Beans Mature Seeds Raw ☛ 1 cup= 120 g; Calories = 579.5

Yellow Canary Or Peruvian Beans Canned Drained Fat Added In Cooking Ns As To Type Of Fat ☛ 1 slice (2-3/4" x 1" x 1/2")= 29 g; Calories = 351

Yellow Canary Or Peruvian Beans Dry Cooked Fat Added In Cooking Ns As To Type Of Fat ☛ 1 steak with gravy= 92 g; Calories = 351

Yellow Canary Or Peruvian Beans Dry Cooked Fat Not Added In Cooking ☛ 1 pie= 227 g; Calories = 257.4

Yellow Canary Or Peruvian Beans Dry Cooked Made With Animal Fat Or Meat Drippings ☛ 1 cup= 254 g; Calories = 340.2

Yellow Canary Or Peruvian Beans Dry Cooked Made With Margarine ☛ 1 cup= 247 g; Calories = 309.6

Yellow Canary Or Peruvian Beans Dry Cooked Made With Oil ☛ 1 box (3.2 oz), dry, yields= 466 g; Calories = 351

Yellow Canary Or Peruvian Beans Dry Cooked Ns As To Fat Added In Cooking ☛ 1 sandwich= 140 g; Calories = 351

Yokan Prepared From Adzuki Beans And Sugar ☛ 1 cup, cubes= 146 g; Calories = 36.4

10

BEVERAGES

100 Proof Liquor ☞ serving size: 1 fl oz = 27.8 g; Calories = 82

86 Proof Liquor ☞ serving size: 1 fl oz = 27.8 g; Calories = 70

90 Proof Liquor ☞ serving size: 1 fl oz = 27.8 g; Calories = 73

94 Proof Liquor ☞ serving size: 1 fl oz = 27.8 g; Calories = 77

Abbott Eas Soy Protein Powder ☞ serving size: 1 scoop = 44 g; Calories = 178

Abbott Eas Whey Protein Powder ☞ serving size: 2 scoop = 39 g; Calories = 150

Abbott Ensure Nutritional Shake Ready-To-Drink ☞ serving size: 8 fl oz = 254 g; Calories = 267

Abbott Ensure Plus Ready-To-Drink ☞ serving size: 1 cup = 252 g; Calories = 355

Acai Berry Drink Fortified ☞ serving size: 8 fl oz = 266 g; Calories = 165

Alcoholic Beverage Beer Light Budweiser Select ☛ serving size: 1 fl oz = 29.5 g; Calories = 8

Alcoholic Beverage Beer Light Higher Alcohol ☛ serving size: 12 fl oz = 356 g; Calories = 164

Alcoholic Beverage Beer Light Low Carb ☛ serving size: 1 fl oz = 29.5 g; Calories = 8

Alcoholic Beverage Creme De Menthe 72 Proof ☛ serving size: 1 fl oz = 33.6 g; Calories = 125

Alcoholic Beverage Daiquiri Prepared-From-Recipe ☛ serving size: 1 fl oz = 30.2 g; Calories = 56

Alcoholic Beverage Distilled All (Gin Rum Vodka Whiskey) 80 Proof ☛ serving size: 1 fl oz = 27.8 g; Calories = 64

Alcoholic Beverage Liqueur Coffee 63 Proof ☛ serving size: 1 fl oz = 34.8 g; Calories = 107

Alcoholic Beverage Malt Beer Hard Lemonade ☛ serving size: fl oz = 335 g; Calories = 228

Alcoholic Beverage Pina Colada Canned ☛ serving size: 1 fl oz = 32.6 g; Calories = 77

Alcoholic Beverage Pina Colada Prepared-From-Recipe ☛ serving size: 1 fl oz = 31.4 g; Calories = 55

Alcoholic Beverage Rice (Sake) ☛ serving size: 1 fl oz = 29.1 g; Calories = 39

Alcoholic Beverage Whiskey Sour ☛ serving size: 1 fl oz = 30.4 g; Calories = 45

Alcoholic Beverage Whiskey Sour Canned ☛ serving size: 1 fl oz = 30.8 g; Calories = 37

Alcoholic Beverage Whiskey Sour Prepared From Item 14028 ☛ serving size: 1 fl oz = 30.4 g; Calories = 47

Alcoholic Beverage Whiskey Sour Prepared With Water Whiskey And Powder Mix ☞ serving size: 1 fl oz = 29.4 g; Calories = 48

Alcoholic Beverage Wine Cooking ☞ serving size: 1 tsp = 4.9 g; Calories = 3

Alcoholic Beverage Wine Light ☞ serving size: 1 fl oz = 29.5 g; Calories = 15

Alcoholic Beverage Wine Table White Muller Thurgau ☞ serving size: 1 fl oz = 29.5 g; Calories = 22

Alcoholic Malt Beverage Higher Alcohol Sweetened ☞ serving size: 1 fl oz = 30 g; Calories = 26

Aloe Vera Juice Drink Fortified With Vitamin C ☞ serving size: 8 fl oz = 240 g; Calories = 36

Amber Hard Cider ☞ serving size: 12 fl oz = 355 g; Calories = 199

Arizona Tea Ready-To-Drink Lemon ☞ serving size: 1 fl oz = 30.6 g; Calories = 12

Barbera ☞ serving size: 1 fl oz = 29.4 g; Calories = 25

Beer ☞ serving size: 1 fl oz = 29.7 g; Calories = 13

Black Tea (Brewed) ☞ serving size: 1 fl oz = 29.6 g; Calories = 0

Black Tea (Ready To Drink) ☞ serving size: 16 fl oz = 473 g; Calories = 0

Bottled Water ☞ serving size: 1 fl oz = 29.6 g; Calories = 0

Brandy And Cola ☞ serving size: 1 fl oz = 30 g; Calories = 27

Budweiser Beer ☞ serving size: 1 fl oz = 29.8 g; Calories = 12

Budweiser Light Beer ☞ serving size: 1 fl oz = 29.5 g; Calories = 9

Burgundy ☞ serving size: 1 fl oz = 29.5 g; Calories = 25

Cabernet Franc ☞ serving size: 1 fl oz = 29.4 g; Calories = 24

📖 Cabernet Sauvignon 🐾 serving size: 1 fl oz = 29.4 g; Calories = 24

📖 Caffeine Free Cola 🐾 serving size: 1 fl oz = 30.7 g; Calories = 13

📖 Carbonated Beverage Chocolate-Flavored Soda 🐾 serving size: 1 fl oz = 31 g; Calories = 13

📖 Carbonated Beverage Low Calorie Other Than Cola Or Pepper With Sodium Saccharin Without Caffeine 🐾 serving size: 1 fl oz = 29.6 g; Calories = 0

📖 Carbonated Cola Fast-Food Cola 🐾 serving size: 1 serving child 12 fl oz, without ice = 258 g; Calories = 96

📖 Carbonated Lemon-Lime Soda No Caffeine 🐾 serving size: 1 fl oz = 30.8 g; Calories = 13

📖 Carbonated Limeade High Caffeine 🐾 serving size: 1 cup = 253 g; Calories = 43

📖 Carbonated Low Calorie Cola Or Pepper-Type With Aspartame Contains Caffeine 🐾 serving size: 1 fl oz = 29.6 g; Calories = 1

📖 Carbonated Low Calorie Other Than Cola Or Pepper Without Caffeine 🐾 serving size: 1 fl oz = 29.6 g; Calories = 0

📖 Carbonated Low Calorie Other Than Cola Or Pepper With Aspartame Contains Caffeine 🐾 serving size: 1 fl oz = 29.6 g; Calories = 0

📖 Carignane 🐾 serving size: 1 fl oz = 29.4 g; Calories = 22

📖 Carob-Flavor Beverage Mix Powder 🐾 serving size: 1 tbsp = 12 g; Calories = 45

📖 Carob-Flavor Beverage Mix Powder Prepared With Whole Milk 🐾 serving size: 1 cup (8 fl oz) = 256 g; Calories = 192

📖 Cereal Beverage 🐾 serving size: 1 fl oz = 30 g; Calories = 2

📖 Cereal Beverage With Beet Roots From Powdered Instant 🐾 serving size: 1 fl oz = 30 g; Calories = 2

Champagne Punch ☞ serving size: 1 fl oz = 30 g; Calories = 38

Chardonnay ☞ serving size: 1 fl oz = 29.3 g; Calories = 25

Chenin Blanc ☞ serving size: 1 fl oz = 29.5 g; Calories = 24

Chicory Beverage ☞ serving size: 1 fl oz = 30 g; Calories = 2

Chocolate Almond Milk ☞ serving size: 8 fl oz = 240 g; Calories = 120

Chocolate Drink Powder ☞ serving size: 2 tbsp = 11 g; Calories = 39

Chocolate Malt Powder Prepared With 1% Milk Fortified ☞ serving size: 1 cup dry mix = 98 g; Calories = 56

Chocolate Malt Powder Prepared With Fat Free Milk ☞ serving size: 1 serving = 256 g; Calories = 125

Chocolate Syrup ☞ serving size: 1 serving 2 tbsp = 39 g; Calories = 109

Chocolate Syrup Prepared With Whole Milk ☞ serving size: 1 cup (8 fl oz) = 282 g; Calories = 254

Chocolate-Flavor Beverage Mix For Milk Powder With Added Nutrients ☞ serving size: 1 serving = 22 g; Calories = 88

Chocolate-Flavor Beverage Mix For Milk Powder With Added Nutrients Prepared With Whole Milk ☞ serving size: 1 serving = 266 g; Calories = 237

Chocolate-Flavor Beverage Mix Powder Prepared With Whole Milk ☞ serving size: 1 cup (8 fl oz) = 266 g; Calories = 226

Chocolate-Flavored Drink Whey And Milk Based ☞ serving size: 1 cup = 244 g; Calories = 120

Citrus Energy Drink ☞ serving size: 8 fl oz = 240 g; Calories = 108

Citrus Fruit Juice Drink Frozen Concentrate ☞ serving size: 1 fl oz = 35.2 g; Calories = 57

Citrus Fruit Juice Drink Frozen Concentrate Prepared With Water serving size: 1 fl oz = 31 g; Calories = 14

Citrus Green Tea serving size: 1 cup = 265 g; Calories = 3

Clam And Tomato Juice Canned serving size: 1 fl oz = 30.2 g; Calories = 15

Claret serving size: 1 fl oz = 29.4 g; Calories = 24

Club Soda serving size: 1 fl oz = 29.6 g; Calories = 0

Coca-Cola Powerade Lemon-Lime Flavored Ready-To-Drink serving size: 1 fl oz = 30.5 g; Calories = 10

Cocktail Mix Non-Alcoholic Concentrated Frozen serving size: 1 fl oz = 36 g; Calories = 103

Cocoa Mix Low Calorie Powder With Added Calcium Phosphorus Aspartame Without Added Sodium Or Vitamin A serving size: 1 envelope swiss miss (.53 oz) = 15 g; Calories = 54

Cocoa Mix Nestle Hot Cocoa Mix Rich Chocolate With Marshmallows serving size: 1 serving 1 envelope = 20 g; Calories = 80

Cocoa Mix Nestle Rich Chocolate Hot Cocoa Mix serving size: 1 serving 1 envelope = 20 g; Calories = 80

Cocoa Mix No Sugar Added Powder serving size: 1 envelope alba (.675 oz) = 19 g; Calories = 72

Cocoa Mix Powder serving size: 1 serving (3 heaping tsp or 1 envelope) = 28 g; Calories = 111

Cocoa Mix Powder Prepared With Water serving size: 1 fl oz = 34.3 g; Calories = 19

Cocoa Mix With Aspartame Powder Prepared With Water serving size: 1 fl oz = 32.1 g; Calories = 9

Coconut Milk Sweetened Fortified With Calcium Vitamins A B12 D2 serving size: 1 cup = 240 g; Calories = 74

Coconut Water Ready-To-Drink Unsweetened ☞ serving size: 1 cup = 245 g; Calories = 44

Coffee ☞ serving size: 1 fl oz = 29.6 g; Calories = 0

Coffee And Cocoa Instant Decaffeinated With Whitener And Low Calorie Sweetener ☞ serving size: 1 tsp dry = 6.4 g; Calories = 28

Coffee Bottled/canned Light ☞ serving size: 1 fl oz = 30 g; Calories = 11

Coffee Brewed Blend Of Regular And Decaffeinated ☞ serving size: 1 fl oz = 30 g; Calories = 0

Coffee Brewed Breakfast Blend ☞ serving size: 1 cup = 248 g; Calories = 5

Coffee Brewed Espresso Restaurant-Prepared Decaffeinated ☞ serving size: 1 fl oz = 29.6 g; Calories = 3

Coffee Cafe Con Leche ☞ serving size: 1 fl oz = 31 g; Calories = 12

Coffee Cafe Con Leche Decaffeinated ☞ serving size: 1 fl oz = 31 g; Calories = 12

Coffee Cafe Mocha ☞ serving size: 1 fl oz = 31 g; Calories = 20

Coffee Cafe Mocha Decaffeinated ☞ serving size: 1 fl oz = 31 g; Calories = 20

Coffee Cafe Mocha Decaffeinated Nonfat ☞ serving size: 1 fl oz = 31 g; Calories = 16

Coffee Cafe Mocha Decaffeinated With Non-Dairy Milk ☞ serving size: 1 fl oz = 31 g; Calories = 18

Coffee Cafe Mocha Nonfat ☞ serving size: 1 fl oz = 31 g; Calories = 16

Coffee Cafe Mocha With Non-Dairy Milk ☞ serving size: 1 fl oz = 31 g; Calories = 18

Coffee Cappuccino ☞ serving size: 1 fl oz = 30 g; Calories = 8

Coffee Cappuccino Decaffeinated ☞ serving size: 1 fl oz = 30 g; Calories = 8

Coffee Cappuccino Decaffeinated Nonfat ☞ serving size: 1 fl oz = 30 g; Calories = 6

Coffee Cappuccino Decaffeinated With Non-Dairy Milk ☞ serving size: 1 fl oz = 30 g; Calories = 7

Coffee Cappuccino Nonfat ☞ serving size: 1 fl oz = 30 g; Calories = 6

Coffee Cappuccino With Non-Dairy Milk ☞ serving size: 1 fl oz = 30 g; Calories = 7

Coffee Cream Liqueur ☞ serving size: 1 fl oz = 31.1 g; Calories = 102

Coffee Cuban ☞ serving size: 1 fl oz = 31 g; Calories = 10

Coffee Decaffeinated Pre-Lightened ☞ serving size: 1 fl oz = 30 g; Calories = 4

Coffee Decaffeinated Pre-Lightened And Pre-Sweetened With Low Calorie Sweetener ☞ serving size: 1 fl oz = 30 g; Calories = 5

Coffee Decaffeinated Pre-Lightened And Pre-Sweetened With Sugar ☞ serving size: 1 fl oz = 31 g; Calories = 8

Coffee Decaffeinated Pre-Sweetened With Low Calorie Sweetener ☞ serving size: 1 fl oz = 30 g; Calories = 2

Coffee Decaffeinated Pre-Sweetened With Sugar ☞ serving size: 1 fl oz = 31 g; Calories = 5

Coffee Iced Cafe Mocha ☞ serving size: 1 fl oz = 31 g; Calories = 16

Coffee Iced Cafe Mocha Decaffeinated ☞ serving size: 1 fl oz = 31 g; Calories = 16

Coffee Iced Cafe Mocha Decaffeinated Nonfat ☛ serving size: 1 fl oz = 31 g; Calories = 13

Coffee Iced Cafe Mocha Decaffeinated With Non-Dairy Milk ☛ serving size: 1 fl oz = 31 g; Calories = 14

Coffee Iced Cafe Mocha Nonfat ☛ serving size: 1 fl oz = 31 g; Calories = 13

Coffee Iced Cafe Mocha With Non-Dairy Milk ☛ serving size: 1 fl oz = 31 g; Calories = 14

Coffee Iced Latte ☛ serving size: 1 fl oz = 30 g; Calories = 8

Coffee Iced Latte Decaffeinated ☛ serving size: 1 fl oz = 30 g; Calories = 8

Coffee Iced Latte Decaffeinated Flavored ☛ serving size: 1 fl oz = 31 g; Calories = 12

Coffee Iced Latte Decaffeinated Nonfat ☛ serving size: 1 fl oz = 30 g; Calories = 6

Coffee Iced Latte Decaffeinated Nonfat Flavored ☛ serving size: 1 fl oz = 31 g; Calories = 10

Coffee Iced Latte Decaffeinated With Non-Dairy Milk ☛ serving size: 1 fl oz = 30 g; Calories = 7

Coffee Iced Latte Decaffeinated With Non-Dairy Milk Flavored ☛ serving size: 1 fl oz = 31 g; Calories = 11

Coffee Iced Latte Flavored ☛ serving size: 1 fl oz = 31 g; Calories = 12

Coffee Iced Latte Nonfat ☛ serving size: 1 fl oz = 30 g; Calories = 6

Coffee Iced Latte Nonfat Flavored ☛ serving size: 1 fl oz = 31 g; Calories = 10

Coffee Iced Latte With Non-Dairy Milk ☛ serving size: 1 fl oz = 30 g; Calories = 7

Coffee Iced Latte With Non-Dairy Milk Flavored ☞ serving size: 1 fl oz = 31 g; Calories = 11

Coffee Instant 50% Less Caffeine Reconstituted ☞ serving size: 1 fl oz = 30 g; Calories = 1

Coffee Instant Chicory ☞ serving size: 1 fl oz = 29.9 g; Calories = 1

Coffee Instant Decaffeinated Powder ☞ serving size: 1 tsp rounded = 1.8 g; Calories = 6

Coffee Instant Decaffeinated Pre-Lightened And Pre-Sweetened With Low Calorie Sweetener Reconstituted ☞ serving size: 1 fl oz = 30 g; Calories = 5

Coffee Instant Decaffeinated Pre-Lightened And Pre-Sweetened With Sugar Reconsititued ☞ serving size: 1 fl oz = 31 g; Calories = 8

Coffee Instant Decaffeinated Prepared With Water ☞ serving size: 1 fl oz = 29.9 g; Calories = 1

Coffee Instant Decaffeinated Reconstituted ☞ serving size: 1 fl oz = 30 g; Calories = 1

Coffee Instant Mocha Sweetened ☞ serving size: 1 serving 2 tbsp = 13 g; Calories = 60

Coffee Instant Pre-Lightened And Pre-Sweetened With Low Calorie Sweetener Reconstituted ☞ serving size: 1 fl oz = 30 g; Calories = 5

Coffee Instant Pre-Lightened And Pre-Sweetened With Sugar Reconstituted ☞ serving size: 1 fl oz = 31 g; Calories = 8

Coffee Instant Pre-Sweetened With Sugar Reconstituted ☞ serving size: 1 fl oz = 31 g; Calories = 5

Coffee Instant Reconstituted ☞ serving size: 1 fl oz = 30 g; Calories = 1

Coffee Instant Regular Half The Caffeine ☛ serving size: 1 tsp = 1 g; Calories = 4

Coffee Instant Regular Powder ☛ serving size: 1 tsp = 1 g; Calories = 4

Coffee Instant Vanilla Sweetened Decaffeinated With Non Dairy Creamer ☛ serving size: 1 serving = 15 g; Calories = 70

Coffee Instant With Chicory ☛ serving size: 1 tsp, rounded = 1.8 g; Calories = 6

Coffee Instant With Whitener Reduced Calorie ☛ serving size: 1 tsp dry = 1.7 g; Calories = 9

Coffee Latte ☛ serving size: 1 fl oz = 30 g; Calories = 13

Coffee Latte Decaffeinated ☛ serving size: 1 fl oz = 30 g; Calories = 13

Coffee Latte Decaffeinated Flavored ☛ serving size: 1 fl oz = 31 g; Calories = 17

Coffee Latte Decaffeinated Nonfat ☛ serving size: 1 fl oz = 30 g; Calories = 9

Coffee Latte Decaffeinated Nonfat Flavored ☛ serving size: 1 fl oz = 31 g; Calories = 13

Coffee Latte Decaffeinated With Non-Dairy Milk ☛ serving size: 1 fl oz = 30 g; Calories = 11

Coffee Latte Decaffeinated With Non-Dairy Milk Flavored ☛ serving size: 1 fl oz = 31 g; Calories = 15

Coffee Latte Flavored ☛ serving size: 1 fl oz = 31 g; Calories = 17

Coffee Latte Nonfat ☛ serving size: 1 fl oz = 30 g; Calories = 9

Coffee Latte Nonfat Flavored ☛ serving size: 1 fl oz = 31 g; Calories = 13

Coffee Latte With Non-Dairy Milk ☛ serving size: 1 fl oz = 30 g; Calories = 11

Coffee Latte With Non-Dairy Milk Flavored ☛ serving size: 1 fl oz = 31 g; Calories = 15

Coffee Liqueur ☛ serving size: 1 fl oz = 34.8 g; Calories = 117

Coffee Macchiato ☛ serving size: 1 fl oz = 30 g; Calories = 7

Coffee Macchiato Sweetened ☛ serving size: 1 fl oz = 31 g; Calories = 12

Coffee Mocha Instant Decaffeinated Pre-Lightened And Pre-Sweetened With Low Calorie Sweetener Reconstituted ☛ serving size: 1 fl oz = 30 g; Calories = 4

Coffee Mocha Instant Pre-Lightened And Pre-Sweetened With Low Calorie Sweetener Reconstituted ☛ serving size: 1 fl oz = 30 g; Calories = 5

Coffee Mocha Instant Pre-Lightened And Pre-Sweetened With Sugar Reconstituted ☛ serving size: 1 fl oz = 31 g; Calories = 14

Coffee Pre-Lightened ☛ serving size: 1 fl oz = 30 g; Calories = 4

Coffee Pre-Lightened And Pre-Sweetened With Low Calorie Sweetener ☛ serving size: 1 fl oz = 30 g; Calories = 5

Coffee Pre-Lightened And Pre-Sweetened With Sugar ☛ serving size: 1 fl oz = 31 g; Calories = 8

Coffee Pre-Sweetened With Low Calorie Sweetener ☛ serving size: 1 fl oz = 30 g; Calories = 2

Coffee Pre-Sweetened With Sugar ☛ serving size: 1 fl oz = 31 g; Calories = 5

Coffee Ready To Drink Milk Based Sweetened ☛ serving size: 1 cup = 262 g; Calories = 186

Coffee Ready To Drink Vanilla Light Milk Based Sweetened ☛ serving size: fl oz = 281 g; Calories = 101

Coffee Substitute Cereal Grain Beverage Powder ☛ serving size: 1 tsp (1 serving) = 3 g; Calories = 11

Coffee Substitute Cereal Grain Beverage Powder Prepared With Whole Milk ☛ serving size: 6 fl oz = 185 g; Calories = 120

Coffee Substitute Cereal Grain Beverage Prepared With Water ☛ serving size: 1 fl oz = 30.1 g; Calories = 2

Coffee Turkish ☛ serving size: 1 fl oz = 31 g; Calories = 8

Cola Soft Drink ☛ serving size: 1 fl oz = 30.7 g; Calories = 13

Corn Beverage ☛ serving size: 1 fl oz = 30 g; Calories = 13

Cornmeal Beverage ☛ serving size: 1 cup = 248 g; Calories = 208

Cranberry Juice Cocktail ☛ serving size: 1 cup = 271 g; Calories = 141

Cranberry Juice Cocktail Bottled ☛ serving size: 1 fl oz = 31.6 g; Calories = 17

Cranberry Juice Cocktail Bottled Low Calorie With Calcium Saccharin And Corn Sweetener ☛ serving size: 1 fl oz = 29.6 g; Calories = 6

Cranberry Juice Cocktail Frozen Concentrate ☛ serving size: 1 fl oz = 36.2 g; Calories = 73

Cranberry Juice Cocktail Frozen Concentrate Prepared With Water ☛ serving size: 1 fl oz = 29.6 g; Calories = 14

Cranberry-Apple Juice Drink Bottled ☛ serving size: 1 fl oz = 30.6 g; Calories = 19

Cranberry-Apple Juice Drink Low Calorie With Vitamin C Added ☛ serving size: 1 cup (8 fl oz) = 240 g; Calories = 46

Cranberry-Apricot Juice Drink Bottled ☛ serving size: 1 fl oz = 30.6 g; Calories = 20

Cranberry-Grape Juice Drink Bottled ☛ serving size: 1 fl oz = 30.6 g; Calories = 17

Cream Soda ☛ serving size: 1 fl oz = 30.9 g; Calories = 16

Cytosport Muscle Milk Ready-To-Drink ☛ serving size: 14 fl oz = 414 g; Calories = 215

Daiquiri ☛ serving size: 1 fl oz = 30.5 g; Calories = 38

Dairy Drink Mix Chocolate Reduced Calorie With Aspartame Powder Prepared With Water And Ice ☛ serving size: 1 serving = 243 g; Calories = 71

Dairy Drink Mix Chocolate Reduced Calorie With Low-Calorie Sweeteners Powder ☛ serving size: 1 packet (.75 oz) = 21 g; Calories = 69

Decaf Coffee ☛ serving size: 1 fl oz = 29.6 g; Calories = 0

Diet Cola ☛ serving size: 1 fl oz = 29.6 g; Calories = 6

Diet Green Tea ☛ serving size: 1 cup = 269 g; Calories = 11

Diet Pepper Cola ☛ serving size: 1 fl oz = 29.6 g; Calories = 0

Drink Mix Quaker Oats Gatorade Orange Flavor Powder ☛ serving size: 1 scoop powder = 23 g; Calories = 89

Dry Dessert Wine ☛ serving size: 1 fl oz = 29.5 g; Calories = 45

Eggnog Alcoholic ☛ serving size: 1 fl oz = 30 g; Calories = 34

Eggnog-Flavor Mix Powder Prepared With Whole Milk ☛ serving size: 1 cup (8 fl oz) = 272 g; Calories = 258

Energy Drink ☛ serving size: 8 fl oz = 240 g; Calories = 149

Energy Drink Amp ☛ serving size: 1 serving = 240 g; Calories = 110

Energy Drink Amp Sugar Free ☛ serving size: 8 fl oz = 240 g; Calories = 5

Energy Drink Full Throttle ☛ serving size: 1 serving 8 fluid oz = 240 g; Calories = 110

Energy Drink Monster Fortified With Vitamins C B2 B3 B6 B12 ☛ serving size: 1 serving = 240 g; Calories = 113

Energy Drink Red Bull ☛ serving size: 1 can 8.4 fl oz = 258 g; Calories = 111

Energy Drink Red Bull Sugar Free With Added Caffeine Niacin Pantothenic Acid Vitamins B6 And B12 ☛ serving size: 1 serving 8.3 fl oz can = 250 g; Calories = 13

Energy Drink Rockstar ☛ serving size: 1 fl oz = 31 g; Calories = 18

Energy Drink Rockstar Sugar Free ☛ serving size: 8 fl oz = 240 g; Calories = 10

Energy Drink Sugar Free ☛ serving size: 8 fl oz = 240 g; Calories = 10

Energy Drink Vault Citrus Flavor ☛ serving size: 1 oz = 31 g; Calories = 15

Energy Drink Vault Zero Sugar-Free Citrus Flavor ☛ serving size: 1 serving (8 fl oz) = 246 g; Calories = 3

Espresso ☛ serving size: 1 fl oz = 29.6 g; Calories = 3

Fluid Replacement 5% Glucose In Water ☛ serving size: 1 cup = 240 g; Calories = 43

Frozen Coffee Drink ☛ serving size: 1 fl oz = 31 g; Calories = 21

Frozen Coffee Drink Decaffeinated ☛ serving size: 1 fl oz = 31 g; Calories = 21

Frozen Coffee Drink Decaffeinated Nonfat ☛ serving size: 1 fl oz = 31 g; Calories = 19

Frozen Coffee Drink Decaffeinated Nonfat With Whipped Cream serving size: 1 fl oz = 31 g; Calories = 23

Frozen Coffee Drink Decaffeinated With Non-Dairy Milk serving size: 1 fl oz = 31 g; Calories = 20

Frozen Coffee Drink Decaffeinated With Non-Dairy Milk And Whipped Cream serving size: 1 fl oz = 31 g; Calories = 24

Frozen Coffee Drink Decaffeinated With Whipped Cream serving size: 1 fl oz = 31 g; Calories = 25

Frozen Coffee Drink Nonfat serving size: 1 fl oz = 31 g; Calories = 18

Frozen Coffee Drink Nonfat With Whipped Cream serving size: 1 fl oz = 31 g; Calories = 23

Frozen Coffee Drink With Non-Dairy Milk serving size: 1 fl oz = 31 g; Calories = 19

Frozen Coffee Drink With Non-Dairy Milk And Whipped Cream serving size: 1 fl oz = 31 g; Calories = 24

Frozen Coffee Drink With Whipped Cream serving size: 1 fl oz = 31 g; Calories = 25

Frozen Daiquiri serving size: 1 fl oz = 30 g; Calories = 38

Frozen Daiquiri Mix From Frozen Concentrate Reconstituted serving size: 1 fl oz = 29 g; Calories = 19

Frozen Margarita serving size: 1 fl oz = 30 g; Calories = 37

Frozen Mocha Coffee Drink serving size: 1 fl oz = 31 g; Calories = 21

Frozen Mocha Coffee Drink Decaffeinated serving size: 1 fl oz = 31 g; Calories = 21

Frozen Mocha Coffee Drink Decaffeinated Nonfat serving size: 1 fl oz = 31 g; Calories = 18

Frozen Mocha Coffee Drink Decaffeinated Nonfat With Whipped Cream ☛ serving size: 1 fl oz = 31 g; Calories = 23

Frozen Mocha Coffee Drink Decaffeinated With Non-Dairy Milk ☛ serving size: 1 fl oz = 31 g; Calories = 19

Frozen Mocha Coffee Drink Decaffeinated With Non-Dairy Milk And Whipped Cream ☛ serving size: 1 fl oz – 31 g; Calories = 24

Frozen Mocha Coffee Drink Decaffeinated With Whipped Cream ☛ serving size: 1 fl oz = 31 g; Calories = 25

Frozen Mocha Coffee Drink Nonfat ☛ serving size: 1 fl oz = 31 g; Calories = 18

Frozen Mocha Coffee Drink Nonfat With Whipped Cream ☛ serving size: 1 fl oz = 31 g; Calories = 23

Frozen Mocha Coffee Drink With Non-Dairy Milk ☛ serving size: 1 fl oz = 31 g; Calories = 19

Frozen Mocha Coffee Drink With Non-Dairy Milk And Whipped Cream ☛ serving size: 1 fl oz = 31 g; Calories = 24

Frozen Mocha Coffee Drink With Whipped Cream ☛ serving size: 1 fl oz = 31 g; Calories = 25

Fruit And Vegetable Smoothie ☛ serving size: 1 fl oz = 27 g; Calories = 16

Fruit And Vegetable Smoothie Added Protein ☛ serving size: 1 fl oz = 27 g; Calories = 22

Fruit Flavored Drink Containing Less Than 3% Fruit Juice With High Vitamin C ☛ serving size: 1 cup (8 fl oz) = 238 g; Calories = 64

Fruit Flavored Drink Less Than 3% Juice Not Fortified With Vitamin C ☛ serving size: 1 cup (8 fl oz) = 238 g; Calories = 152

Fruit Flavored Drink Reduced Sugar Greater Than 3% Fruit Juice

High Vitamin C Added Calcium ☛ serving size: 8 fl oz = 240 g; Calories = 70

🍹 Fruit Flavored Drink With High Vitamin C Powdered Reconstituted ☛ serving size: 1 fl oz (no ice) = 31 g; Calories = 13

🍹 Fruit Flavored Smoothie Drink Frozen Light No Dairy ☛ serving size: 1 fl oz = 30 g; Calories = 4

🍹 Fruit Flavored Smoothie Drink Frozen No Dairy ☛ serving size: 1 fl oz = 30 g; Calories = 8

🍹 Fruit Juice Drink Citrus Carbonated ☛ serving size: 1 fl oz (no ice) = 31 g; Calories = 9

🍹 Fruit Juice Drink Diet ☛ serving size: 1 fl oz (no ice) = 30 g; Calories = 0

🍹 Fruit Juice Drink Greater Than 3% Fruit Juice High Vitamin C And Added Thiamin ☛ serving size: 8 fl oz = 237 g; Calories = 128

🍹 Fruit Juice Drink Greater Than 3% Juice High Vitamin C ☛ serving size: 1 cup (8 fl oz) = 238 g; Calories = 110

🍹 Fruit Juice Drink Noncitrus Carbonated ☛ serving size: 1 fl oz (no ice) = 31 g; Calories = 10

🍹 Fruit Juice Drink Reduced Sugar (Sunny D) ☛ serving size: 1 fl oz (no ice) = 31 g; Calories = 1

🍹 Fruit Juice Drink Reduced Sugar With Vitamin E Added ☛ serving size: 1 container = 209 g; Calories = 82

🍹 Fruit Punch Drink Frozen Concentrate ☛ serving size: 1 fl oz = 34.8 g; Calories = 56

🍹 Fruit Punch Drink Frozen Concentrate Prepared With Water ☛ serving size: 1 fl oz = 30.9 g; Calories = 14

🍹 Fruit Punch Drink With Added Nutrients Canned ☛ serving size: 1 fl oz = 31 g; Calories = 15

🍹 Fruit Punch Drink Without Added Nutrients Canned ☛ serving size: 6 (3/4) fl oz = 210 g; Calories = 101

🍹 Fruit Punch Juice Drink Frozen Concentrate ☛ serving size: 1 fl oz = 35.2 g; Calories = 62

🍹 Fruit Punch Juice Drink Frozen Concentrate Prepared With Water ☛ serving size: 1 fl oz = 29.3 g; Calories = 12

🍹 Fruit Punch-Flavor Drink Powder Without Added Sodium Prepared With Water ☛ serving size: 1 fl oz = 32.7 g; Calories = 12

🍹 Fruit Smoothie Juice Drink No Dairy ☛ serving size: 1 fl oz = 27 g; Calories = 14

🍹 Fruit Smoothie Light ☛ serving size: 1 fl oz = 27 g; Calories = 14

🍹 Fruit Smoothie Nfs ☛ serving size: 1 fl oz = 27 g; Calories = 17

🍹 Fruit Smoothie With Whole Fruit And Dairy ☛ serving size: 1 fl oz = 27 g; Calories = 17

🍹 Fruit Smoothie With Whole Fruit And Dairy Added Protein ☛ serving size: 1 fl oz = 27 g; Calories = 21

🍹 Fruit Smoothie With Whole Fruit No Dairy ☛ serving size: 1 fl oz = 27 g; Calories = 14

🍹 Fruit Smoothie With Whole Fruit No Dairy Added Protein ☛ serving size: 1 fl oz = 27 g; Calories = 20

🍹 Fruit-Flavored Drink Dry Powdered Mix Low Calorie With Aspartame ☛ serving size: 1 tsp = 8 g; Calories = 17

🍹 Fruit-Flavored Drink Powder With High Vitamin C With Other Added Vitamins Low Calorie ☛ serving size: 1 tsp = 2 g; Calories = 5

🍹 Fume Blanc ☛ serving size: 1 fl oz = 29.3 g; Calories = 24

🍹 Fuze Orange Mango Fortified With Vitamins A C E B6 ☛ serving size: 1 bottle = 500 g; Calories = 190

Gamay (Red Wine) ☛ serving size: 1 fl oz = 29.4 g; Calories = 23

Gelatin Shot Alcoholic ☛ serving size: 1 shot = 42 g; Calories = 69

Gerolsteiner Brunnen Gmbh & Co. Kggerolsteiner Naturally Sparkling Mineral Water ☛ serving size: 8 fl oz = 240 g; Calories = 0

Gewurztraminer ☛ serving size: 1 fl oz = 29.5 g; Calories = 24

Gewurztraminer (Late Harvest) ☛ serving size: 1 fl oz = 30.5 g; Calories = 33

Ginger Ale ☛ serving size: 1 fl oz = 30.5 g; Calories = 10

Grape Drink Canned ☛ serving size: 1 fl oz = 31.3 g; Calories = 19

Grape Juice Drink Canned ☛ serving size: 1 fl oz = 31.3 g; Calories = 18

Grape Juice Drink Light ☛ serving size: 1 fl oz (no ice) = 30 g; Calories = 6

Grape Soda ☛ serving size: 1 fl oz = 31 g; Calories = 13

Green Tea ☛ serving size: 16 fl oz = 473 g; Calories = 0

Greyhound ☛ serving size: 1 fl oz = 30 g; Calories = 25

High Alcohol Beer ☛ serving size: 1 fl oz = 30.6 g; Calories = 18

Horchata ☛ serving size: 1 cup = 228 g; Calories = 123

Horchata Beverage Made With Milk ☛ serving size: 1 cup = 248 g; Calories = 223

Horchata Beverage Made With Water ☛ serving size: 1 cup = 248 g; Calories = 216

Ice Mocha ☛ serving size: 1 cup = 265 g; Calories = 159

Iced Coffee Brewed ☛ serving size: 1 fl oz = 30 g; Calories = 0

Iced Coffee Brewed Decaffeinated ☛ serving size: 1 fl oz = 30 g; Calories = 0

Iced Coffee Pre-Lightened And Pre-Sweetened ☞ serving size: 1 fl oz = 31 g; Calories = 9

Iced Tea / Lemonade Juice Drink ☞ serving size: 1 fl oz (no ice) = 30 g; Calories = 10

Iced Tea / Lemonade Juice Drink Diet ☞ serving size: 1 fl oz (no ice) = 30 g; Calories = 1

Iced Tea / Lemonade Juice Drink Light ☞ serving size: 1 fl oz (no ice) = 30 g; Calories = 6

Instant Coffee (Prepared With Water) ☞ serving size: 1 fl oz = 29.8 g; Calories = 1

Irish Coffee ☞ serving size: 1 fl oz = 30 g; Calories = 26

Jagerbomb ☞ serving size: 1 fl oz = 30 g; Calories = 38

Kiwi Strawberry Juice Drink ☞ serving size: 16 fl oz = 473 g; Calories = 222

Kraft Coffee Instant French Vanilla Cafe ☞ serving size: 1 nlea serving = 14 g; Calories = 67

Late Harvest White Wine ☞ serving size: 1 fl oz = 30.8 g; Calories = 35

Lemberger ☞ serving size: 1 fl oz = 29.4 g; Calories = 24

Lemonade Frozen Concentrate Pink ☞ serving size: 1 fl oz = 36.4 g; Calories = 70

Lemonade Frozen Concentrate Pink Prepared With Water ☞ serving size: 1 fl oz = 30.9 g; Calories = 13

Lemonade Frozen Concentrate White ☞ serving size: 1 fl oz = 36.5 g; Calories = 72

Lemonade Frozen Concentrate White Prepared With Water ☞ serving size: 1 fl oz = 30.9 g; Calories = 12

Lemonade Fruit Flavored Drink ☛ serving size: 1 fl oz (no ice) = 31 g; Calories = 8

Lemonade Fruit Juice Drink Light Fortified With Vitamin E And C ☛ serving size: 8 fl oz = 240 g; Calories = 50

Lemonade Powder ☛ serving size: 1 serving = 18 g; Calories = 68

Lemonade Powder Prepared With Water ☛ serving size: 1 fl oz = 33 g; Calories = 5

Lemonade-Flavor Drink Powder ☛ serving size: 1 serving = 18 g; Calories = 68

Lemonade-Flavor Drink Powder Prepared With Water ☛ serving size: 1 fl oz = 31.8 g; Calories = 9

Licuado Or Batido ☛ serving size: 1 fl oz = 27 g; Calories = 19

Light Beer ☛ serving size: 1 fl oz = 29.5 g; Calories = 9

Limeade Frozen Concentrate Prepared With Water ☛ serving size: 1 fl oz = 30.9 g; Calories = 16

Lipton Brisk Tea Black Ready-To-Drink Lemon ☛ serving size: 1 fl oz = 30.6 g; Calories = 11

Low Calorie Cola ☛ serving size: 1 fl oz = 29.6 g; Calories = 0

Low Carb Monster Energy Drink ☛ serving size: 8 fl oz = 240 g; Calories = 12

Malt Beverage Includes Non-Alcoholic Beer ☛ serving size: 1 fl oz = 29.6 g; Calories = 11

Malt Liquor Beverage ☛ serving size: 1 bottle = 1184 g; Calories = 474

Malted Drink Mix Chocolate Powder ☛ serving size: 1 serving (3 heaping tsp or 1 envelope) = 21 g; Calories = 86

Malted Drink Mix Chocolate Powder Prepared With Whole Milk ☛ serving size: 1 cup (8 fl oz) = 265 g; Calories = 225

Malted Drink Mix Chocolate With Added Nutrients Powder Prepared With Whole Milk ☛ serving size: 1 cup (8 fl oz) = 265 g; Calories = 231

Malted Drink Mix Natural Powder Dairy Based. ☛ serving size: 1 serving (3 heaping tsp or 1 envelope) = 21 g; Calories = 90

Malted Drink Mix Natural Powder Prepared With Whole Milk ☛ serving size: 1 cup (8 fl oz) = 265 g; Calories = 233

Malted Drink Mix Natural With Added Nutrients Powder Prepared With Whole Milk ☛ serving size: 1 cup (8 fl oz) = 265 g; Calories = 228

Martini Flavored ☛ serving size: 1 fl oz = 30 g; Calories = 57

Meal Supplement Drink Canned Peanut Flavor ☛ serving size: 1 cup = 158 g; Calories = 160

Merlot ☛ serving size: 1 fl oz = 29.4 g; Calories = 24

Milk And Soy Chocolate Drink ☛ serving size: 8 fl oz = 237 g; Calories = 239

Milk Beverage Reduced Fat Flavored And Sweetened Ready-To-Drink Added Calcium Vitamin A And Vitamin D ☛ serving size: 1 cup = 244 g; Calories = 188

Minute Maid Lemonada Limeade ☛ serving size: 8 fl oz = 240 g; Calories = 120

Minute Maid Lemonade ☛ serving size: 8 fl oz = 240 g; Calories = 110

Mixed Berry Powerade Zero ☛ serving size: 12 fl oz = 360 g; Calories = 0

Mixed Vegetable And Fruit Juice Drink With Added Nutrients ☛ serving size: 8 fl oz = 247 g; Calories = 72

Motts Light Apple Juice ☛ serving size: 8 fl oz = 240 g; Calories = 53

Mouvedre Wine ☛ serving size: 1 fl oz = 29.4 g; Calories = 26

Muscat Wine ☛ serving size: 1 fl oz = 30 g; Calories = 25

Nestea ☛ serving size: 1 fl oz = 30.6 g; Calories = 11

Nestle Boost Plus Nutritional Drink Ready-To-Drink ☛ serving size: 1 bottle = 237 g; Calories = 327

Nutritional Drink Or Shake High Protein Ready-To-Drink (Slim Fast) ☛ serving size: 1 cup = 248 g; Calories = 144

Nutritional Drink Or Shake High Protein Ready-To-Drink Nfs ☛ serving size: 1 cup = 256 g; Calories = 149

Nutritional Drink Or Shake Ready-To-Drink (Carnation Instant Breakfast) ☛ serving size: 1 cup = 248 g; Calories = 226

Nutritional Drink Or Shake Ready-To-Drink (Kellogg's Special K Protein) ☛ serving size: 1 fl oz = 32 g; Calories = 21

Nutritional Drink Or Shake Ready-To-Drink (Muscle Milk) ☛ serving size: 1 cup = 256 g; Calories = 125

Nutritional Drink Or Shake Ready-To-Drink Light (Muscle Milk) ☛ serving size: 1 cup = 256 g; Calories = 97

Nutritional Shake Mix High Protein Powder ☛ serving size: 1 tbsp = 10 g; Calories = 39

Oatmeal Beverage With Milk ☛ serving size: 1 cup = 248 g; Calories = 203

Oatmeal Beverage With Water ☛ serving size: 1 fl oz = 31 g; Calories = 13

Ocean Spray Cran Cherry ☛ serving size: 8 fl oz = 248 g; Calories = 114

Ocean Spray Cran Grape ☛ serving size: 8 fl oz = 240 g; Calories = 130

Ocean Spray Cran Lemonade ☛ serving size: 8 fl oz = 247 g; Calories = 111

Ocean Spray Cran Pomegranate ☛ serving size: 8 fl oz = 248 g; Calories = 117

Ocean Spray Cran Raspberry Juice Drink ☛ serving size: 8 fl oz = 248 g; Calories = 122

Ocean Spray Cran-Energy Cranberry Energy Juice Drink ☛ serving size: 1 can = 250 g; Calories = 38

Ocean Spray Cranberry-Apple Juice Drink Bottled ☛ serving size: 8 fl oz = 249 g; Calories = 139

Ocean Spray Diet Cran Cherry ☛ serving size: 8 fl oz = 237 g; Calories = 10

Ocean Spray Diet Cranberry Juice ☛ serving size: 8 fl oz = 237 g; Calories = 10

Ocean Spray Light Cranberry ☛ serving size: 8 fl oz = 248 g; Calories = 47

Ocean Spray Light Cranberry And Raspberry Flavored Juice ☛ serving size: 8 fl oz = 242 g; Calories = 63

Ocean Spray Light Cranberry Concord Grape ☛ serving size: 8 fl oz = 248 g; Calories = 57

Ocean Spray Ruby Red Cranberry ☛ serving size: 8 fl oz = 227 g; Calories = 102

Ocean Spray White Cranberry Peach ☛ serving size: 8 fl oz = 247 g; Calories = 111

Ocean Spray White Cranberry Strawberry Flavored Juice Drink ☛ serving size: 8 fl oz = 247 g; Calories = 121

Orange And Apricot Juice Drink Canned ☛ serving size: 1 fl oz = 31.2 g; Calories = 16

Orange Blossom ☛ serving size: 1 fl oz = 30 g; Calories = 30

Orange Breakfast Drink Ready-To-Drink With Added Nutrients ☛ serving size: 1 fl oz = 31.6 g; Calories = 17

Orange Drink Breakfast Type With Juice And Pulp Frozen Concentrate ☛ serving size: 1 fl oz = 36.3 g; Calories = 56

Orange Drink Breakfast Type With Juice And Pulp Frozen Concentrate Prepared With Water ☛ serving size: 1 fl oz = 31.3 g; Calories = 14

Orange Drink Canned With Added Vitamin C ☛ serving size: 1 fl oz = 31 g; Calories = 15

Orange Juice Drink ☛ serving size: 1 cup = 249 g; Calories = 135

Orange Juice Light No Pulp ☛ serving size: 8 fl oz = 240 g; Calories = 50

Orange Soda ☛ serving size: 1 fl oz = 31 g; Calories = 15

Orange-Flavor Drink Breakfast Type Low Calorie Powder ☛ serving size: 1 portion, amount of dry mix to make 8 fl oz prepared = 2.5 g; Calories = 5

Orange-Flavor Drink Breakfast Type Powder ☛ serving size: 1 serving 2 tbsp = 26 g; Calories = 100

Orange-Flavor Drink Breakfast Type Powder Prepared With Water ☛ serving size: 1 fl oz = 33.9 g; Calories = 17

Orange-Flavor Drink Breakfast Type With Pulp Frozen Concentrate Prepared With Water ☛ serving size: 1 fl oz = 31 g; Calories = 15

Orange-Flavor Drink Breakfast Type With Pulp Frozen Concentrate. Not Manufactured Anymore. ☛ serving size: 1 fl oz = 35.3 g; Calories = 61

Ovaltine Chocolate Malt Powder ☛ serving size: 1 cup = 78 g; Calories = 290

Ovaltine Classic Malt Powder ☛ serving size: 1 serving (4 tbsp or 1 envelope) = 21 g; Calories = 78

Pepper Soda ☛ serving size: 1 fl oz = 30.7 g; Calories = 13

Pepsico Quaker Gatorade G Performance O 2 Ready-To-Drink. ☛ serving size: 1 fl oz = 30.5 g; Calories = 8

Pepsico Quaker Gatorade G2 Low Calorie ☛ serving size: 8 fl oz = 237 g; Calories = 19

Petite Sirah ☛ serving size: 1 fl oz = 29.5 g; Calories = 25

Pina Colada Nonalcoholic ☛ serving size: 1 fl oz = 30 g; Calories = 28

Pineapple And Grapefruit Juice Drink Canned ☛ serving size: 1 fl oz = 31.3 g; Calories = 15

Pineapple And Orange Juice Drink Canned ☛ serving size: 1 fl oz = 31.3 g; Calories = 16

Pinot Blanc ☛ serving size: 1 fl oz = 29.3 g; Calories = 24

Pinot Gris (Grigio) ☛ serving size: 1 fl oz = 29.3 g; Calories = 24

Pinot Noir ☛ serving size: 1 fl oz = 29.4 g; Calories = 24

Powerade Zero Ion4 Calorie-Free Assorted Flavors ☛ serving size: 8 fl oz = 237 g; Calories = 0

Propel Zero Fruit-Flavored Non-Carbonated ☛ serving size: 1 fl oz = 29.6 g; Calories = 2

Protein Powder Soy Based ☛ serving size: 1 scoop = 45 g; Calories = 175

Protein Powder Whey Based ☛ serving size: 1/3 cup = 32 g; Calories = 113

Red Wine ☛ serving size: 1 fl oz – 29.4 g; Calories = 25

Rich Chocolate Powder ☛ serving size: 2 tbsp = 11 g; Calories = 41

Riesling ☛ serving size: 1 fl oz = 29.6 g; Calories = 24

Root Beer ☛ serving size: 1 fl oz = 30.8 g; Calories = 13

Rose Wine ☛ serving size: 1 fl oz = 30.3 g; Calories = 25

Rum ☛ serving size: 1 fl oz = 27.8 g; Calories = 64

Rum And Diet Cola ☛ serving size: 1 fl oz = 30 g; Calories = 18

Rum Hot Buttered ☛ serving size: 1 fl oz = 30 g; Calories = 48

Sangiovese ☛ serving size: 1 fl oz = 29.4 g; Calories = 25

Sangria Red ☛ serving size: 1 fl oz = 30 g; Calories = 29

Sangria White ☛ serving size: 1 fl oz = 30 g; Calories = 28

Sauvignon Blanc ☛ serving size: 1 fl oz = 29.3 g; Calories = 24

Semillon ☛ serving size: 1 fl oz = 29.5 g; Calories = 24

Shake Fast Food Strawberry ☛ serving size: 1 fl oz = 23.5 g; Calories = 27

Shake Fast Food Vanilla ☛ serving size: 1 fl oz = 20.8 g; Calories = 31

Slimfast Meal Replacement High Protein Shake Ready-To-Drink 3-2-1 Plan ☛ serving size: 1 bottle = 295 g; Calories = 180

Soft Drink Fruit Flavored Caffeine Containing ☛ serving size: 1 fl oz (no ice) = 31 g; Calories = 15

Sprite ☛ serving size: 1 fl oz = 30.8 g; Calories = 12

Strawberry-Flavor Beverage Mix Powder ☛ serving size: 1 serving (2-3 heaping tsp) = 22 g; Calories = 86

Strawberry-Flavor Beverage Mix Powder Prepared With Whole Milk ☛ serving size: 1 cup (8 fl oz) = 266 g; Calories = 234

Sweet Dessert Wine ☛ serving size: 1 fl oz = 29.5 g; Calories = 47

Sweetened Vanilla Almond Milk ☛ serving size: 8 fl oz = 240 g; Calories = 91

Syrah ☛ serving size: 1 fl oz = 29.4 g; Calories = 24

Table Wine ☛ serving size: 1 serving (5 fl oz) = 148 g; Calories = 123

Tap Water ☛ serving size: 1 fl oz = 29.6 g; Calories = 0

Tea Black Brewed Prepared With Distilled Water ☛ serving size: 1 fl oz = 29.6 g; Calories = 0

Tea Black Brewed Prepared With Tap Water Decaffeinated ☛ serving size: 1 fl oz = 29.6 g; Calories = 0

Tea Black Ready To Drink Decaffeinated ☛ serving size: 1 cup = 240 g; Calories = 91

Tea Black Ready To Drink Decaffeinated Diet ☛ serving size: 1 cup = 240 g; Calories = 0

Tea Black Ready-To-Drink Lemon Diet ☛ serving size: 1 cup = 265 g; Calories = 3

Tea Black Ready-To-Drink Lemon Sweetened ☛ serving size: 1 cup = 271 g; Calories = 122

Tea Black Ready-To-Drink Peach Diet ☛ serving size: 1 cup = 268 g; Calories = 3

Tea Green Brewed Decaffeinated ☛ serving size: ml = 240 g; Calories = 0

Tea Green Brewed Regular ☛ serving size: 1 cup = 245 g; Calories = 3

Tea Green Instant Decaffeinated Lemon Unsweetened Fortified With Vitamin C ☛ serving size: 2 tbsp = 4.5 g; Calories = 17

Tea Green Ready To Drink Ginseng And Honey Sweetened ☛ serving size: 1 cup = 260 g; Calories = 78

Tea Green Ready-To-Drink Sweetened ☛ serving size: 1 cup = 270 g; Calories = 73

Tea Herb Brewed Chamomile ☛ serving size: 1 fl oz = 29.6 g; Calories = 0

Tea Herb Other Than Chamomile Brewed ☛ serving size: 1 fl oz = 29.6 g; Calories = 0

Tea Hibiscus Brewed ☛ serving size: 8 fl oz = 237 g; Calories = 0

Tea Hot Chai With Milk ☛ serving size: 1 fl oz = 30 g; Calories = 15

Tea Iced Brewed Black Decaffeinated Pre-Sweetened With Low Calorie Sweetener ☛ serving size: 1 fl oz (no ice) = 30 g; Calories = 1

Tea Iced Brewed Black Decaffeinated Pre-Sweetened With Sugar ☛ serving size: 1 fl oz (no ice) = 31 g; Calories = 10

Tea Iced Brewed Black Pre-Sweetened With Low Calorie Sweetener ☛ serving size: 1 fl oz (no ice) = 30 g; Calories = 1

Tea Iced Brewed Black Pre-Sweetened With Sugar ☛ serving size: 1 fl oz (no ice) = 31 g; Calories = 10

Tea Iced Brewed Green Decaffeinated Pre-Sweetened With Low Calorie Sweetener ☛ serving size: 1 fl oz (no ice) = 30 g; Calories = 0

Tea Iced Brewed Green Decaffeinated Pre-Sweetened With Sugar ☛ serving size: 1 fl oz (no ice) = 31 g; Calories = 9

Tea Iced Brewed Green Pre-Sweetened With Low Calorie Sweetener ☛ serving size: 1 fl oz (no ice) = 30 g; Calories = 1

Tea Iced Brewed Green Pre-Sweetened With Sugar ☛ serving size: 1 fl oz (no ice) = 31 g; Calories = 10

Tea Instant Decaffeinated Lemon Diet ☛ serving size: 2 tsp = 1.6 g; Calories = 5

Tea Instant Decaffeinated Lemon Sweetened ☛ serving size: 1 serving (3 heaping tsp) = 23 g; Calories = 92

Tea Instant Decaffeinated Unsweetened ☛ serving size: 1 serving 2 tsp = 0.7 g; Calories = 2

Tea Instant Lemon Diet ☛ serving size: 1 fl oz = 29.8 g; Calories = 1

Tea Instant Lemon Sweetened Powder ☛ serving size: 1 serving (3 heaping tsp) = 23 g; Calories = 92

Tea Instant Lemon Sweetened Prepared With Water ☛ serving size: 1 cup (8 fl oz) = 259 g; Calories = 91

Tea Instant Lemon Unsweetened ☛ serving size: 1 tsp, rounded = 1.4 g; Calories = 5

Tea Instant Lemon With Added Ascorbic Acid ☛ serving size: 1 serving (3 heaping tsp) = 23 g; Calories = 89

Tea Instant Sweetened With Sodium Saccharin Lemon-Flavored Powder ☛ serving size: 2 tsp = 1.6 g; Calories = 5

Tea Instant Unsweetened Powder ☛ serving size: 1 serving 1 tsp = 0.7 g; Calories = 2

Tea Instant Unsweetened Prepared With Water ☛ serving size: 1 fl oz = 29.7 g; Calories = 0

Tea Ready-To-Drink Lemon Diet ☛ serving size: 1 cup = 266 g; Calories = 5

Tequila Sunrise ☛ serving size: 1 fl oz = 31.1 g; Calories = 34

The Coca-Cola Company Dasani Water Bottled Non-Carbonated ☛ serving size: 1 fl oz = 29.6 g; Calories = 0

📖 The Coca-Cola Company Glaceau Vitamin Water Revive Fruit Punch Fortified 🖝 serving size: 20 fl oz = 591 g; Calories = 0

📖 The Coca-Cola Company Hi-C Flashin Fruit Punch 🖝 serving size: 6 (3/4) fl oz = 200 g; Calories = 90

📖 The Coca-Cola Company Nos Energy Drink Original Grape Loaded Cherry Charged Citrus Fortified With Vitamins B6 And B12 🖝 serving size: 16 fl oz = 480 g; Calories = 211

📖 The Coca-Cola Company Nos Zero Energy Drink Sugar-Free With Guarana Fortified With Vitamins B6 And B12 🖝 serving size: 16 fl oz = 480 g; Calories = 19

📖 Tonic Water 🖝 serving size: 1 fl oz = 30.5 g; Calories = 10

📖 Tropical Punch Ready-To-Drink 🖝 serving size: 1 nlea serving = 210 g; Calories = 21

📖 Unilever Slimfast Meal Replacement Regular Ready-To-Drink 3-2-1 Plan 🖝 serving size: 1 bottle = 295 g; Calories = 168

📖 Unilever Slimfast Shake Mix High Protein Whey Powder 3-2-1 Plan 🖝 serving size: 1 scoop = 26 g; Calories = 113

📖 Unilever Slimfast Shake Mix Powder 3-2-1 Plan 🖝 serving size: 1 scoop = 26 g; Calories = 117

📖 Unsweetened Almond Milk 🖝 serving size: 1 cup = 262 g; Calories = 39

📖 Unsweetened Chocolate Almond Milk 🖝 serving size: 1 cup = 240 g; Calories = 50

📖 Unsweetened Rice Milk 🖝 serving size: 8 fl oz (approximate weight, 1 serving) = 240 g; Calories = 113

📖 V8 Splash Juice Drinks Berry Blend 🖝 serving size: 1 serving 8 oz = 243 g; Calories = 71

V8 Splash Juice Drinks Diet Berry Blend ☞ serving size: 8 fl oz = 243 g; Calories = 10

V8 Splash Juice Drinks Diet Fruit Medley ☞ serving size: 1 serving 8 oz = 238 g; Calories = 10

V8 Splash Juice Drinks Diet Strawberry Kiwi ☞ serving size: 1 serving = 238 g; Calories = 10

V8 Splash Juice Drinks Diet Tropical Blend ☞ serving size: 1 serving 8 oz = 238 g; Calories = 10

V8 Splash Juice Drinks Fruit Medley ☞ serving size: 1 serving 8 oz = 243 g; Calories = 80

V8 Splash Juice Drinks Guava Passion Fruit ☞ serving size: 1 serving 8 oz = 243 g; Calories = 80

V8 Splash Juice Drinks Mango Peach ☞ serving size: 1 serving 8 oz = 243 g; Calories = 80

V8 Splash Juice Drinks Orange Pineapple ☞ serving size: 1 serving 8 oz = 243 g; Calories = 71

V8 Splash Juice Drinks Orchard Blend ☞ serving size: 1 serving 8 oz = 243 g; Calories = 80

V8 Splash Juice Drinks Strawberry Banana ☞ serving size: 1 serving 8 oz = 243 g; Calories = 71

V8 Splash Juice Drinks Strawberry Kiwi ☞ serving size: 1 serving 8 oz = 243 g; Calories = 71

V8 Splash Juice Drinks Tropical Blend ☞ serving size: 1 serving 8 oz = 243 g; Calories = 71

V8 Splash Smoothies Peach Mango ☞ serving size: 1 serving 8 oz = 245 g; Calories = 91

V8 Splash Smoothies Strawberry Banana ☞ serving size: 1 serving 8 oz = 245 g; Calories = 91

V8 Splash Smoothies Tropical Colada ☛ serving size: 1 serving 8 oz = 246 g; Calories = 101

V8 V- Fusion Juices Acai Berry ☛ serving size: 1 serving 8 oz = 246 g; Calories = 111

V8 V-Fusion Juices Peach Mango ☛ serving size: 1 serving 8 oz = 246 g; Calories = 121

V8 V-Fusion Juices Strawberry Banana ☛ serving size: 1 serving 8 oz = 246 g; Calories = 121

V8 V-Fusion Juices Tropical ☛ serving size: 1 serving 8 oz = 246 g; Calories = 121

Vegetable And Fruit Juice Blend 100% Juice With Added Vitamins A C E ☛ serving size: 1 serving 8 oz = 246 g; Calories = 113

Vegetable And Fruit Juice Drink Reduced Calorie With Low-Calorie Sweetener Added Vitamin C ☛ serving size: 1 serving = 238 g; Calories = 10

Vitamin Fortified Water ☛ serving size: 8 fl oz = 240 g; Calories = 12

Vodka ☛ serving size: 1 fl oz = 27.8 g; Calories = 64

Vodka And Cola ☛ serving size: 1 fl oz = 30 g; Calories = 27

Vodka And Diet Cola ☛ serving size: 1 fl oz = 30 g; Calories = 18

Vodka And Energy Drink ☛ serving size: 1 fl oz = 30 g; Calories = 27

Vodka And Lemonade ☛ serving size: 1 fl oz = 30 g; Calories = 28

Vodka And Soda ☛ serving size: 1 fl oz = 30 g; Calories = 18

Vodka And Tonic ☛ serving size: 1 fl oz = 30 g; Calories = 25

Vodka And Water ☛ serving size: 1 fl oz = 30 g; Calories = 18

Water Bottled Non-Carbonated Calistoga ☞ serving size: 1 fl oz = 29.6 g; Calories = 0

Water Bottled Non-Carbonated Crystal Geyser ☞ serving size: 1 fl oz = 29.6 g; Calories = 0

Water Bottled Non-Carbonated Dannon ☞ serving size: 1 fl oz = 29.6 g; Calories = 0

Water Bottled Non-Carbonated Dannon Fluoride To Go ☞ serving size: 1 fl oz = 29.6 g; Calories = 0

Water Bottled Non-Carbonated Evian ☞ serving size: 1 fl oz = 29.6 g; Calories = 0

Water Bottled Non-Carbonated Naya ☞ serving size: 1 fl oz = 29.6 g; Calories = 0

Water Bottled Non-Carbonated Pepsi Aquafina ☞ serving size: 1 fl oz = 29.6 g; Calories = 0

Water Bottled Perrier ☞ serving size: 1 fl oz = 29.6 g; Calories = 0

Water Bottled Poland Spring ☞ serving size: 1 fl oz = 29.6 g; Calories = 0

Water Non-Carbonated Bottles Natural Fruit Flavors Sweetened With Low Calorie Sweetener ☞ serving size: 1 fl oz = 29.6 g; Calories = 0

Water Tap Municipal ☞ serving size: 1 fl oz = 29.6 g; Calories = 0

Water With Added Vitamins And Minerals Bottles Sweetened Assorted Fruit Flavors ☞ serving size: 8 fl oz (1 nlea serving) = 237 g; Calories = 52

Water With Corn Syrup And/or Sugar And Low Calorie Sweetener Fruit Flavored ☞ serving size: 1 pouch = 200 g; Calories = 36

Well Water ☞ serving size: 1 fl oz = 29.6 g; Calories = 0

Wendys Tea Ready-To-Drink Unsweetened ☛ serving size: 1 fl oz = 29.6 g; Calories = 0

Whey Protein Powder Isolate ☛ serving size: 3 scoop = 86 g; Calories = 309

Whiskey ☛ serving size: 1 fl oz = 27.8 g; Calories = 70

Whiskey And Cola ☛ serving size: 1 fl oz = 30 g; Calories = 27

Whiskey And Diet Cola ☛ serving size: 1 fl oz = 30 g; Calories = 18

Whiskey And Ginger Ale ☛ serving size: 1 fl oz = 30 g; Calories = 25

Whiskey And Water ☛ serving size: 1 fl oz = 30 g; Calories = 18

Whiskey Sour Mix ☛ serving size: 1 packet = 17 g; Calories = 65

Whiskey Sour Mix Bottled ☛ serving size: 1 fl oz = 32.3 g; Calories = 28

Whiskey Sour Mix Bottled With Added Potassium And Sodium ☛ serving size: 1 fl oz = 32.3 g; Calories = 27

White Wine ☛ serving size: 1 fl oz = 29.4 g; Calories = 24

Wine Non-Alcoholic ☛ serving size: 1 fl oz = 29 g; Calories = 2

Yellow Green Colored Citrus Soft Drink With Caffeine ☛ serving size: 16 fl oz = 473 g; Calories = 232

Zevia Cola ☛ serving size: 1 can = 355 g; Calories = 0

Zevia Cola Caffeine Free ☛ serving size: 1 can = 355 g; Calories = 0

Zinfandel ☛ serving size: 1 fl oz = 29.4 g; Calories = 26

11

BREAKFAST CEREALS

🥣 Alpen ☞ serving size: 2/3 cup (1 nlea serving) = 55 g; Calories = 194

🥣 Barbaras Puffins Original ☞ serving size: 3/4 cup (1 nlea serving) = 27 g; Calories = 90

🥣 Cereal (General Mills 25% Less Sugar Cocoa Puffs) ☞ serving size: 1 cup = 32 g; Calories = 122

🥣 Cereal (General Mills 25% Less Sugar Trix) ☞ serving size: 1 cup = 30 g; Calories = 115

🥣 Cereal (General Mills Basic 4) ☞ serving size: 1 cup = 55 g; Calories = 197

🥣 Cereal (General Mills Boo Berry) ☞ serving size: 1 cup = 33 g; Calories = 127

🥣 Cereal (General Mills Cheerios Apple Cinnamon) ☞ serving size: 1 cup = 40 g; Calories = 154

🥣 Cereal (General Mills Cheerios Banana Nut) ☞ serving size: 1 cup = 37 g; Calories = 139

🥣 Cereal (General Mills Cheerios Berry Burst) ☛ serving size: 1 cup = 36 g; Calories = 136

🥣 Cereal (General Mills Cheerios Chocolate) ☛ serving size: 1 cup = 36 g; Calories = 137

🥣 Cereal (General Mills Cheerios Frosted) ☛ serving size: 1 cup = 37 g; Calories = 139

🥣 Cereal (General Mills Cheerios Fruity) ☛ serving size: 1 cup = 36 g; Calories = 137

🥣 Cereal (General Mills Cheerios Honey Nut) ☛ serving size: 1 cup = 37 g; Calories = 139

🥣 Cereal (General Mills Cheerios Multigrain) ☛ serving size: 1 cup = 30 g; Calories = 111

🥣 Cereal (General Mills Cheerios Oat Cluster Crunch) ☛ serving size: 1 cup = 36 g; Calories = 136

🥣 Cereal (General Mills Cheerios Protein) ☛ serving size: 1 cup = 28 g; Calories = 106

🥣 Cereal (General Mills Cheerios Yogurt Burst) ☛ serving size: 1 cup = 40 g; Calories = 160

🥣 Cereal (General Mills Cheerios) ☛ serving size: 10 cheerios = 1 g; Calories = 4

🥣 Cereal (General Mills Chex Chocolate) ☛ serving size: 1 cup = 43 g; Calories = 177

🥣 Cereal (General Mills Chex Cinnamon) ☛ serving size: 1 cup = 39 g; Calories = 157

🥣 Cereal (General Mills Chex Corn) ☛ serving size: 1 piece = 0 g; Calories = 0

🥣 Cereal (General Mills Chex Honey Nut) ☛ serving size: 1 piece = 0 g; Calories = 0

Cereal (General Mills Chex Rice) ☛ serving size: 1 cup = 27 g; Calories = 101

Cereal (General Mills Cinnamon Toast Crunch) ☛ serving size: 1 cup = 40 g; Calories = 164

Cereal (General Mills Cocoa Puffs) ☛ serving size: 1 cup = 36 g; Calories = 138

Cereal (General Mills Cookie Crisp) ☛ serving size: 1 cup = 35 g; Calories = 133

Cereal (General Mills Count Chocula) ☛ serving size: 1 cup = 36 g; Calories = 138

Cereal (General Mills Frankenberry) ☛ serving size: 1 cup = 33 g; Calories = 127

Cereal (General Mills Golden Grahams) ☛ serving size: 1 cup = 40 g; Calories = 150

Cereal (General Mills Honey Nut Clusters) ☛ serving size: 1 cup = 55 g; Calories = 206

Cereal (General Mills Kix Berry Berry) ☛ serving size: 1 cup = 33 g; Calories = 124

Cereal (General Mills Lucky Charms Chocolate) ☛ serving size: 1 cup = 37 g; Calories = 141

Cereal (General Mills Lucky Charms) ☛ serving size: 1 cup = 36 g; Calories = 137

Cereal (General Mills Oatmeal Crisp With Almonds) ☛ serving size: 1 cup = 60 g; Calories = 234

Cereal (General Mills Oatmeal Crisp With Raisins) ☛ serving size: 1 cup = 62 g; Calories = 231

Cereal (General Mills Reese's Puffs) ☛ serving size: 1 cup = 40 g; Calories = 165

 Cereal (General Mills Trix) serving size: 1 cup = 32 g; Calories = 123

 Cereal (Kashi Heart To Heart Oat Flakes And Blueberry Clusters) serving size: 1 cup = 55 g; Calories = 207

 Cereal (Kellogg's Cinnabon) serving size: 1 cup = 30 g; Calories = 123

 Cereal (Kellogg's Cocoa Krispies) serving size: 1 cup = 41 g; Calories = 160

 Cereal (Kellogg's Corn Flakes) serving size: 1 cup = 28 g; Calories = 100

 Cereal (Kellogg's Corn Pops) serving size: 1 cup = 29 g; Calories = 112

 Cereal (Kellogg's Crispix) serving size: 1 cup = 29 g; Calories = 110

 Cereal (Kellogg's Froot Loops Marshmallow) serving size: 1 cup = 29 g; Calories = 109

 Cereal (Kellogg's Frosted Flakes Reduced Sugar) serving size: 1 cup = 31 g; Calories = 111

 Cereal (Kellogg's Frosted Flakes) serving size: 1 cup = 41 g; Calories = 151

 Cereal (Kellogg's Frosted Krispies) serving size: 1 cup = 40 g; Calories = 154

 Cereal (Kellogg's Honey Crunch Corn Flakes) serving size: 1 cup = 40 g; Calories = 154

 Cereal (Kellogg's Honey Smacks) serving size: 1 cup = 36 g; Calories = 137

 Cereal (Kellogg's Low Fat Granola With Raisins) serving size: 1 cup = 90 g; Calories = 343

Cereal (Kellogg's Low Fat Granola) ☞ serving size: 1 cup = 98 g; Calories = 381

Cereal (Kellogg's Product 19) ☞ serving size: 1 cup = 30 g; Calories = 112

Cereal (Kellogg's Rice Krispies Treats Cereal) ☞ serving size: 1 cup = 40 g; Calories = 158

Cereal (Kellogg's Rice Krispies) ☞ serving size: 1 cup = 26 g; Calories = 99

Cereal (Kellogg's Smart Start Strong) ☞ serving size: 1 cup = 50 g; Calories = 186

Cereal (Kellogg's Special K Blueberry) ☞ serving size: 1 cup = 40 g; Calories = 145

Cereal (Kellogg's Special K Low Fat Granola) ☞ serving size: 1 cup = 104 g; Calories = 405

Cereal (Kellogg's Special K) ☞ serving size: 1 cup = 31 g; Calories = 117

Cereal (Malt-O-Meal Blueberry Muffin Tops) ☞ serving size: 1 cup = 40 g; Calories = 150

Cereal (Malt-O-Meal Crispy Rice) ☞ serving size: 1 cup = 28 g; Calories = 107

Cereal (Malt-O-Meal Golden Puffs) ☞ serving size: 1 cup = 32 g; Calories = 122

Cereal (Malt-O-Meal Honey Graham Squares) ☞ serving size: 1 cup = 40 g; Calories = 150

Cereal (Malt-O-Meal Honey Nut Toasty O's) ☞ serving size: 1 cup = 38 g; Calories = 143

Cereal (Malt-O-Meal Toasted Oat Cereal) ☞ serving size: 1 cup = 22 g; Calories = 83

🥣 Cereal (Nature Valley Granola) ☛ serving size: 1 cup = 82 g; Calories = 312

🥣 Cereal Cooked Nfs ☛ serving size: 1 cup, cooked = 240 g; Calories = 154

🥣 Cereal Corn Flakes ☛ serving size: 1 cup = 25 g; Calories = 89

🥣 Cereal Crispy Brown Rice ☛ serving size: 1 cup = 32 g; Calories = 126

🥣 Cereal Frosted Corn Flakes ☛ serving size: 1 cup = 40 g; Calories = 148

🥣 Cereal Frosted Rice ☛ serving size: 1 cup = 45 g; Calories = 173

🥣 Cereal Granola ☛ serving size: 1 cup = 111 g; Calories = 423

🥣 Cereal Muesli ☛ serving size: 1 cup = 85 g; Calories = 302

🥣 Cereal Oat Nfs ☛ serving size: 1 cup, nfs = 33 g; Calories = 124

🥣 Cereal Puffed Wheat Sweetened ☛ serving size: 1 cup = 38 g; Calories = 144

🥣 Cereal Ready-To-Eat Nfs ☛ serving size: 1 cup = 40 g; Calories = 150

🥣 Cereal Rice Flakes ☛ serving size: 1 cup = 27 g; Calories = 106

🥣 Chocolate-Flavored Frosted Puffed Corn ☛ serving size: 1 cup = 30 g; Calories = 122

🥣 Corn Grits White Regular And Quick Enriched Cooked With Water With Salt ☛ serving size: 1 cup = 257 g; Calories = 183

🥣 Corn Grits White Regular And Quick Enriched Dry ☛ serving size: 1 tbsp = 9.7 g; Calories = 36

🥣 Corn Grits Yellow Regular And Quick Unenriched Dry ☛ serving size: 1 tbsp = 9.7 g; Calories = 36

Corn Grits Yellow Regular Quick Enriched Cooked With Water With Salt ☛ serving size: 1 cup = 233 g; Calories = 152

Cornmeal Mush Fat Added In Cooking ☛ serving size: 1 cup, cooked = 240 g; Calories = 168

Cornmeal Mush Fat Not Added In Cooking ☛ serving size: 1 cup, cooked = 240 g; Calories = 139

Cornmeal Mush Ns As To Fat Added In Cooking ☛ serving size: 1 cup, cooked = 240 g; Calories = 168

Cornmeal Puerto Rican Style ☛ serving size: 1 cup, cooked = 240 g; Calories = 355

Cream Of Rice Cooked With Water With Salt ☛ serving size: 1 cup = 244 g; Calories = 127

Cream Of Rice Dry ☛ serving size: 1/4 cup (1 nlea serving) = 45 g; Calories = 167

Cream Of Rye ☛ serving size: 1 cup, cooked = 240 g; Calories = 98

Cream Of Wheat 1 Minute Cook Time Cooked With Water Microwaved Without Salt ☛ serving size: 1 cup = 237 g; Calories = 130

Cream Of Wheat 1 Minute Cook Time Cooked With Water Stove-Top Without Salt ☛ serving size: 1 cup = 245 g; Calories = 137

Cream Of Wheat 1 Minute Cook Time Dry ☛ serving size: 3 tablespoon (1 serving) = 33 g; Calories = 119

Cream Of Wheat 2 1/2 Minute Cook Time Cooked With Water Microwaved Without Salt ☛ serving size: 1 cup = 231 g; Calories = 120

Cream Of Wheat 2 1/2 Minute Cook Time Cooked With Water Stove-Top Without Salt ☛ serving size: 1 cup = 244 g; Calories = 137

Cream Of Wheat 2 1/2 Minute Cook Time Dry ☛ serving size: 3 tablespoon (1 nlea serving) = 33 g; Calories = 117

Cream Of Wheat Instant Dry ☛ serving size: 1 tbsp = 11.5 g; Calories = 42

Cream Of Wheat Instant Made With Milk Fat Added In Cooking ☛ serving size: 1 cup, cooked = 240 g; Calories = 290

Cream Of Wheat Instant Made With Milk Fat Not Added In Cooking ☛ serving size: 1 cup, cooked = 240 g; Calories = 259

Cream Of Wheat Instant Made With Milk Ns As To Fat Added In Cooking ☛ serving size: 1 cup, cooked = 240 g; Calories = 290

Cream Of Wheat Instant Made With Non-Dairy Milk Fat Added In Cooking ☛ serving size: 1 cup, cooked = 240 g; Calories = 254

Cream Of Wheat Instant Made With Non-Dairy Milk Fat Not Added In Cooking ☛ serving size: 1 cup, cooked = 240 g; Calories = 221

Cream Of Wheat Instant Made With Non-Dairy Milk Ns As To Fat Added In Cooking ☛ serving size: 1 cup, cooked = 240 g; Calories = 254

Cream Of Wheat Instant Made With Water Fat Added In Cooking ☛ serving size: 1 cup, cooked = 240 g; Calories = 194

Cream Of Wheat Instant Made With Water Fat Not Added In Cooking ☛ serving size: 1 cup, cooked = 240 g; Calories = 158

Cream Of Wheat Instant Made With Water Ns As To Fat Added In Cooking ☛ serving size: 1 cup, cooked = 240 g; Calories = 194

Cream Of Wheat Instant Prepared With Water Without Salt ☛ serving size: 1 cup = 241 g; Calories = 149

Cream Of Wheat Ns As To Regular Quick Or Instant Fat Added In Cooking ☛ serving size: 1 cup, cooked = 240 g; Calories = 154

Cream Of Wheat Ns As To Regular Quick Or Instant Fat Not Added In Cooking ☛ serving size: 1 cup, cooked = 240 g; Calories = 122

Cream Of Wheat Ns As To Regular Quick Or Instant Ns As To Fat Added In Cooking ☞ serving size: 1 cup, cooked = 240 g; Calories = 154

Cream Of Wheat Regular (10 Minute) Cooked With Water With Salt ☞ serving size: 1 cup (1 serving) = 251 g; Calories = 126

Cream Of Wheat Regular (10 Minute) Cooked With Water Without Salt ☞ serving size: 1 cup (1 serving) = 251 g; Calories = 126

Cream Of Wheat Regular 10 Minute Cooking Dry ☞ serving size: 1 tbsp = 10.6 g; Calories = 39

Cream Of Wheat Regular Or Quick Made With Milk Fat Added In Cooking ☞ serving size: 1 cup, cooked = 240 g; Calories = 276

Cream Of Wheat Regular Or Quick Made With Milk Fat Not Added In Cooking ☞ serving size: 1 cup, cooked = 240 g; Calories = 250

Cream Of Wheat Regular Or Quick Made With Milk Ns As To Fat Added In Cooking ☞ serving size: 1 cup, cooked = 240 g; Calories = 276

Cream Of Wheat Regular Or Quick Made With Non-Dairy Milk Fat Added In Cooking ☞ serving size: 1 cup, cooked = 240 g; Calories = 230

Cream Of Wheat Regular Or Quick Made With Non-Dairy Milk Fat Not Added In Cooking ☞ serving size: 1 cup, cooked = 240 g; Calories = 202

Cream Of Wheat Regular Or Quick Made With Non-Dairy Milk Ns As To Fat Added In Cooking ☞ serving size: 1 cup, cooked = 240 g; Calories = 230

Cream Of Wheat Regular Or Quick Made With Water Fat Added In Cooking ☞ serving size: 1 cup, cooked = 240 g; Calories = 154

Cream Of Wheat Regular Or Quick Made With Water Fat Not

Added In Cooking ☞ serving size: 1 cup, cooked = 240 g; Calories = 122

🥣 Cream Of Wheat Regular Or Quick Made With Water Ns As To Fat Added In Cooking ☞ serving size: 1 cup, cooked = 240 g; Calories = 154

🥣 Familia ☞ serving size: 1 cup = 122 g; Calories = 473

🥣 Farina Enriched Assorted Brands Including Cream Of Wheat Quick (1-3 Minutes) Cooked With Wat ☞ serving size: 1 cup = 240 g; Calories = 132

🥣 Farina Enriched Assorted Brands Including Cream Of Wheat Quick (1-3 Minutes) Dry ☞ serving size: 1 tbsp = 11 g; Calories = 40

🥣 Farina Enriched Cooked With Water With Salt ☞ serving size: 1 cup = 233 g; Calories = 124

🥣 Farina Unenriched Dry ☞ serving size: 1 tbsp = 10.9 g; Calories = 40

🥣 Frosted Oat Cereal With Marshmallows ☞ serving size: 3/4 cup (1 nlea serving) = 30 g; Calories = 120

🥣 General Mills Cheerios ☞ serving size: 1 cup (1 nlea serving) = 28 g; Calories = 104

🥣 Granola Homemade ☞ serving size: 1 cup = 122 g; Calories = 597

🥣 Grits Instant Made With Milk Fat Added In Cooking ☞ serving size: 1 cup, cooked = 240 g; Calories = 298

🥣 Grits Instant Made With Milk Fat Not Added In Cooking ☞ serving size: 1 cup, cooked = 240 g; Calories = 254

🥣 Grits Instant Made With Milk Ns As To Fat Added In Cooking ☞ serving size: 1 cup, cooked = 240 g; Calories = 298

🥣 Grits Instant Made With Non-Dairy Milk Fat Added In Cooking ☞ serving size: 1 cup, cooked = 240 g; Calories = 262

Grits Instant Made With Non-Dairy Milk Ns As To Fat Added In Cooking ☛ serving size: 1 cup, cooked = 240 g; Calories = 262

Grits Instant Made With Water Fat Added In Cooking ☛ serving size: 1 cup, cooked = 240 g; Calories = 202

Grits Instant Made With Water Fat Not Added In Cooking ☛ serving size: 1 cup, cooked = 240 g; Calories = 156

Grits Instant Made With Water Ns As To Fat Added In Cooking ☛ serving size: 1 cup, cooked = 240 g; Calories = 202

Grits Ns As To Regular Quick Or Instant Fat Added In Cooking ☛ serving size: 1 cup, cooked = 240 g; Calories = 168

Grits Ns As To Regular Quick Or Instant Fat Not Added In Cooking ☛ serving size: 1 cup, cooked = 240 g; Calories = 139

Grits Ns As To Regular Quick Or Instant Ns As To Fat Added In Cooking ☛ serving size: 1 cup, cooked = 240 g; Calories = 168

Grits Regular Or Quick Made With Milk Fat Added In Cooking ☛ serving size: 1 cup, cooked = 240 g; Calories = 290

Grits Regular Or Quick Made With Milk Fat Not Added In Cooking ☛ serving size: 1 cup, cooked = 240 g; Calories = 264

Grits Regular Or Quick Made With Milk Ns As To Fat Added In Cooking ☛ serving size: 1 cup, cooked = 240 g; Calories = 290

Grits Regular Or Quick Made With Non-Dairy Milk Fat Added In Cooking ☛ serving size: 1 cup, cooked = 240 g; Calories = 245

Grits Regular Or Quick Made With Non-Dairy Milk Fat Not Added In Cooking ☛ serving size: 1 cup, cooked = 240 g; Calories = 216

Grits Regular Or Quick Made With Non-Dairy Milk Ns As To Fat Added In Cooking ☛ serving size: 1 cup, cooked = 240 g; Calories = 245

 Grits Regular Or Quick Made With Water Fat Added In Cooking ☞ serving size: 1 cup, cooked = 240 g; Calories = 168

 Grits Regular Or Quick Made With Water Fat Not Added In Cooking ☞ serving size: 1 cup, cooked = 240 g; Calories = 139

 Grits Regular Or Quick Made With Water Ns As To Fat Added In Cooking ☞ serving size: 1 cup, cooked = 240 g; Calories = 168

 Grits With Cheese Fat Added In Cooking ☞ serving size: 1 cup, cooked = 240 g; Calories = 257

 Grits With Cheese Fat Not Added In Cooking ☞ serving size: 1 cup, cooked = 240 g; Calories = 230

 Grits With Cheese Ns As To Fat Added In Cooking ☞ serving size: 1 cup, cooked = 240 g; Calories = 257

 Health Valley Fiber 7 Flakes ☞ serving size: 3/4 cup (1 nlea serving) = 31 g; Calories = 109

 Hominy Cooked Fat Added In Cooking ☞ serving size: 1 cup = 170 g; Calories = 148

 Hominy Cooked Fat Not Added In Cooking ☞ serving size: 1 cup = 165 g; Calories = 119

 Hominy Cooked Ns As To Fat Added In Cooking ☞ serving size: 1 cup = 170 g; Calories = 148

 Incaparina Dry Mix (Corn And Soy Flours) Unprepared ☞ serving size: 1 tbsp = 8.9 g; Calories = 34

 Instant Grits (Made with Vegetable Fat) ☞ serving size: 1 cup, cooked = 240 g; Calories = 218

 Malt-O-Meal Apple Zings ☞ serving size: 1 cup (1 nlea serving) = 33 g; Calories = 129

 Malt-O-Meal Berry Colossal Crunch ☞ serving size: 3/4 cup (1 nlea serving) = 30 g; Calories = 119

🥣 Malt-O-Meal Blueberry Mini Spooners ☛ serving size: 1 cup (1 nlea serving) = 55 g; Calories = 193

🥣 Malt-O-Meal Blueberry Muffin Tops Cereal ☛ serving size: 3/4 cup (1 nlea serving) = 30 g; Calories = 133

🥣 Malt-O-Meal Chocolate Dry ☛ serving size: 3 tbsp (1 nlea serving) = 35 g; Calories = 127

🥣 Malt-O-Meal Chocolate Marshmallow Mateys ☛ serving size: 3/4 cup (1 nlea serving) = 30 g; Calories = 118

🥣 Malt-O-Meal Chocolate Prepared With Water Without Salt ☛ serving size: 1 serving (3 t dry cereal plus 1 cup water) = 268 g; Calories = 126

🥣 Malt-O-Meal Cinnamon Toasters ☛ serving size: 3/4 cup (1 nlea serving) = 30 g; Calories = 128

🥣 Malt-O-Meal Coco-Roos ☛ serving size: 3/4 cup (1 nlea serving) = 30 g; Calories = 117

🥣 Malt-O-Meal Cocoa Dyno-Bites ☛ serving size: 3/4 cup (1 nlea serving) = 29 g; Calories = 115

🥣 Malt-O-Meal Colossal Crunch ☛ serving size: 3/4 cup (1 nlea serving) = 30 g; Calories = 120

🥣 Malt-O-Meal Corn Bursts ☛ serving size: 1 cup (1 nlea serving) = 31 g; Calories = 119

🥣 Malt-O-Meal Crispy Rice ☛ serving size: 1 (1/4) cup (1 nlea serving) = 33 g; Calories = 114

🥣 Malt-O-Meal Farina Hot Wheat Cereal Dry ☛ serving size: 3 tbsp (1 nlea serving) = 35 g; Calories = 128

🥣 Malt-O-Meal Frosted Flakes ☛ serving size: 3/4 cup (1 nlea serving) = 31 g; Calories = 121

🥣 Malt-O-Meal Frosted Mini Spooners ☛ serving size: 1 cup (1 nlea serving) = 55 g; Calories = 195

🥣 Malt-O-Meal Fruity Dyno-Bites ☛ serving size: 3/4 cup = 27 g; Calories = 109

🥣 Malt-O-Meal Golden Puffs ☛ serving size: 3/4 cup (1 nlea serving) = 27 g; Calories = 100

🥣 Malt-O-Meal Honey Buzzers ☛ serving size: 1 (1/3) cup = 29 g; Calories = 110

🥣 Malt-O-Meal Honey Graham Squares ☛ serving size: 3/4 cup (1 nlea serving) = 30 g; Calories = 119

🥣 Malt-O-Meal Honey Nut Scooters ☛ serving size: 1 cup (1 nlea serving) = 30 g; Calories = 116

🥣 Malt-O-Meal Maple & Brown Sugar Hot Wheat Cereal Dry ☛ serving size: 1/4 cup (1 nlea serving) = 45 g; Calories = 166

🥣 Malt-O-Meal Marshmallow Mateys ☛ serving size: 1 cup = 30 g; Calories = 116

🥣 Malt-O-Meal Oat Blenders With Honey ☛ serving size: 3/4 cup (1 nlea serving) = 30 g; Calories = 119

🥣 Malt-O-Meal Oat Blenders With Honey & Almonds ☛ serving size: 3/4 cup (1 nlea serving) = 30 g; Calories = 114

🥣 Malt-O-Meal Original Plain Dry ☛ serving size: 3 tbsp (1 nlea serving) = 35 g; Calories = 128

🥣 Malt-O-Meal Original Plain Prepared With Water Without Salt ☛ serving size: 1 serving (3 t dry cereal plus 1 cup water) = 268 g; Calories = 129

🥣 Malt-O-Meal Raisin Bran Cereal ☛ serving size: 1 cup (1 nlea serving) = 59 g; Calories = 202

🥣 Malt-O-Meal Tootie Fruities ☛ serving size: 1 cup (1 nlea serving) = 32 g; Calories = 125

◡ Masa Harina Cooked ☛ serving size: 1 cup, cooked = 240 g; Calories = 233

◡ Millet Puffed ☛ serving size: 1 cup = 21 g; Calories = 74

◡ Moms Best Honey Nut Toasty Os ☛ serving size: 1 cup (1 nlea serving) = 30 g; Calories = 116

◡ Moms Best Sweetened Wheat-Fuls ☛ serving size: 1 cup (1 nlea serving) = 55 g; Calories = 205

◡ Natures Path Organic Flax Plus Flakes ☛ serving size: 3/4 cup (1 nlea serving) = 30 g; Calories = 105

◡ Natures Path Organic Flax Plus Pumpkin Granola ☛ serving size: 3/4 cup (1 nlea serving) = 55 g; Calories = 257

◡ Oat Bran Flakes Health Valley ☛ serving size: 1 cup (1 nlea serving) = 50 g; Calories = 190

◡ Oatmeal Instant Plain Made With Milk Fat Added In Cooking ☛ serving size: 1 cup, cooked = 240 g; Calories = 305

◡ Oatmeal From Fast Food Fruit Flavored ☛ serving size: 1 cup, cooked = 240 g; Calories = 293

◡ Oatmeal From Fast Food Maple Flavored ☛ serving size: 1 cup, cooked = 240 g; Calories = 262

◡ Oatmeal From Fast Food Other Flavors ☛ serving size: 1 cup, cooked = 240 g; Calories = 262

◡ Oatmeal From Fast Food Plain ☛ serving size: 1 cup, cooked = 240 g; Calories = 190

◡ Oatmeal Instant Fruit Flavored Fat Added In Cooking ☛ serving size: 1 cup, cooked = 240 g; Calories = 269

◡ Oatmeal Instant Fruit Flavored Fat Not Added In Cooking ☛ serving size: 1 cup, cooked = 240 g; Calories = 230

Oatmeal Instant Fruit Flavored Ns As To Fat Added In Cooking ☞ serving size: 1 cup, cooked = 240 g; Calories = 269

Oatmeal Instant Maple Flavored Fat Added In Cooking ☞ serving size: 1 cup, cooked = 240 g; Calories = 271

Oatmeal Instant Maple Flavored Fat Not Added In Cooking ☞ serving size: 1 cup, cooked = 240 g; Calories = 233

Oatmeal Instant Maple Flavored Ns As To Fat Added In Cooking ☞ serving size: 1 cup, cooked = 240 g; Calories = 271

Oatmeal Instant Other Flavors Fat Added In Cooking ☞ serving size: 1 cup, cooked = 240 g; Calories = 271

Oatmeal Instant Other Flavors Fat Not Added In Cooking ☞ serving size: 1 cup, cooked = 240 g; Calories = 233

Oatmeal Instant Other Flavors Ns As To Fat Added In Cooking ☞ serving size: 1 cup, cooked = 240 g; Calories = 271

Oatmeal Instant Plain Made With Milk Fat Not Added In Cooking ☞ serving size: 1 cup, cooked = 240 g; Calories = 264

Oatmeal Instant Plain Made With Milk Ns As To Fat Added In Cooking ☞ serving size: 1 cup, cooked = 240 g; Calories = 305

Oatmeal Instant Plain Made With Non-Dairy Milk Fat Added In Cooking ☞ serving size: 1 cup, cooked = 240 g; Calories = 269

Oatmeal Instant Plain Made With Non-Dairy Milk Fat Not Added In Cooking ☞ serving size: 1 cup, cooked = 240 g; Calories = 226

Oatmeal Instant Plain Made With Non-Dairy Milk Ns As To Fat Added In Cooking ☞ serving size: 1 cup, cooked = 240 g; Calories = 269

Oatmeal Instant Plain Made With Water Fat Added In Cooking ☞ serving size: 1 cup, cooked = 240 g; Calories = 209

Oatmeal Instant Plain Made With Water Fat Not Added In Cooking ☞ serving size: 1 cup, cooked = 240 g; Calories = 163

Oatmeal Instant Plain Made With Water Ns As To Fat Added In Cooking ☞ serving size: 1 cup, cooked = 240 g; Calories = 209

Oatmeal Made With Milk And Sugar Puerto Rican Style ☞ serving size: 1 cup, cooked = 240 g; Calories = 348

Oatmeal Multigrain Fat Added In Cooking ☞ serving size: 1 cup, cooked = 240 g; Calories = 163

Oatmeal Multigrain Fat Not Added In Cooking ☞ serving size: 1 cup, cooked = 240 g; Calories = 134

Oatmeal Multigrain Ns As To Fat Added In Cooking ☞ serving size: 1 cup, cooked = 240 g; Calories = 163

Oatmeal Ns As To Regular Quick Or Instant Fat Added In Cooking ☞ serving size: 1 cup, cooked = 240 g; Calories = 182

Oatmeal Ns As To Regular Quick Or Instant Fat Not Added In Cooking ☞ serving size: 1 cup, cooked = 240 g; Calories = 154

Oatmeal Ns As To Regular Quick Or Instant Ns As To Fat Added In Cooking ☞ serving size: 1 cup, cooked = 240 g; Calories = 182

Oatmeal Reduced Sugar Flavored Fat Added In Cooking ☞ serving size: 1 cup, cooked = 240 g; Calories = 240

Oatmeal Reduced Sugar Flavored Fat Not Added In Cooking ☞ serving size: 1 cup, cooked = 240 g; Calories = 199

Oatmeal Reduced Sugar Flavored Ns As To Fat Added In Cooking ☞ serving size: 1 cup, cooked = 240 g; Calories = 240

Oatmeal Reduced Sugar Plain Fat Added In Cooking ☞ serving size: 1 cup, cooked = 240 g; Calories = 240

Oatmeal Reduced Sugar Plain Fat Not Added In Cooking ☞ serving size: 1 cup, cooked = 240 g; Calories = 199

🥣 Oatmeal Reduced Sugar Plain Ns As To Fat Added In Cooking ☞ serving size: 1 cup, cooked = 240 g; Calories = 240

🥣 Oatmeal Regular Or Quick Made With Milk Fat Added In Cooking ☞ serving size: 1 cup, cooked = 240 g; Calories = 302

🥣 Oatmeal Regular Or Quick Made With Milk Fat Not Added In Cooking ☞ serving size: 1 cup, cooked = 240 g; Calories = 276

🥣 Oatmeal Regular Or Quick Made With Milk Ns As To Fat Added In Cooking ☞ serving size: 1 cup, cooked = 240 g; Calories = 302

🥣 Oatmeal Regular Or Quick Made With Non-Dairy Milk Fat Added In Cooking ☞ serving size: 1 cup, cooked = 240 g; Calories = 257

🥣 Oatmeal Regular Or Quick Made With Non-Dairy Milk Fat Not Added In Cooking ☞ serving size: 1 cup, cooked = 240 g; Calories = 230

🥣 Oatmeal Regular Or Quick Made With Non-Dairy Milk Ns As To Fat Added In Cooking ☞ serving size: 1 cup, cooked = 240 g; Calories = 257

🥣 Oatmeal Regular Or Quick Made With Water Fat Added In Cooking ☞ serving size: 1 cup, cooked = 240 g; Calories = 182

🥣 Oatmeal Regular Or Quick Made With Water Fat Not Added In Cooking ☞ serving size: 1 cup, cooked = 240 g; Calories = 154

🥣 Oatmeal Regular Or Quick Made With Water Ns As To Fat Added In Cooking ☞ serving size: 1 cup, cooked = 240 g; Calories = 182

🥣 Oats Instant Fortified Maple And Brown Sugar Dry ☞ serving size: 1 packet = 43 g; Calories = 166

🥣 Oats Instant Fortified Plain Dry ☞ serving size: 1 packet = 28 g; Calories = 101

🥣 Oats Instant Fortified Plain Prepared With Water (Boiling Water Added Or Microwaved) ☞ serving size: 1 cup, cooked = 234 g; Calories = 159

🥣 Oats Instant Fortified With Cinnamon And Spice Dry ☛ serving size: 1 packet = 45 g; Calories = 166

🥣 Oats Instant Fortified With Cinnamon And Spice Prepared With Water ☛ serving size: 1 cup = 240 g; Calories = 230

🥣 Oats Instant Fortified With Raisins And Spice Prepared With Water ☛ serving size: 1 cup = 240 g; Calories = 211

🥣 Oats Regular And Quick And Instant Unenriched Cooked With Water (Includes Boiling And Microw ☛ serving size: 1 cup = 234 g; Calories = 166

🥣 Oats Regular And Quick Not Fortified Dry ☛ serving size: 1 cup = 81 g; Calories = 307

🥣 Post Alpha-Bits ☛ serving size: 1 cup (1 nlea serving for adults) = 30 g; Calories = 117

🥣 Post Bran Flakes ☛ serving size: 3/4 cup (1 nlea serving) = 30 g; Calories = 98

🥣 Post Cocoa Pebbles ☛ serving size: 3/4 cup (1 nlea serving) = 29 g; Calories = 115

🥣 Post Fruity Pebbles ☛ serving size: 3/4 cup (1 nlea serving) = 27 g; Calories = 109

🥣 Post Golden Crisp ☛ serving size: 3/4 cup (1 nlea serving) = 27 g; Calories = 103

🥣 Post Grape-Nuts Cereal ☛ serving size: 1/2 cup (1 nlea serving) = 58 g; Calories = 209

🥣 Post Grape-Nuts Flakes ☛ serving size: 3/4 cup (1 nlea serving) = 29 g; Calories = 109

🥣 Post Great Grains Banana Nut Crunch ☛ serving size: 1 cup (1 nlea serving) = 59 g; Calories = 230

Post Great Grains Cranberry Almond Crunch ☞ serving size: 3/4 cup (1 nlea serving) = 48 g; Calories = 184

Post Great Grains Crunchy Pecan Cereal ☞ serving size: 3/4 cup (1 nlea serving) = 52 g; Calories = 210

Post Great Grains Raisin Date & Pecan ☞ serving size: 3/4 cup (1 nlea serving) = 55 g; Calories = 208

Post Honey Bunches Of Oats Honey Roasted ☞ serving size: 3/4 cup (1 nlea serving) = 30 g; Calories = 120

Post Honey Bunches Of Oats Pecan Bunches ☞ serving size: 3/4 cup (1 nlea serving) = 29 g; Calories = 116

Post Honey Bunches Of Oats With Almonds ☞ serving size: 3/4 cup (1 nlea serving) = 32 g; Calories = 131

Post Honey Bunches Of Oats With Cinnamon Bunches ☞ serving size: 3/4 cup (1 nlea serving) = 30 g; Calories = 120

Post Honey Bunches Of Oats With Real Strawberries ☞ serving size: 3/4 cup (1 nlea serving) = 31 g; Calories = 124

Post Honey Bunches Of Oats With Vanilla Bunches ☞ serving size: 1 cup (1 nlea serving) = 56 g; Calories = 221

Post Honey Nut Shredded Wheat ☞ serving size: 1 cup (1 nlea serving) = 59 g; Calories = 220

Post Honeycomb Cereal ☞ serving size: 1 (1/2) cup (1 nlea serving) = 32 g; Calories = 126

Post Raisin Bran Cereal ☞ serving size: 1 cup (1 nlea serving) = 59 g; Calories = 191

Post Selects Blueberry Morning ☞ serving size: 1 (1/4) cup (1 nlea serving) = 55 g; Calories = 217

Post Selects Maple Pecan Crunch ☞ serving size: 3/4 cup (1 nlea serving) = 52 g; Calories = 215

Post Shredded Wheat Lightly Frosted Spoon-Size ☛ serving size: 1 cup (1 nlea serving) = 52 g; Calories = 183

Post Shredded Wheat N Bran Spoon-Size ☛ serving size: 1 (1/4) cup (1 nlea serving) = 59 g; Calories = 200

Post Shredded Wheat Original Big Biscuit ☛ serving size: 2 biscuits (1 nlea serving) = 47 g; Calories = 158

Post Shredded Wheat Original Spoon-Size ☛ serving size: 1 cup (1 nlea serving) = 49 g; Calories = 172

Post Waffle Crisp ☛ serving size: 1 cup (1 nlea serving) = 30 g; Calories = 117

Quaker 100% Natural Granola Oats Wheat And Honey ☛ serving size: 1/2 cup (1 nlea serving) = 48 g; Calories = 202

Quaker Capn Crunch ☛ serving size: 3/4 cup (1 nlea serving) = 27 g; Calories = 108

Quaker Capn Crunch With Crunchberries ☛ serving size: 3/4 cup (1 nlea serving) = 26 g; Calories = 103

Quaker Capn Crunchs Halloween Crunch ☛ serving size: 3/4 cup (1 nlea serving) = 26 g; Calories = 105

Quaker Capn Crunchs Oops! All Berries Cereal ☛ serving size: 1 cup (1 nlea serving) = 32 g; Calories = 126

Quaker Capn Crunchs Peanut Butter Crunch ☛ serving size: 3/4 cup (1 nlea serving) = 27 g; Calories = 113

Quaker Christmas Crunch ☛ serving size: 3/4 cup (1 nlea serving) = 26 g; Calories = 103

Quaker Corn Grits Instant Cheddar Cheese Flavor Dry ☛ serving size: 1 packet (1 nlea serving) = 28 g; Calories = 102

Quaker Corn Grits Instant Plain Dry ☛ serving size: 1 packet = 29 g; Calories = 100

Quaker Corn Grits Instant Plain Prepared (Microwaved Or Boiling Water Added) Without Salt ☞ serving size: 1 cup = 219 g; Calories = 162

Quaker Hominy Grits White Quick Dry ☞ serving size: 1/4 cup = 37 g; Calories = 129

Quaker Hominy Grits White Regular Dry ☞ serving size: 1/4 cup (1 nlea serving) = 41 g; Calories = 148

Quaker Honey Graham Oh!s ☞ serving size: 3/4 cup (1 nlea serving) = 27 g; Calories = 111

Quaker Instant Grits Butter Flavor Dry ☞ serving size: 1 packet (1 nlea serving) = 28 g; Calories = 103

Quaker Instant Grits Country Bacon Flavor Dry ☞ serving size: 1 packet (1 nlea serving) = 28 g; Calories = 95

Quaker Instant Grits Ham N Cheese Flavor Dry ☞ serving size: 1 packet (1 nlea serving) = 28 g; Calories = 99

Quaker Instant Grits Product With American Cheese Flavor Dry ☞ serving size: 1 packet (1 nlea serving) = 28 g; Calories = 101

Quaker Instant Grits Redeye Gravy & Country Ham Flavor Dry ☞ serving size: 1 packet (1 nlea serving) = 28 g; Calories = 96

Quaker Instant Oatmeal Apple And Cinnamon Reduced Sugar ☞ serving size: 1 packet (1 nlea serving) = 31 g; Calories = 111

Quaker Instant Oatmeal Apples And Cinnamon Dry ☞ serving size: 1 packet (1 nlea serving) = 43 g; Calories = 157

Quaker Instant Oatmeal Banana Bread Dry ☞ serving size: 1 packet (1 nlea serving) = 41 g; Calories = 151

Quaker Instant Oatmeal Cinnamon Spice Reduced Sugar ☞ serving size: 1 packet (1 nlea serving) = 34 g; Calories = 122

Quaker Instant Oatmeal Cinnamon Swirl High Fiber ☛ serving size: 1 packet (1 nlea serving) = 45 g; Calories = 165

Quaker Instant Oatmeal Cinnamon-Spice Dry ☛ serving size: 1 packet (1 nlea serving) = 43 g; Calories = 159

Quaker Instant Oatmeal Dinosaur Eggs Brown Sugar Dry ☛ serving size: 1 packet (1 nlea serving) = 50 g; Calories = 192

Quaker Instant Oatmeal Fruit And Cream Variety Dry ☛ serving size: 1 packet = 35 g; Calories = 133

Quaker Instant Oatmeal Fruit And Cream Variety Of Flavors Reduced Sugar ☛ serving size: 1 packet = 33 g; Calories = 124

Quaker Instant Oatmeal Maple And Brown Sugar Dry ☛ serving size: 1 packet = 43 g; Calories = 158

Quaker Instant Oatmeal Organic Regular ☛ serving size: 1 packet = 41 g; Calories = 151

Quaker Instant Oatmeal Raisin And Spice Dry ☛ serving size: 1 packet (1 nlea serving) = 43 g; Calories = 155

Quaker Instant Oatmeal Raisins Dates And Walnuts Dry ☛ serving size: 1 packet = 37 g; Calories = 137

Quaker Instant Oatmeal Weight Control Cinnamon ☛ serving size: 1 packet (1 nlea serving) = 45 g; Calories = 163

Quaker King Vitaman ☛ serving size: 1 (1/2) cup (1 nlea serving) = 31 g; Calories = 118

Quaker Low Fat 100% Natural Granola With Raisins ☛ serving size: 2/3 cup (1 nlea serving) = 55 g; Calories = 213

Quaker Maple Brown Sugar Life Cereal ☛ serving size: 3/4 cup (1 nlea serving) = 32 g; Calories = 119

Quaker Mothers Cinnamon Oat Crunch ☛ serving size: 1 cup (1 nlea serving) = 60 g; Calories = 229

👄 Quaker Mothers Cocoa Bumpers ☛ serving size: 1 cup (1 nlea serving) = 33 g; Calories = 126

👄 Quaker Mothers Graham Bumpers ☛ serving size: 3/4 cup (1 nlea serving) = 28 g; Calories = 106

👄 Quaker Mothers Peanut Butter Bumpers Cereal ☛ serving size: 1 cup (1 nlea serving) = 33 g; Calories = 134

👄 Quaker Mothers Toasted Oat Bran Cereal ☛ serving size: 3/4 cup (1 nlea serving) = 32 g; Calories = 119

👄 Quaker Natural Granola Apple Cranberry Almond ☛ serving size: 1/2 cup (1 nlea serving) = 49 g; Calories = 205

👄 Quaker Oat Bran Quaker/mothers Oat Bran Dry ☛ serving size: 1/2 cup (1 nlea serving) = 40 g; Calories = 146

👄 Quaker Oatmeal Real Medleys Apple Walnut Dry ☛ serving size: 1 package (1 nlea serving) = 75 g; Calories = 293

👄 Quaker Oatmeal Real Medleys Blueberry Hazelnut Dry ☛ serving size: 1 package (1 nlea serving) = 70 g; Calories = 270

👄 Quaker Oatmeal Real Medleys Cherry Pistachio Dry ☛ serving size: 1 package (1 nlea serving) = 73 g; Calories = 288

👄 Quaker Oatmeal Real Medleys Peach Almond Dry ☛ serving size: 1 package (1 nlea serving) = 75 g; Calories = 290

👄 Quaker Oatmeal Real Medleys Summer Berry Dry ☛ serving size: 1 package (1 nlea serving) = 70 g; Calories = 247

👄 Quaker Oatmeal Squares ☛ serving size: 1 cup (1 nlea serving) = 56 g; Calories = 212

👄 Quaker Oatmeal Squares Cinnamon ☛ serving size: 1 cup (1 nlea serving) = 56 g; Calories = 212

👄 Quaker Oatmeal Squares Golden Maple ☛ serving size: 1 cup (1 nlea serving) = 56 g; Calories = 213

Quaker Quaker 100% Natural Granola With Oats Wheat Honey And Raisins ☞ serving size: 1/2 cup (1 nlea serving) = 51 g; Calories = 210

Quaker Quaker Crunchy Bran ☞ serving size: 3/4 cup (1 nlea serving) = 27 g; Calories = 89

Quaker Quaker Honey Graham Life Cereal ☞ serving size: 3/4 cup (1 nlea serving) = 32 g; Calories = 119

Quaker Quaker Multigrain Oatmeal Dry ☞ serving size: 1/2 cup (1 nlea serving) = 40 g; Calories = 134

Quaker Quaker Oat Cinnamon Life ☞ serving size: 3/4 cup (1 nlea serving) = 32 g; Calories = 120

Quaker Quaker Oat Life Plain ☞ serving size: 3/4 cup (1 nlea serving) = 32 g; Calories = 120

Quaker Quaker Puffed Rice ☞ serving size: 3/4 cup (1 nlea serving) = 14 g; Calories = 54

Quaker Quaker Puffed Wheat ☞ serving size: 1 cup (1 nlea serving) = 15 g; Calories = 55

Quaker Quick Oats Dry ☞ serving size: 1/2 cup = 40 g; Calories = 148

Quaker Quick Oats With Iron Dry ☞ serving size: 1/2 cup = 40 g; Calories = 148

Quaker Shredded Wheat Bagged Cereal ☞ serving size: 3 biscuits (1 nlea serving) = 63 g; Calories = 219

Quaker Sweet Crunch/quisp ☞ serving size: 1 cup (1 nlea serving) = 27 g; Calories = 110

Quaker Toasted Multigrain Crisps ☞ serving size: 1 (1/4) cup (1 nlea serving) = 57 g; Calories = 212

Quaker Weight Control Instant Oatmeal Banana Bread ☞ serving size: 1 packet (1 nlea serving) = 45 g; Calories = 163

🥣 Quaker Weight Control Instant Oatmeal Maple And Brown Sugar ☛ serving size: 1 packet (1 nlea serving) = 45 g; Calories = 163

🥣 Quaker Whole Hearts Oat Cereal ☛ serving size: 3/4 cup (1 nlea serving) = 28 g; Calories = 105

🥣 Quaker Whole Wheat Natural Cereal Dry ☛ serving size: 1/2 cup = 40 g; Calories = 133

🥣 Ralston Corn Biscuits ☛ serving size: 1 cup (nlea serving) = 30 g; Calories = 113

🥣 Ralston Corn Flakes ☛ serving size: 1 cup (1 nlea serving) = 28 g; Calories = 108

🥣 Ralston Crisp Rice ☛ serving size: 1 (1/4) cup (1 nlea serving) = 33 g; Calories = 126

🥣 Ralston Crispy Hexagons ☛ serving size: 1 cup (1 nlea serving) = 29 g; Calories = 110

🥣 Ralston Enriched Bran Flakes ☛ serving size: 1 serving (nlea serving size = 0.75 cup) = 29 g; Calories = 113

🥣 Ralston Tasteeos ☛ serving size: 1 cup (1 nlea serving) = 28 g; Calories = 111

🥣 Rice Cream Of Cooked Fat Added In Cooking ☛ serving size: 1 cup, cooked = 240 g; Calories = 192

🥣 Rice Cream Of Cooked Fat Not Added In Cooking ☛ serving size: 1 cup, cooked = 240 g; Calories = 166

🥣 Rice Cream Of Cooked Made With Milk ☛ serving size: 1 cup, cooked = 240 g; Calories = 312

🥣 Rice Cream Of Cooked Ns As To Fat Added In Cooking ☛ serving size: 1 cup, cooked = 240 g; Calories = 192

Rice Creamed Made With Milk And Sugar Puerto Rican Style ☛ serving size: 1 cup, cooked = 245 g; Calories = 216

Rice Puffed Fortified ☛ serving size: 1 cup = 14 g; Calories = 56

Sun Country Kretschmer Honey Crunch Wheat Germ ☛ serving size: 2 tbsp (1 nlea serving) = 14 g; Calories = 52

Sun Country Kretschmer Toasted Wheat Bran ☛ serving size: 1/4 cup (1 nlea serving) = 16 g; Calories = 32

Sun Country Kretschmer Wheat Germ Regular ☛ serving size: 2 tbsp (1 nlea serving) = 14 g; Calories = 51

Toasted Wheat Germ ☛ serving size: 1 oz = 28.4 g; Calories = 109

Uncle Sam Cereal ☛ serving size: 3/4 cup (1 nlea serving) = 55 g; Calories = 190

Upma Indian Breakfast Dish ☛ serving size: 1 cup, cooked = 170 g; Calories = 148

Weetabix Whole Grain Cereal ☛ serving size: 2 biscuits (1 nlea serving) = 35 g; Calories = 130

Wheat And Bran Presweetened With Nuts And Fruits ☛ serving size: 1 cup (1 nlea serving) = 55 g; Calories = 212

Wheat Cereal Chocolate Flavored Cooked ☛ serving size: 1 cup, cooked = 240 g; Calories = 118

Wheat Cream Of Cooked Made With Milk And Sugar Puerto Rican Style ☛ serving size: 1 cup, cooked = 245 g; Calories = 267

Wheat Puffed Fortified ☛ serving size: 1 cup = 12 g; Calories = 44

Wheatena Cooked With Water ☛ serving size: 1 cup = 243 g; Calories = 136

Wheatena Cooked With Water With Salt ☛ serving size: 1 cup = 243 g; Calories = 143

🥣 Wheatena Dry ☛ serving size: 1/3 cup (1 nlea serving) = 40 g; Calories = 143

🥣 White Cornmeal (Grits) ☛ serving size: 1 cup = 257 g; Calories = 183

🥣 Whole Wheat Cereal Cooked Fat Added In Cooking ☛ serving size: 1 cup, cooked = 240 g; Calories = 144

🥣 Whole Wheat Cereal Cooked Fat Not Added In Cooking ☛ serving size: 1 cup, cooked = 240 g; Calories = 113

🥣 Whole Wheat Cereal Cooked Ns As To Fat Added In Cooking ☛ serving size: 1 cup, cooked = 240 g; Calories = 144

🥣 Whole Wheat Hot Natural Cereal Cooked With Water With Salt ☛ serving size: 1 cup = 242 g; Calories = 150

🥣 Whole Wheat Hot Natural Cereal Cooked With Water Without Salt ☛ serving size: 1 cup = 242 g; Calories = 150

🥣 Whole Wheat Hot Natural Cereal Dry ☛ serving size: 1 cup = 94 g; Calories = 322

12

DAIRY AND EGG PRODUCTS

⊍ Almond Milk Unsweetened ☛ serving size: 1 cup = 244 g; Calories = 37

⊍ American Cheese ☛ serving size: 1 cup = 113 g; Calories = 373

⊍ American Cheese Spread ☛ serving size: 1 cup, diced = 140 g; Calories = 406

⊍ Baked Alaska ☛ serving size: 1 baked alaska = 820 g; Calories = 2034

⊍ Beverage Instant Breakfast Powder Chocolate Not Reconstituted ☛ serving size: 1 tbsp = 7.4 g; Calories = 26

⊍ Beverage Instant Breakfast Powder Chocolate Sugar-Free Not Reconstituted ☛ serving size: 1 tbsp = 5.6 g; Calories = 20

⊍ Blue Cheese ☛ serving size: 1 oz = 28.4 g; Calories = 100

⊍ Breast Milk (Human) ☛ serving size: 1 fl oz = 30.8 g; Calories = 22

⊍ Brick Cheese ☛ serving size: 1 cup, diced = 132 g; Calories = 490

⊍ Brie Cheese ☛ serving size: 1 oz = 28.4 g; Calories = 95

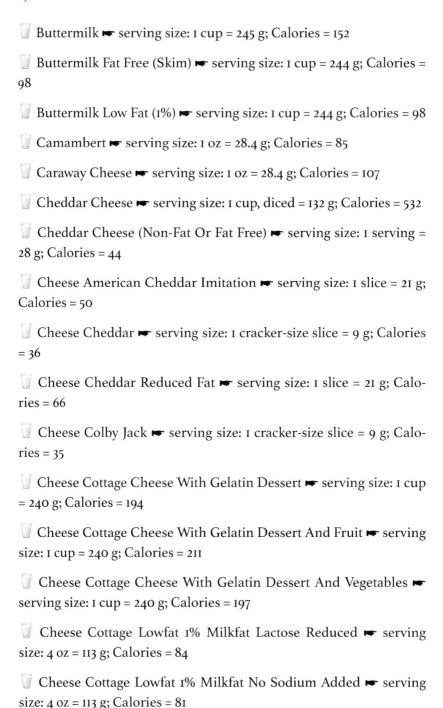

Buttermilk ☞ serving size: 1 cup = 245 g; Calories = 152

Buttermilk Fat Free (Skim) ☞ serving size: 1 cup = 244 g; Calories = 98

Buttermilk Low Fat (1%) ☞ serving size: 1 cup = 244 g; Calories = 98

Camambert ☞ serving size: 1 oz = 28.4 g; Calories = 85

Caraway Cheese ☞ serving size: 1 oz = 28.4 g; Calories = 107

Cheddar Cheese ☞ serving size: 1 cup, diced = 132 g; Calories = 532

Cheddar Cheese (Non-Fat Or Fat Free) ☞ serving size: 1 serving = 28 g; Calories = 44

Cheese American Cheddar Imitation ☞ serving size: 1 slice = 21 g; Calories = 50

Cheese Cheddar ☞ serving size: 1 cracker-size slice = 9 g; Calories = 36

Cheese Cheddar Reduced Fat ☞ serving size: 1 slice = 21 g; Calories = 66

Cheese Colby Jack ☞ serving size: 1 cracker-size slice = 9 g; Calories = 35

Cheese Cottage Cheese With Gelatin Dessert ☞ serving size: 1 cup = 240 g; Calories = 194

Cheese Cottage Cheese With Gelatin Dessert And Fruit ☞ serving size: 1 cup = 240 g; Calories = 211

Cheese Cottage Cheese With Gelatin Dessert And Vegetables ☞ serving size: 1 cup = 240 g; Calories = 197

Cheese Cottage Lowfat 1% Milkfat Lactose Reduced ☞ serving size: 4 oz = 113 g; Calories = 84

Cheese Cottage Lowfat 1% Milkfat No Sodium Added ☞ serving size: 4 oz = 113 g; Calories = 81

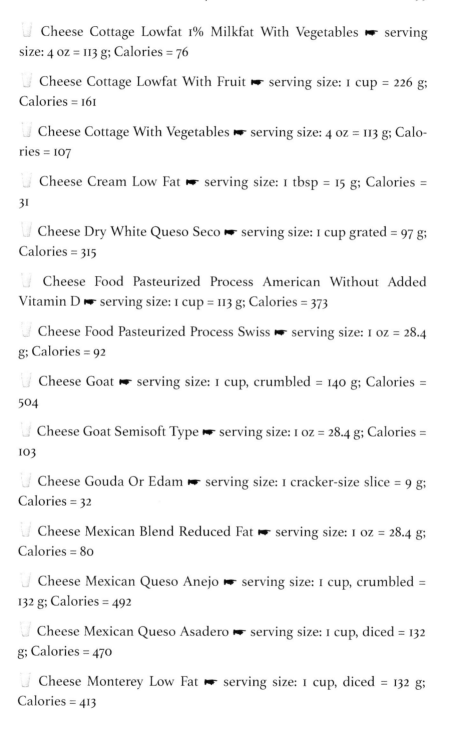

Cheese Cottage Lowfat 1% Milkfat With Vegetables ☛ serving size: 4 oz = 113 g; Calories = 76

Cheese Cottage Lowfat With Fruit ☛ serving size: 1 cup = 226 g; Calories = 161

Cheese Cottage With Vegetables ☛ serving size: 4 oz = 113 g; Calories = 107

Cheese Cream Low Fat ☛ serving size: 1 tbsp = 15 g; Calories = 31

Cheese Dry White Queso Seco ☛ serving size: 1 cup grated = 97 g; Calories = 315

Cheese Food Pasteurized Process American Without Added Vitamin D ☛ serving size: 1 cup = 113 g; Calories = 373

Cheese Food Pasteurized Process Swiss ☛ serving size: 1 oz = 28.4 g; Calories = 92

Cheese Goat ☛ serving size: 1 cup, crumbled = 140 g; Calories = 504

Cheese Goat Semisoft Type ☛ serving size: 1 oz = 28.4 g; Calories = 103

Cheese Gouda Or Edam ☛ serving size: 1 cracker-size slice = 9 g; Calories = 32

Cheese Mexican Blend Reduced Fat ☛ serving size: 1 oz = 28.4 g; Calories = 80

Cheese Mexican Queso Anejo ☛ serving size: 1 cup, crumbled = 132 g; Calories = 492

Cheese Mexican Queso Asadero ☛ serving size: 1 cup, diced = 132 g; Calories = 470

Cheese Monterey Low Fat ☛ serving size: 1 cup, diced = 132 g; Calories = 413

Cheese Mozzarella Low Moisture Part-Skim Shredded ☞ serving size: 1 cup = 86 g; Calories = 261

Cheese Mozzarella Low Sodium ☞ serving size: 1 cup, diced = 132 g; Calories = 370

Cheese Muenster Low Fat ☞ serving size: 1 cup, shredded = 113 g; Calories = 306

Cheese Nfs ☞ serving size: 1 cracker-size slice = 9 g; Calories = 33

Cheese Parmesan Dry Grated Reduced Fat ☞ serving size: 1 cup = 100 g; Calories = 265

Cheese Pasteurized Process American Low Fat ☞ serving size: 1 cup, diced = 140 g; Calories = 252

Cheese Pasteurized Process American Without Added Vitamin D ☞ serving size: 1 oz = 28.4 g; Calories = 105

Cheese Pasteurized Process Cheddar Or American Low Sodium ☞ serving size: 1 cup, diced = 140 g; Calories = 526

Cheese Product Pasteurized Process American Reduced Fat Fortified With Vitamin D ☞ serving size: 1 slice 3/4 oz = 21 g; Calories = 50

Cheese Product Pasteurized Process American Vitamin D Fortified ☞ serving size: 1 slice (2/3 oz) = 19 g; Calories = 58

Cheese Ricotta ☞ serving size: 1 cup = 246 g; Calories = 384

Cheese Sauce Prepared From Recipe ☞ serving size: 2 tbsp = 30 g; Calories = 59

Cheese Souffle ☞ serving size: 1 cup = 95 g; Calories = 194

Cheese Spread American Or Cheddar Cheese Base Reduced Fat ☞ serving size: 1 piece = 21 g; Calories = 37

Cheese Spread Cream Cheese Base ☞ serving size: 1 oz = 28.4 g; Calories = 84

Cheese Substitute Mozzarella ☞ serving size: 1 cup, shredded = 113 g; Calories = 280

Cheese Swiss Low Fat ☞ serving size: 1 slice (1 oz) = 28 g; Calories = 50

Cheese Swiss Low Sodium ☞ serving size: 1 slice = 28 g; Calories = 105

Cheese With Nuts ☞ serving size: 1 tablespoon = 15 g; Calories = 64

Chesire Cheese ☞ serving size: 1 oz = 28.4 g; Calories = 110

Chicken Or Turkey Souffle ☞ serving size: 1 cup = 159 g; Calories = 269

Chocolate Milk Made From Dry Mix Ns As To Type Of Milk ☞ serving size: 1 cup = 248 g; Calories = 179

Chocolate Milk Made From Dry Mix Ns As To Type Of Milk (Nesquik) ☞ serving size: 1 cup = 248 g; Calories = 179

Chocolate Milk Made From Dry Mix With Fat Free Milk ☞ serving size: 1 cup = 248 g; Calories = 141

Chocolate Milk Made From Dry Mix With Fat Free Milk (Nesquik) ☞ serving size: 1 cup = 248 g; Calories = 141

Chocolate Milk Made From Dry Mix With Low Fat Milk ☞ serving size: 1 cup = 248 g; Calories = 159

Chocolate Milk Made From Dry Mix With Low Fat Milk (Nesquik) ☞ serving size: 1 cup = 248 g; Calories = 159

Chocolate Milk Made From Dry Mix With Non-Dairy Milk ☞ serving size: 1 cup = 248 g; Calories = 156

Chocolate Milk Made From Dry Mix With Non-Dairy Milk (Nesquik) ☞ serving size: 1 cup = 248 g; Calories = 156

Chocolate Milk Made From Dry Mix With Reduced Fat Milk ☞ serving size: 1 cup = 248 g; Calories = 179

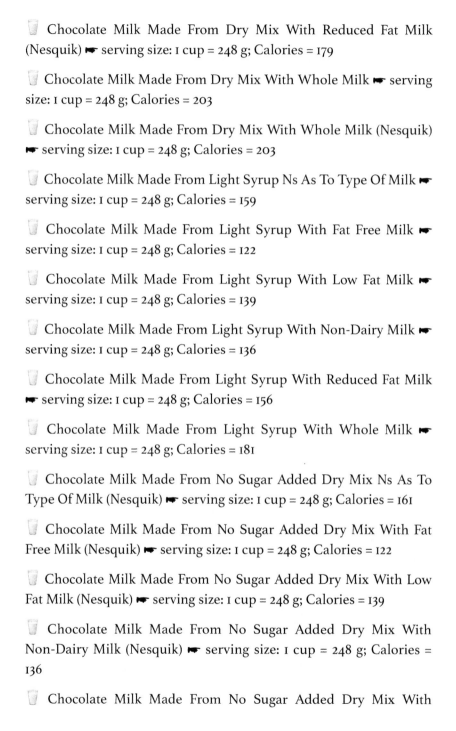

Chocolate Milk Made From Dry Mix With Reduced Fat Milk (Nesquik) ☞ serving size: 1 cup = 248 g; Calories = 179

Chocolate Milk Made From Dry Mix With Whole Milk ☞ serving size: 1 cup = 248 g; Calories = 203

Chocolate Milk Made From Dry Mix With Whole Milk (Nesquik) ☞ serving size: 1 cup = 248 g; Calories = 203

Chocolate Milk Made From Light Syrup Ns As To Type Of Milk ☞ serving size: 1 cup = 248 g; Calories = 159

Chocolate Milk Made From Light Syrup With Fat Free Milk ☞ serving size: 1 cup = 248 g; Calories = 122

Chocolate Milk Made From Light Syrup With Low Fat Milk ☞ serving size: 1 cup = 248 g; Calories = 139

Chocolate Milk Made From Light Syrup With Non-Dairy Milk ☞ serving size: 1 cup = 248 g; Calories = 136

Chocolate Milk Made From Light Syrup With Reduced Fat Milk ☞ serving size: 1 cup = 248 g; Calories = 156

Chocolate Milk Made From Light Syrup With Whole Milk ☞ serving size: 1 cup = 248 g; Calories = 181

Chocolate Milk Made From No Sugar Added Dry Mix Ns As To Type Of Milk (Nesquik) ☞ serving size: 1 cup = 248 g; Calories = 161

Chocolate Milk Made From No Sugar Added Dry Mix With Fat Free Milk (Nesquik) ☞ serving size: 1 cup = 248 g; Calories = 122

Chocolate Milk Made From No Sugar Added Dry Mix With Low Fat Milk (Nesquik) ☞ serving size: 1 cup = 248 g; Calories = 139

Chocolate Milk Made From No Sugar Added Dry Mix With Non-Dairy Milk (Nesquik) ☞ serving size: 1 cup = 248 g; Calories = 136

Chocolate Milk Made From No Sugar Added Dry Mix With

Reduced Fat Milk (Nesquik) ☞ serving size: 1 cup = 248 g; Calories = 159

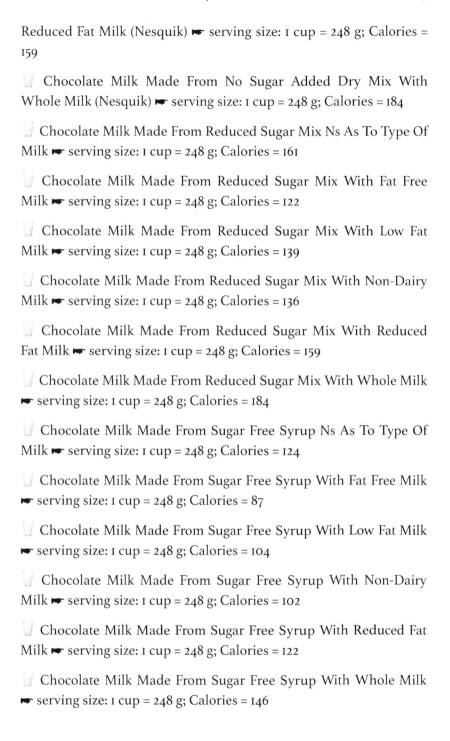 Chocolate Milk Made From No Sugar Added Dry Mix With Whole Milk (Nesquik) ☞ serving size: 1 cup = 248 g; Calories = 184

Chocolate Milk Made From Reduced Sugar Mix Ns As To Type Of Milk ☞ serving size: 1 cup = 248 g; Calories = 161

Chocolate Milk Made From Reduced Sugar Mix With Fat Free Milk ☞ serving size: 1 cup = 248 g; Calories = 122

Chocolate Milk Made From Reduced Sugar Mix With Low Fat Milk ☞ serving size: 1 cup = 248 g; Calories = 139

Chocolate Milk Made From Reduced Sugar Mix With Non-Dairy Milk ☞ serving size: 1 cup = 248 g; Calories = 136

Chocolate Milk Made From Reduced Sugar Mix With Reduced Fat Milk ☞ serving size: 1 cup = 248 g; Calories = 159

Chocolate Milk Made From Reduced Sugar Mix With Whole Milk ☞ serving size: 1 cup = 248 g; Calories = 184

Chocolate Milk Made From Sugar Free Syrup Ns As To Type Of Milk ☞ serving size: 1 cup = 248 g; Calories = 124

Chocolate Milk Made From Sugar Free Syrup With Fat Free Milk ☞ serving size: 1 cup = 248 g; Calories = 87

Chocolate Milk Made From Sugar Free Syrup With Low Fat Milk ☞ serving size: 1 cup = 248 g; Calories = 104

Chocolate Milk Made From Sugar Free Syrup With Non-Dairy Milk ☞ serving size: 1 cup = 248 g; Calories = 102

Chocolate Milk Made From Sugar Free Syrup With Reduced Fat Milk ☞ serving size: 1 cup = 248 g; Calories = 122

Chocolate Milk Made From Sugar Free Syrup With Whole Milk ☞ serving size: 1 cup = 248 g; Calories = 146

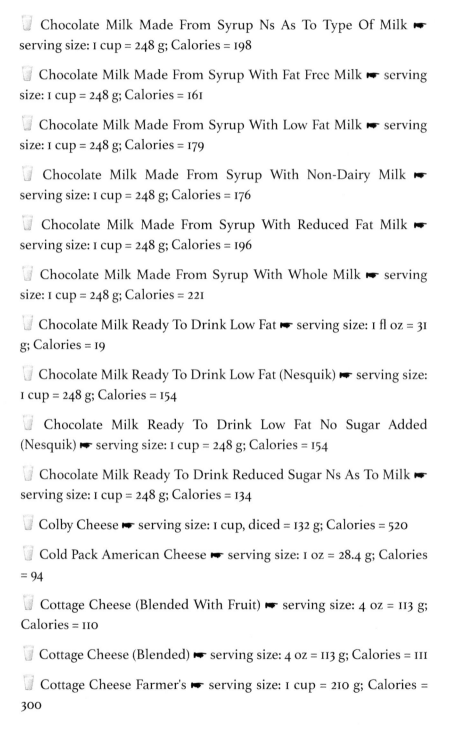

Chocolate Milk Made From Syrup Ns As To Type Of Milk ☞ serving size: 1 cup = 248 g; Calories = 198

Chocolate Milk Made From Syrup With Fat Free Milk ☞ serving size: 1 cup = 248 g; Calories = 161

Chocolate Milk Made From Syrup With Low Fat Milk ☞ serving size: 1 cup = 248 g; Calories = 179

Chocolate Milk Made From Syrup With Non-Dairy Milk ☞ serving size: 1 cup = 248 g; Calories = 176

Chocolate Milk Made From Syrup With Reduced Fat Milk ☞ serving size: 1 cup = 248 g; Calories = 196

Chocolate Milk Made From Syrup With Whole Milk ☞ serving size: 1 cup = 248 g; Calories = 221

Chocolate Milk Ready To Drink Low Fat ☞ serving size: 1 fl oz = 31 g; Calories = 19

Chocolate Milk Ready To Drink Low Fat (Nesquik) ☞ serving size: 1 cup = 248 g; Calories = 154

Chocolate Milk Ready To Drink Low Fat No Sugar Added (Nesquik) ☞ serving size: 1 cup = 248 g; Calories = 154

Chocolate Milk Ready To Drink Reduced Sugar Ns As To Milk ☞ serving size: 1 cup = 248 g; Calories = 134

Colby Cheese ☞ serving size: 1 cup, diced = 132 g; Calories = 520

Cold Pack American Cheese ☞ serving size: 1 oz = 28.4 g; Calories = 94

Cottage Cheese (Blended With Fruit) ☞ serving size: 4 oz = 113 g; Calories = 110

Cottage Cheese (Blended) ☞ serving size: 4 oz = 113 g; Calories = 111

Cottage Cheese Farmer's ☞ serving size: 1 cup = 210 g; Calories = 300

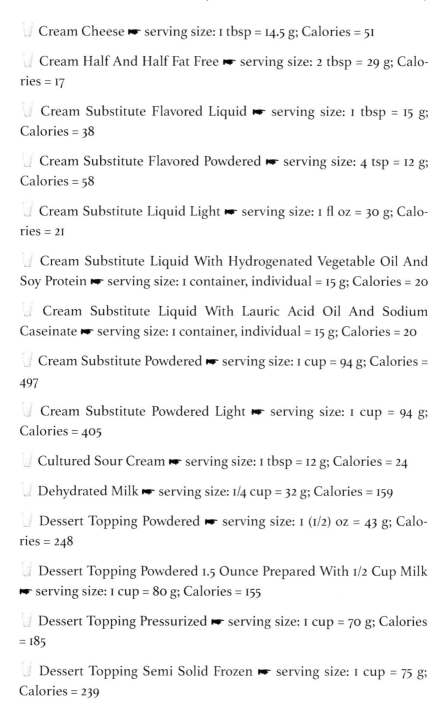

Cream Cheese ☛ serving size: 1 tbsp = 14.5 g; Calories = 51

Cream Half And Half Fat Free ☛ serving size: 2 tbsp = 29 g; Calories = 17

Cream Substitute Flavored Liquid ☛ serving size: 1 tbsp = 15 g; Calories = 38

Cream Substitute Flavored Powdered ☛ serving size: 4 tsp = 12 g; Calories = 58

Cream Substitute Liquid Light ☛ serving size: 1 fl oz = 30 g; Calories = 21

Cream Substitute Liquid With Hydrogenated Vegetable Oil And Soy Protein ☛ serving size: 1 container, individual = 15 g; Calories = 20

Cream Substitute Liquid With Lauric Acid Oil And Sodium Caseinate ☛ serving size: 1 container, individual = 15 g; Calories = 20

Cream Substitute Powdered ☛ serving size: 1 cup = 94 g; Calories = 497

Cream Substitute Powdered Light ☛ serving size: 1 cup = 94 g; Calories = 405

Cultured Sour Cream ☛ serving size: 1 tbsp = 12 g; Calories = 24

Dehydrated Milk ☛ serving size: 1/4 cup = 32 g; Calories = 159

Dessert Topping Powdered ☛ serving size: 1 (1/2) oz = 43 g; Calories = 248

Dessert Topping Powdered 1.5 Ounce Prepared With 1/2 Cup Milk ☛ serving size: 1 cup = 80 g; Calories = 155

Dessert Topping Pressurized ☛ serving size: 1 cup = 70 g; Calories = 185

Dessert Topping Semi Solid Frozen ☛ serving size: 1 cup = 75 g; Calories = 239

Dried Eggs ☛ serving size: 1 cup, sifted = 85 g; Calories = 503

Dried Sweet Whey Powder ☛ serving size: 1 cup = 145 g; Calories = 512

Dried Whey Powder (Acid) ☛ serving size: 1 cup = 57 g; Calories = 193

Duck Egg Cooked ☛ serving size: 1 egg = 70 g; Calories = 146

Dulce De Leche ☛ serving size: 1 tbsp = 19 g; Calories = 60

Edam Cheese ☛ serving size: 1 oz = 28.4 g; Calories = 101

Egg Benedict ☛ serving size: 1 medium egg = 149 g; Calories = 428

Egg Casserole With Bread Cheese Milk And Meat ☛ serving size: 1 cup = 164 g; Calories = 315

Egg Creamed ☛ serving size: 1 medium egg = 139 g; Calories = 209

Egg Deviled ☛ serving size: 1/2 small egg = 24 g; Calories = 48

Egg Duck Whole Fresh Raw ☛ serving size: 1 egg = 70 g; Calories = 130

Egg Goose Whole Fresh Raw ☛ serving size: 1 egg = 144 g; Calories = 266

Egg Omelet ☛ serving size: 1 tbsp = 15 g; Calories = 23

Egg Substitute Liquid Or Frozen Fat Free ☛ serving size: 1/4 cup = 60 g; Calories = 29

Egg Substitute Powder ☛ serving size: 7/20 oz = 9.9 g; Calories = 44

Egg Turkey Whole Fresh Raw ☛ serving size: 1 egg = 79 g; Calories = 135

Egg White Cooked Ns As To Fat Added In Cooking ☛ serving size: 1 small egg white = 24 g; Calories = 27

Egg White Dried ☛ serving size: 1 oz = 28 g; Calories = 107

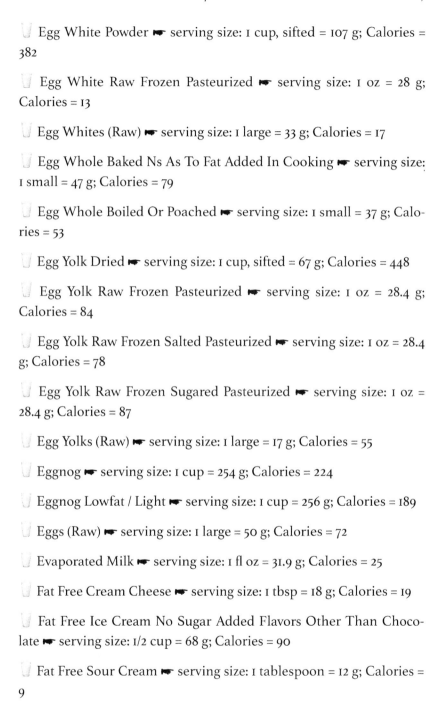

Egg White Powder ☞ serving size: 1 cup, sifted = 107 g; Calories = 382

Egg White Raw Frozen Pasteurized ☞ serving size: 1 oz = 28 g; Calories = 13

Egg Whites (Raw) ☞ serving size: 1 large = 33 g; Calories = 17

Egg Whole Baked Ns As To Fat Added In Cooking ☞ serving size: 1 small = 47 g; Calories = 79

Egg Whole Boiled Or Poached ☞ serving size: 1 small = 37 g; Calories = 53

Egg Yolk Dried ☞ serving size: 1 cup, sifted = 67 g; Calories = 448

Egg Yolk Raw Frozen Pasteurized ☞ serving size: 1 oz = 28.4 g; Calories = 84

Egg Yolk Raw Frozen Salted Pasteurized ☞ serving size: 1 oz = 28.4 g; Calories = 78

Egg Yolk Raw Frozen Sugared Pasteurized ☞ serving size: 1 oz = 28.4 g; Calories = 87

Egg Yolks (Raw) ☞ serving size: 1 large = 17 g; Calories = 55

Eggnog ☞ serving size: 1 cup = 254 g; Calories = 224

Eggnog Lowfat / Light ☞ serving size: 1 cup = 256 g; Calories = 189

Eggs (Raw) ☞ serving size: 1 large = 50 g; Calories = 72

Evaporated Milk ☞ serving size: 1 fl oz = 31.9 g; Calories = 25

Fat Free Cream Cheese ☞ serving size: 1 tbsp = 18 g; Calories = 19

Fat Free Ice Cream No Sugar Added Flavors Other Than Chocolate ☞ serving size: 1/2 cup = 68 g; Calories = 90

Fat Free Sour Cream ☞ serving size: 1 tablespoon = 12 g; Calories = 9

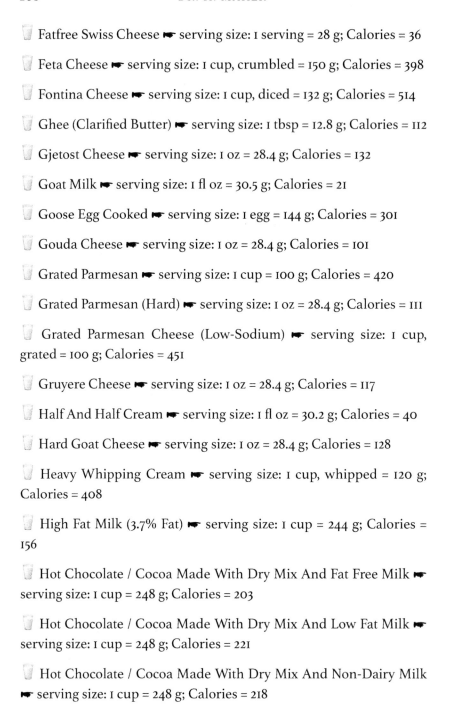

Fatfree Swiss Cheese ☛ serving size: 1 serving = 28 g; Calories = 36

Feta Cheese ☛ serving size: 1 cup, crumbled = 150 g; Calories = 398

Fontina Cheese ☛ serving size: 1 cup, diced = 132 g; Calories = 514

Ghee (Clarified Butter) ☛ serving size: 1 tbsp = 12.8 g; Calories = 112

Gjetost Cheese ☛ serving size: 1 oz = 28.4 g; Calories = 132

Goat Milk ☛ serving size: 1 fl oz = 30.5 g; Calories = 21

Goose Egg Cooked ☛ serving size: 1 egg = 144 g; Calories = 301

Gouda Cheese ☛ serving size: 1 oz = 28.4 g; Calories = 101

Grated Parmesan ☛ serving size: 1 cup = 100 g; Calories = 420

Grated Parmesan (Hard) ☛ serving size: 1 oz = 28.4 g; Calories = 111

Grated Parmesan Cheese (Low-Sodium) ☛ serving size: 1 cup, grated = 100 g; Calories = 451

Gruyere Cheese ☛ serving size: 1 oz = 28.4 g; Calories = 117

Half And Half Cream ☛ serving size: 1 fl oz = 30.2 g; Calories = 40

Hard Goat Cheese ☛ serving size: 1 oz = 28.4 g; Calories = 128

Heavy Whipping Cream ☛ serving size: 1 cup, whipped = 120 g; Calories = 408

High Fat Milk (3.7% Fat) ☛ serving size: 1 cup = 244 g; Calories = 156

Hot Chocolate / Cocoa Made With Dry Mix And Fat Free Milk ☛ serving size: 1 cup = 248 g; Calories = 203

Hot Chocolate / Cocoa Made With Dry Mix And Low Fat Milk ☛ serving size: 1 cup = 248 g; Calories = 221

Hot Chocolate / Cocoa Made With Dry Mix And Non-Dairy Milk ☛ serving size: 1 cup = 248 g; Calories = 218

Hot Chocolate / Cocoa Made With Dry Mix And Reduced Fat Milk ☞ serving size: 1 cup = 248 g; Calories = 238

Hot Chocolate / Cocoa Made With Dry Mix And Whole Milk ☞ serving size: 1 cup = 248 g; Calories = 263

Hot Chocolate / Cocoa Made With No Sugar Added Dry Mix And Fat Free Milk ☞ serving size: 1 packet, reconstituted = 199 g; Calories = 123

Hot Chocolate / Cocoa Made With No Sugar Added Dry Mix And Low Fat Milk ☞ serving size: 1 packet, reconstituted = 199 g; Calories = 137

Hot Chocolate / Cocoa Made With No Sugar Added Dry Mix And Non-Dairy Milk ☞ serving size: 1 packet, reconstituted = 199 g; Calories = 133

Hot Chocolate / Cocoa Made With No Sugar Added Dry Mix And Reduced Fat Milk ☞ serving size: 1 packet, reconstituted = 199 g; Calories = 151

Hot Chocolate / Cocoa Made With No Sugar Added Dry Mix And Water ☞ serving size: 1 packet, reconstituted = 194 g; Calories = 60

Hot Chocolate / Cocoa Made With No Sugar Added Dry Mix And Whole Milk ☞ serving size: 1 packet, reconstituted = 199 g; Calories = 171

Hot Chocolate / Cocoa Ready To Drink ☞ serving size: 1 cup = 248 g; Calories = 226

Hot Chocolate / Cocoa Ready To Drink Made With Non-Dairy Milk ☞ serving size: 1 cup = 248 g; Calories = 206

Hot Chocolate / Cocoa Ready To Drink Made With Non-Dairy Milk And Whipped Cream ☞ serving size: 1 cup = 248 g; Calories = 236

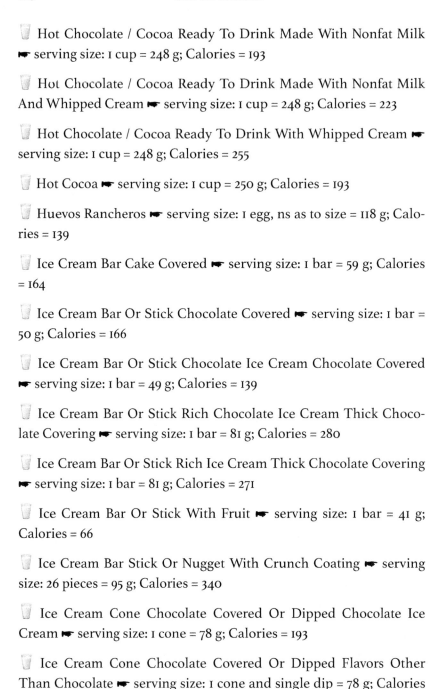

Hot Chocolate / Cocoa Ready To Drink Made With Nonfat Milk ☛ serving size: 1 cup = 248 g; Calories = 193

Hot Chocolate / Cocoa Ready To Drink Made With Nonfat Milk And Whipped Cream ☛ serving size: 1 cup = 248 g; Calories = 223

Hot Chocolate / Cocoa Ready To Drink With Whipped Cream ☛ serving size: 1 cup = 248 g; Calories = 255

Hot Cocoa ☛ serving size: 1 cup = 250 g; Calories = 193

Huevos Rancheros ☛ serving size: 1 egg, ns as to size = 118 g; Calories = 139

Ice Cream Bar Cake Covered ☛ serving size: 1 bar = 59 g; Calories = 164

Ice Cream Bar Or Stick Chocolate Covered ☛ serving size: 1 bar = 50 g; Calories = 166

Ice Cream Bar Or Stick Chocolate Ice Cream Chocolate Covered ☛ serving size: 1 bar = 49 g; Calories = 139

Ice Cream Bar Or Stick Rich Chocolate Ice Cream Thick Chocolate Covering ☛ serving size: 1 bar = 81 g; Calories = 280

Ice Cream Bar Or Stick Rich Ice Cream Thick Chocolate Covering ☛ serving size: 1 bar = 81 g; Calories = 271

Ice Cream Bar Or Stick With Fruit ☛ serving size: 1 bar = 41 g; Calories = 66

Ice Cream Bar Stick Or Nugget With Crunch Coating ☛ serving size: 26 pieces = 95 g; Calories = 340

Ice Cream Cone Chocolate Covered Or Dipped Chocolate Ice Cream ☛ serving size: 1 cone = 78 g; Calories = 193

Ice Cream Cone Chocolate Covered Or Dipped Flavors Other Than Chocolate ☛ serving size: 1 cone and single dip = 78 g; Calories = 191

Ice Cream Cone Chocolate Covered With Nuts Chocolate Ice Cream ☛ serving size: 1 cone = 78 g; Calories = 225

Ice Cream Cone Chocolate Covered With Nuts Flavors Other Than Chocolate ☛ serving size: 1 unit = 96 g; Calories = 340

Ice Cream Cone No Topping Chocolate Ice Cream ☛ serving size: 1 cone and single dip (or 1 small cone) = 78 g; Calories = 176

Ice Cream Cone No Topping Flavors Other Than Chocolate ☛ serving size: 1 cone and single dip (or 1 small cone) = 78 g; Calories = 171

Ice Cream Cone No Topping Ns As To Flavor ☛ serving size: 1 cone and single dip (or 1 small cone) = 78 g; Calories = 173

Ice Cream Cone With Nuts Chocolate Ice Cream ☛ serving size: 1 cone = 78 g; Calories = 214

Ice Cream Cone With Nuts Flavors Other Than Chocolate ☛ serving size: 1 cone = 78 g; Calories = 208

Ice Cream Cookie Sandwich ☛ serving size: 1 serving = 82 g; Calories = 197

Ice Cream Fried ☛ serving size: 1 cup = 133 g; Calories = 375

Ice Cream Light Soft Serve Chocolate ☛ serving size: 1 medium = 298 g; Calories = 420

Ice Cream Pie No Crust ☛ serving size: 1 pie (8" dia) = 794 g; Calories = 1779

Ice Cream Pie With Cookie Crust Fudge Topping And Whipped Cream ☛ serving size: 1 pie (8" dia) = 1836 g; Calories = 5563

Ice Cream Sandwich ☛ serving size: 1 serving = 70 g; Calories = 166

Ice Cream Sandwich Made With Light Chocolate Ice Cream ☛ serving size: 1 sandwich = 68 g; Calories = 161

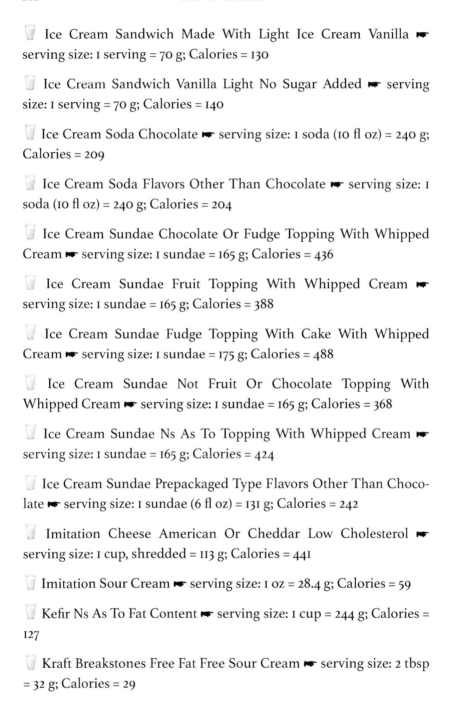

Ice Cream Sandwich Made With Light Ice Cream Vanilla ☛ serving size: 1 serving = 70 g; Calories = 130

Ice Cream Sandwich Vanilla Light No Sugar Added ☛ serving size: 1 serving = 70 g; Calories = 140

Ice Cream Soda Chocolate ☛ serving size: 1 soda (10 fl oz) = 240 g; Calories = 209

Ice Cream Soda Flavors Other Than Chocolate ☛ serving size: 1 soda (10 fl oz) = 240 g; Calories = 204

Ice Cream Sundae Chocolate Or Fudge Topping With Whipped Cream ☛ serving size: 1 sundae = 165 g; Calories = 436

Ice Cream Sundae Fruit Topping With Whipped Cream ☛ serving size: 1 sundae = 165 g; Calories = 388

Ice Cream Sundae Fudge Topping With Cake With Whipped Cream ☛ serving size: 1 sundae = 175 g; Calories = 488

Ice Cream Sundae Not Fruit Or Chocolate Topping With Whipped Cream ☛ serving size: 1 sundae = 165 g; Calories = 368

Ice Cream Sundae Ns As To Topping With Whipped Cream ☛ serving size: 1 sundae = 165 g; Calories = 424

Ice Cream Sundae Prepackaged Type Flavors Other Than Chocolate ☛ serving size: 1 sundae (6 fl oz) = 131 g; Calories = 242

Imitation Cheese American Or Cheddar Low Cholesterol ☛ serving size: 1 cup, shredded = 113 g; Calories = 441

Imitation Sour Cream ☛ serving size: 1 oz = 28.4 g; Calories = 59

Kefir Ns As To Fat Content ☛ serving size: 1 cup = 244 g; Calories = 127

Kraft Breakstones Free Fat Free Sour Cream ☛ serving size: 2 tbsp = 32 g; Calories = 29

Kraft Breakstones Reduced Fat Sour Cream ☞ serving size: 2 tbsp = 31 g; Calories = 47

Kraft Cheez Whiz Light Pasteurized Process Cheese Product ☞ serving size: 2 tbsp = 35 g; Calories = 75

Kraft Cheez Whiz Pasteurized Process Cheese Sauce ☞ serving size: 2 tbsp = 33 g; Calories = 91

Kraft Free Singles American Nonfat Pasteurized Process Cheese Product ☞ serving size: 1 slice = 21 g; Calories = 31

Kraft Velveeta Light Reduced Fat Pasteurized Process Cheese Product ☞ serving size: 1 oz = 28 g; Calories = 62

Kraft Velveeta Pasteurized Process Cheese Spread ☞ serving size: 1 oz = 28 g; Calories = 85

Light Cream (Coffe Cream) ☞ serving size: 1 fl oz = 30 g; Calories = 59

Light Ice Cream Bar Or Stick Chocolate Coated ☞ serving size: 1 bar (3 fl oz) = 56 g; Calories = 162

Light Ice Cream Bar Or Stick Chocolate Covered With Nuts ☞ serving size: 1 bar = 149 g; Calories = 490

Light Ice Cream Cone Chocolate ☞ serving size: 1 cone and single dip (or 1 small cone) = 78 g; Calories = 131

Light Ice Cream Cone Flavors Other Than Chocolate ☞ serving size: 1 cone and single dip (or 1 small cone) = 78 g; Calories = 115

Light Ice Cream Cone Nfs ☞ serving size: 1 cone and single dip (or 1 small cone) = 78 g; Calories = 115

Light Ice Cream Creamsicle Or Dreamsicle No Sugar Added ☞ serving size: 1 sicle = 40 g; Calories = 20

Light Ice Cream Fudgesicle ☞ serving size: 1 sicle (2.5 fl oz) = 73 g; Calories = 133

Light Ice Cream No Sugar Added Cone Chocolate ☛ serving size: 1 cone and single dip (or 1 small cone) = 78 g; Calories = 177

Light Ice Cream No Sugar Added Cone Ns As To Flavor ☛ serving size: 1 cone and single dip (or 1 small cone) = 78 g; Calories = 175

Light Ice Cream Soft Serve Blended With Candy Or Cookies ☛ serving size: 1 small dairy queen blizzard = 298 g; Calories = 525

Light Ice Cream Soft Serve Cone Chocolate ☛ serving size: 1 small fast food cone (include dairy queen) = 142 g; Calories = 236

Light Ice Cream Sundae Soft Serve Chocolate Or Fudge Topping With Whipped Cream ☛ serving size: 1 sundae = 165 g; Calories = 421

Light Ice Cream Sundae Soft Serve Chocolate Or Fudge Topping Without Whipped Cream ☛ serving size: 1 sundae = 179 g; Calories = 326

Light Ice Cream Sundae Soft Serve Fruit Topping With Whipped Cream ☛ serving size: 1 sundae = 165 g; Calories = 368

Light Ice Cream Sundae Soft Serve Fruit Topping Without Whipped Cream ☛ serving size: 1 sundae = 178 g; Calories = 281

Light Ice Cream Sundae Soft Serve Not Fruit Or Chocolate Topping With Whipped Cream ☛ serving size: 1 sundae = 165 g; Calories = 335

Light Ice Cream Sundae Soft Serve Not Fruit Or Chocolate Topping Without Whipped Cream ☛ serving size: 1 sundae = 182 g; Calories = 269

Light Whipping Cream ☛ serving size: 1 cup, whipped = 120 g; Calories = 350

Limburger Cheese ☛ serving size: 1 cup = 134 g; Calories = 438

Low Fat Fruit Yogurt (With Vitamin D) ☛ serving size: 1 container (6 oz) = 170 g; Calories = 173

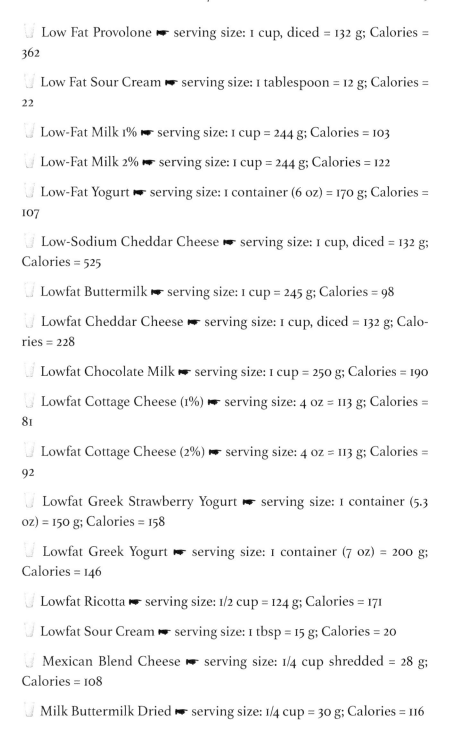

Low Fat Provolone ☞ serving size: 1 cup, diced = 132 g; Calories = 362

Low Fat Sour Cream ☞ serving size: 1 tablespoon = 12 g; Calories = 22

Low-Fat Milk 1% ☞ serving size: 1 cup = 244 g; Calories = 103

Low-Fat Milk 2% ☞ serving size: 1 cup = 244 g; Calories = 122

Low-Fat Yogurt ☞ serving size: 1 container (6 oz) = 170 g; Calories = 107

Low-Sodium Cheddar Cheese ☞ serving size: 1 cup, diced = 132 g; Calories = 525

Lowfat Buttermilk ☞ serving size: 1 cup = 245 g; Calories = 98

Lowfat Cheddar Cheese ☞ serving size: 1 cup, diced = 132 g; Calories = 228

Lowfat Chocolate Milk ☞ serving size: 1 cup = 250 g; Calories = 190

Lowfat Cottage Cheese (1%) ☞ serving size: 4 oz = 113 g; Calories = 81

Lowfat Cottage Cheese (2%) ☞ serving size: 4 oz = 113 g; Calories = 92

Lowfat Greek Strawberry Yogurt ☞ serving size: 1 container (5.3 oz) = 150 g; Calories = 158

Lowfat Greek Yogurt ☞ serving size: 1 container (7 oz) = 200 g; Calories = 146

Lowfat Ricotta ☞ serving size: 1/2 cup = 124 g; Calories = 171

Lowfat Sour Cream ☞ serving size: 1 tbsp = 15 g; Calories = 20

Mexican Blend Cheese ☞ serving size: 1/4 cup shredded = 28 g; Calories = 108

Milk Buttermilk Dried ☞ serving size: 1/4 cup = 30 g; Calories = 116

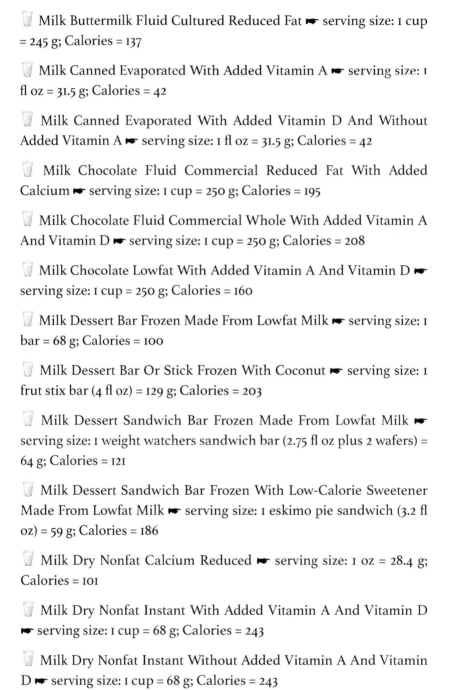

⬜ Milk Buttermilk Fluid Cultured Reduced Fat ☛ serving size: 1 cup = 245 g; Calories = 137

⬜ Milk Canned Evaporated With Added Vitamin A ☛ serving size: 1 fl oz = 31.5 g; Calories = 42

⬜ Milk Canned Evaporated With Added Vitamin D And Without Added Vitamin A ☛ serving size: 1 fl oz = 31.5 g; Calories = 42

⬜ Milk Chocolate Fluid Commercial Reduced Fat With Added Calcium ☛ serving size: 1 cup = 250 g; Calories = 195

⬜ Milk Chocolate Fluid Commercial Whole With Added Vitamin A And Vitamin D ☛ serving size: 1 cup = 250 g; Calories = 208

⬜ Milk Chocolate Lowfat With Added Vitamin A And Vitamin D ☛ serving size: 1 cup = 250 g; Calories = 160

⬜ Milk Dessert Bar Frozen Made From Lowfat Milk ☛ serving size: 1 bar = 68 g; Calories = 100

⬜ Milk Dessert Bar Or Stick Frozen With Coconut ☛ serving size: 1 frut stix bar (4 fl oz) = 129 g; Calories = 203

⬜ Milk Dessert Sandwich Bar Frozen Made From Lowfat Milk ☛ serving size: 1 weight watchers sandwich bar (2.75 fl oz plus 2 wafers) = 64 g; Calories = 121

⬜ Milk Dessert Sandwich Bar Frozen With Low-Calorie Sweetener Made From Lowfat Milk ☛ serving size: 1 eskimo pie sandwich (3.2 fl oz) = 59 g; Calories = 186

⬜ Milk Dry Nonfat Calcium Reduced ☛ serving size: 1 oz = 28.4 g; Calories = 101

⬜ Milk Dry Nonfat Instant With Added Vitamin A And Vitamin D ☛ serving size: 1 cup = 68 g; Calories = 243

⬜ Milk Dry Nonfat Instant Without Added Vitamin A And Vitamin D ☛ serving size: 1 cup = 68 g; Calories = 243

Milk Dry Nonfat Regular With Added Vitamin A And Vitamin D serving size: 1/4 cup = 30 g; Calories = 109

Milk Dry Nonfat Regular Without Added Vitamin A And Vitamin D serving size: 1/4 cup = 30 g; Calories = 109

Milk Dry Reconstituted Fat Free (Skim) serving size: 1 cup = 244 g; Calories = 78

Milk Dry Reconstituted Low Fat (1%) serving size: 1 cup = 244 g; Calories = 98

Milk Dry Reconstituted Ns As To Fat Content serving size: 1 cup = 244 g; Calories = 78

Milk Dry Reconstituted Whole serving size: 1 cup = 244 g; Calories = 185

Milk Dry Whole Without Added Vitamin D serving size: 1 cup = 128 g; Calories = 635

Milk Evaporated 2% Fat With Added Vitamin A And Vitamin D serving size: 1 cup = 252 g; Calories = 270

Milk Evaporated Reduced Fat (2%) serving size: 1 cup = 252 g; Calories = 232

Milk Filled Fluid With Blend Of Hydrogenated Vegetable Oils serving size: 1 cup = 244 g; Calories = 154

Milk Filled Fluid With Lauric Acid Oil serving size: 1 cup = 244 g; Calories = 154

Milk Fluid 1% Fat Without Added Vitamin A And Vitamin D serving size: 1 cup = 244 g; Calories = 103

Milk Fluid Nonfat Calcium Fortified (Fat Free Or Skim) serving size: 1 cup = 247 g; Calories = 87

Milk Imitation Non-Soy serving size: 1 cup = 244 g; Calories = 112

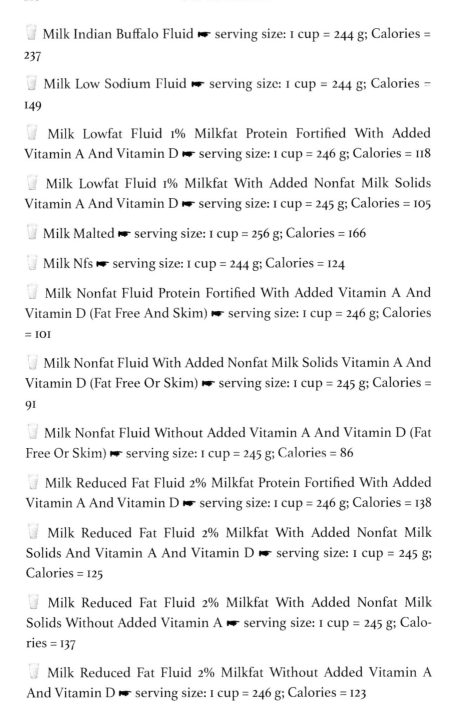

Milk Indian Buffalo Fluid ☞ serving size: 1 cup = 244 g; Calories = 237

Milk Low Sodium Fluid ☞ serving size: 1 cup = 244 g; Calories = 149

Milk Lowfat Fluid 1% Milkfat Protein Fortified With Added Vitamin A And Vitamin D ☞ serving size: 1 cup = 246 g; Calories = 118

Milk Lowfat Fluid 1% Milkfat With Added Nonfat Milk Solids Vitamin A And Vitamin D ☞ serving size: 1 cup = 245 g; Calories = 105

Milk Malted ☞ serving size: 1 cup = 256 g; Calories = 166

Milk Nfs ☞ serving size: 1 cup = 244 g; Calories = 124

Milk Nonfat Fluid Protein Fortified With Added Vitamin A And Vitamin D (Fat Free And Skim) ☞ serving size: 1 cup = 246 g; Calories = 101

Milk Nonfat Fluid With Added Nonfat Milk Solids Vitamin A And Vitamin D (Fat Free Or Skim) ☞ serving size: 1 cup = 245 g; Calories = 91

Milk Nonfat Fluid Without Added Vitamin A And Vitamin D (Fat Free Or Skim) ☞ serving size: 1 cup = 245 g; Calories = 86

Milk Reduced Fat Fluid 2% Milkfat Protein Fortified With Added Vitamin A And Vitamin D ☞ serving size: 1 cup = 246 g; Calories = 138

Milk Reduced Fat Fluid 2% Milkfat With Added Nonfat Milk Solids And Vitamin A And Vitamin D ☞ serving size: 1 cup = 245 g; Calories = 125

Milk Reduced Fat Fluid 2% Milkfat With Added Nonfat Milk Solids Without Added Vitamin A ☞ serving size: 1 cup = 245 g; Calories = 137

Milk Reduced Fat Fluid 2% Milkfat Without Added Vitamin A And Vitamin D ☞ serving size: 1 cup = 246 g; Calories = 123

Milk Shake Bottled Chocolate ☛ serving size: 1 fl oz = 31 g; Calories = 47

Milk Shake Home Recipe Chocolate ☛ serving size: 1 fl oz = 28 g; Calories = 34

Milk Shake Home Recipe Chocolate Light ☛ serving size: 1 fl oz = 28 g; Calories = 27

Milk Shake Home Recipe Flavors Other Than Chocolate ☛ serving size: 1 fl oz = 28 g; Calories = 33

Milk Shake Home Recipe Flavors Other Than Chocolate Light ☛ serving size: 1 fl oz = 28 g; Calories = 26

Milk Shake With Malt ☛ serving size: 1 fl oz = 28 g; Calories = 36

Milk Shakes Thick Chocolate ☛ serving size: 1 fl oz = 28.4 g; Calories = 34

Milk Shakes Thick Vanilla ☛ serving size: 1 fl oz = 28.4 g; Calories = 32

Milk Sheep Fluid ☛ serving size: 1 cup = 245 g; Calories = 265

Milk Substitutes Fluid With Lauric Acid Oil ☛ serving size: 1 cup = 244 g; Calories = 149

Milk Whole 3.25% Milkfat Without Added Vitamin A And Vitamin D ☛ serving size: 1 cup = 244 g; Calories = 149

Monterey Cheese ☛ serving size: 1 cup, diced = 132 g; Calories = 492

Mozzarella ☛ serving size: 1 cup, shredded = 112 g; Calories = 335

Mozzarella (Hard And Lowfat) ☛ serving size: 1 cup, diced = 132 g; Calories = 389

Mozzarella (Hard) ☛ serving size: 1 oz = 28.4 g; Calories = 90

Mozzarella (Lowfat) ☛ serving size: 1 oz = 28.4 g; Calories = 72

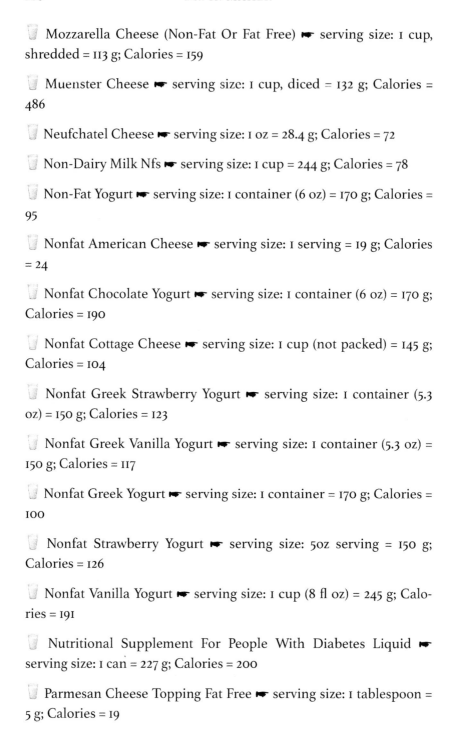

Mozzarella Cheese (Non-Fat Or Fat Free) ☞ serving size: 1 cup, shredded = 113 g; Calories = 159

Muenster Cheese ☞ serving size: 1 cup, diced = 132 g; Calories = 486

Neufchatel Cheese ☞ serving size: 1 oz = 28.4 g; Calories = 72

Non-Dairy Milk Nfs ☞ serving size: 1 cup = 244 g; Calories = 78

Non-Fat Yogurt ☞ serving size: 1 container (6 oz) = 170 g; Calories = 95

Nonfat American Cheese ☞ serving size: 1 serving = 19 g; Calories = 24

Nonfat Chocolate Yogurt ☞ serving size: 1 container (6 oz) = 170 g; Calories = 190

Nonfat Cottage Cheese ☞ serving size: 1 cup (not packed) = 145 g; Calories = 104

Nonfat Greek Strawberry Yogurt ☞ serving size: 1 container (5.3 oz) = 150 g; Calories = 123

Nonfat Greek Vanilla Yogurt ☞ serving size: 1 container (5.3 oz) = 150 g; Calories = 117

Nonfat Greek Yogurt ☞ serving size: 1 container = 170 g; Calories = 100

Nonfat Strawberry Yogurt ☞ serving size: 5oz serving = 150 g; Calories = 126

Nonfat Vanilla Yogurt ☞ serving size: 1 cup (8 fl oz) = 245 g; Calories = 191

Nutritional Supplement For People With Diabetes Liquid ☞ serving size: 1 can = 227 g; Calories = 200

Parmesan Cheese Topping Fat Free ☞ serving size: 1 tablespoon = 5 g; Calories = 19

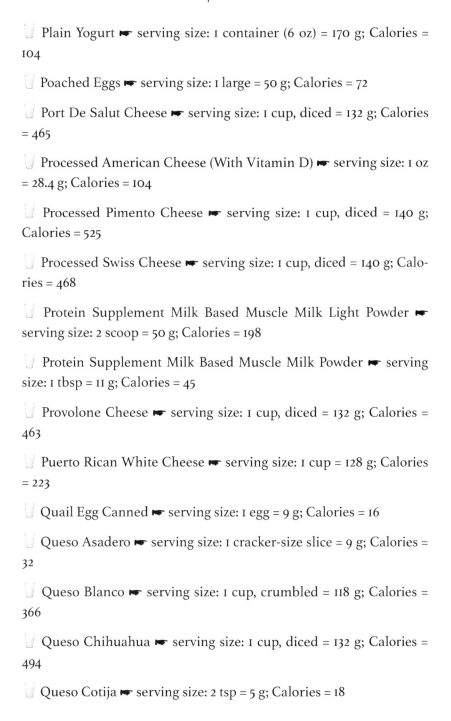

Plain Yogurt ☛ serving size: 1 container (6 oz) = 170 g; Calories = 104

Poached Eggs ☛ serving size: 1 large = 50 g; Calories = 72

Port De Salut Cheese ☛ serving size: 1 cup, diced = 132 g; Calories = 465

Processed American Cheese (With Vitamin D) ☛ serving size: 1 oz = 28.4 g; Calories = 104

Processed Pimento Cheese ☛ serving size: 1 cup, diced = 140 g; Calories = 525

Processed Swiss Cheese ☛ serving size: 1 cup, diced = 140 g; Calories = 468

Protein Supplement Milk Based Muscle Milk Light Powder ☛ serving size: 2 scoop = 50 g; Calories = 198

Protein Supplement Milk Based Muscle Milk Powder ☛ serving size: 1 tbsp = 11 g; Calories = 45

Provolone Cheese ☛ serving size: 1 cup, diced = 132 g; Calories = 463

Puerto Rican White Cheese ☛ serving size: 1 cup = 128 g; Calories = 223

Quail Egg Canned ☛ serving size: 1 egg = 9 g; Calories = 16

Queso Asadero ☛ serving size: 1 cracker-size slice = 9 g; Calories = 32

Queso Blanco ☛ serving size: 1 cup, crumbled = 118 g; Calories = 366

Queso Chihuahua ☛ serving size: 1 cup, diced = 132 g; Calories = 494

Queso Cotija ☛ serving size: 2 tsp = 5 g; Calories = 18

Queso Fresco ☞ serving size: 1 cup, crumbled = 122 g; Calories = 365

Reddi Wip Fat Free Whipped Topping ☞ serving size: 1 tablespoon = 4 g; Calories = 6

Rice Dessert Bar Frozen Chocolate Nondairy Chocolate Covered ☞ serving size: 1 bar (4 oz) = 113 g; Calories = 268

Rice Dessert Bar Frozen Flavors Other Than Chocolate Nondairy Carob Covered ☞ serving size: 1 bar (4 oz) = 113 g; Calories = 249

Rice Frozen Dessert Nondairy Flavors Other Than Chocolate ☞ serving size: 1 cup = 172 g; Calories = 260

Ricotta Cheese ☞ serving size: 1/2 cup = 124 g; Calories = 186

Ripe Plantain Omelet Puerto Rican Style ☞ serving size: 1 medium egg = 79 g; Calories = 177

Romano Cheese ☞ serving size: 1 oz = 28.4 g; Calories = 110

Roquefort ☞ serving size: 1 oz = 28.4 g; Calories = 105

Salted Butter ☞ serving size: 1 pat (1 inch sq, 1/3 inch high) = 5 g; Calories = 36

Scrambled Eggs ☞ serving size: 1 large = 61 g; Calories = 91

Scrambled Eggs With Jerked Beef Puerto Rican Style ☞ serving size: 1 cup = 140 g; Calories = 364

Seafood Souffle ☞ serving size: 1 cup = 159 g; Calories = 240

Sharp Cheddar Cheese ☞ serving size: 1 slice (2/3 oz) = 19 g; Calories = 78

Shredded Parmesan ☞ serving size: 1 tbsp = 5 g; Calories = 21

Shrimp-Egg Patty ☞ serving size: 1 patty (about 2" dia) = 18 g; Calories = 88

Skim Milk ☞ serving size: 1 cup = 245 g; Calories = 83

Soft Goat Cheese ☛ serving size: 1 oz = 28.4 g; Calories = 75

Soft Serve Chocolate Ice Cream ☛ serving size: 1/2 cup = 86 g; Calories = 191

Sour Cream Light ☛ serving size: 1 tablespoon = 12 g; Calories = 16

Sour Dressing Non-Butterfat Cultured Filled Cream-Type ☛ serving size: 1 tbsp = 12 g; Calories = 21

Squash Summer Souffle ☛ serving size: 1 cup = 136 g; Calories = 166

Squash Winter Souffle ☛ serving size: 1 cup = 157 g; Calories = 123

Strawberry Milk Fat Free ☛ serving size: 1 fl oz = 31 g; Calories = 17

Strawberry Milk Low Fat ☛ serving size: 1 cup = 248 g; Calories = 156

Strawberry Milk Nfs ☛ serving size: 1 fl oz = 31 g; Calories = 16

Strawberry Milk Non-Dairy ☛ serving size: 1 cup = 248 g; Calories = 154

Strawberry Milk Reduced Fat ☛ serving size: 1 cup = 248 g; Calories = 176

Strawberry Milk Whole ☛ serving size: 1 cup = 248 g; Calories = 201

Sweet Whey Fluid ☛ serving size: 1 cup = 246 g; Calories = 66

Sweetened Condensed Milk ☛ serving size: 1 fl oz = 38.2 g; Calories = 123

Swiss Cheese ☛ serving size: 1 cup, diced = 132 g; Calories = 519

Tilsit Cheese ☛ serving size: 1 oz = 28.4 g; Calories = 97

Tofu Frozen Dessert Chocolate ☛ serving size: 1 cup = 164 g; Calories = 389

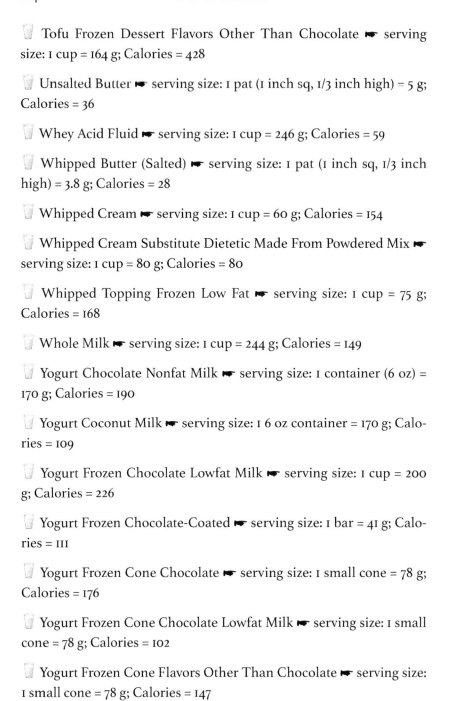

Tofu Frozen Dessert Flavors Other Than Chocolate ☛ serving size: 1 cup = 164 g; Calories = 428

Unsalted Butter ☛ serving size: 1 pat (1 inch sq, 1/3 inch high) = 5 g; Calories = 36

Whey Acid Fluid ☛ serving size: 1 cup = 246 g; Calories = 59

Whipped Butter (Salted) ☛ serving size: 1 pat (1 inch sq, 1/3 inch high) = 3.8 g; Calories = 28

Whipped Cream ☛ serving size: 1 cup = 60 g; Calories = 154

Whipped Cream Substitute Dietetic Made From Powdered Mix ☛ serving size: 1 cup = 80 g; Calories = 80

Whipped Topping Frozen Low Fat ☛ serving size: 1 cup = 75 g; Calories = 168

Whole Milk ☛ serving size: 1 cup = 244 g; Calories = 149

Yogurt Chocolate Nonfat Milk ☛ serving size: 1 container (6 oz) = 170 g; Calories = 190

Yogurt Coconut Milk ☛ serving size: 1 6 oz container = 170 g; Calories = 109

Yogurt Frozen Chocolate Lowfat Milk ☛ serving size: 1 cup = 200 g; Calories = 226

Yogurt Frozen Chocolate-Coated ☛ serving size: 1 bar = 41 g; Calories = 111

Yogurt Frozen Cone Chocolate ☛ serving size: 1 small cone = 78 g; Calories = 176

Yogurt Frozen Cone Chocolate Lowfat Milk ☛ serving size: 1 small cone = 78 g; Calories = 102

Yogurt Frozen Cone Flavors Other Than Chocolate ☛ serving size: 1 small cone = 78 g; Calories = 147

Yogurt Frozen Cone Flavors Other Than Chocolate Lowfat Milk ☛ serving size: 1 small cone = 78 g; Calories = 66

Yogurt Frozen Flavors Not Chocolate Nonfat Milk With Low-Calorie Sweetener ☛ serving size: 1/2 cup = 68 g; Calories = 71

Yogurt Frozen Flavors Other Than Chocolate With Sorbet Or Sorbet-Coated ☛ serving size: 1 haagen-dazs bar (2.3 fl oz) = 75 g; Calories = 114

Yogurt Frozen Ns As To Flavor Nonfat Milk ☛ serving size: 1 cup = 159 g; Calories = 192

Yogurt Frozen Sandwich ☛ serving size: 1 sandwich = 85 g; Calories = 180

Yogurt Fruit Low Fat 10 Grams Protein Per 8 Ounce ☛ serving size: 1 container (6 oz) = 170 g; Calories = 173

Yogurt Fruit Low Fat 11 Grams Protein Per 8 Ounce ☛ serving size: 1 container (6 oz) = 170 g; Calories = 179

Yogurt Fruit Low Fat 9 Grams Protein Per 8 Ounce ☛ serving size: 1 container (6 oz) = 170 g; Calories = 168

Yogurt Fruit Low Fat 9 Grams Protein Per 8 Ounce Fortified With Vitamin D ☛ serving size: 1 container (6 oz) = 170 g; Calories = 168

Yogurt Fruit Lowfat With Low Calorie Sweetener ☛ serving size: 1 container (6 oz) = 170 g; Calories = 179

Yogurt Fruit Lowfat With Low Calorie Sweetener Fortified With Vitamin D ☛ serving size: 1 container (6 oz) = 170 g; Calories = 179

Yogurt Fruit Variety Nonfat ☛ serving size: 1 container (6 oz) = 170 g; Calories = 162

Yogurt Fruit Variety Nonfat Fortified With Vitamin D ☛ serving size: 1 container (6 oz) = 170 g; Calories = 162

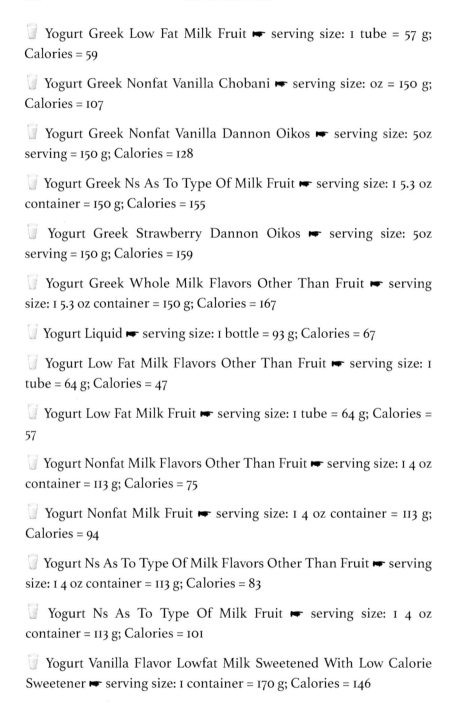

Yogurt Greek Low Fat Milk Fruit ☞ serving size: 1 tube = 57 g; Calories = 59

Yogurt Greek Nonfat Vanilla Chobani ☞ serving size: oz = 150 g; Calories = 107

Yogurt Greek Nonfat Vanilla Dannon Oikos ☞ serving size: 5oz serving = 150 g; Calories = 128

Yogurt Greek Ns As To Type Of Milk Fruit ☞ serving size: 1 5.3 oz container = 150 g; Calories = 155

Yogurt Greek Strawberry Dannon Oikos ☞ serving size: 5oz serving = 150 g; Calories = 159

Yogurt Greek Whole Milk Flavors Other Than Fruit ☞ serving size: 1 5.3 oz container = 150 g; Calories = 167

Yogurt Liquid ☞ serving size: 1 bottle = 93 g; Calories = 67

Yogurt Low Fat Milk Flavors Other Than Fruit ☞ serving size: 1 tube = 64 g; Calories = 47

Yogurt Low Fat Milk Fruit ☞ serving size: 1 tube = 64 g; Calories = 57

Yogurt Nonfat Milk Flavors Other Than Fruit ☞ serving size: 1 4 oz container = 113 g; Calories = 75

Yogurt Nonfat Milk Fruit ☞ serving size: 1 4 oz container = 113 g; Calories = 94

Yogurt Ns As To Type Of Milk Flavors Other Than Fruit ☞ serving size: 1 4 oz container = 113 g; Calories = 83

Yogurt Ns As To Type Of Milk Fruit ☞ serving size: 1 4 oz container = 113 g; Calories = 101

Yogurt Vanilla Flavor Lowfat Milk Sweetened With Low Calorie Sweetener ☞ serving size: 1 container = 170 g; Calories = 146

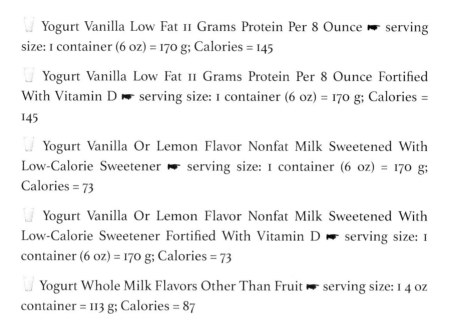

Yogurt Vanilla Low Fat 11 Grams Protein Per 8 Ounce ☛ serving size: 1 container (6 oz) = 170 g; Calories = 145

Yogurt Vanilla Low Fat 11 Grams Protein Per 8 Ounce Fortified With Vitamin D ☛ serving size: 1 container (6 oz) = 170 g; Calories = 145

Yogurt Vanilla Or Lemon Flavor Nonfat Milk Sweetened With Low-Calorie Sweetener ☛ serving size: 1 container (6 oz) = 170 g; Calories = 73

Yogurt Vanilla Or Lemon Flavor Nonfat Milk Sweetened With Low-Calorie Sweetener Fortified With Vitamin D ☛ serving size: 1 container (6 oz) = 170 g; Calories = 73

Yogurt Whole Milk Flavors Other Than Fruit ☛ serving size: 1 4 oz container = 113 g; Calories = 87

13

FAST FOODS

Arbys Roast Beef Sandwich Classic ☞ serving size: 1 sandwich = 149 g; Calories = 361

Bacon And Cheese Sandwich With Spread ☞ serving size: 1 sandwich = 121 g; Calories = 379

Bacon And Egg Sandwich ☞ serving size: 1 sandwich = 177 g; Calories = 420

Bacon Breaded Fried Chicken Fillet And Tomato Club With Lettuce And Spread ☞ serving size: 1 sandwich = 227 g; Calories = 583

Bacon Cheeseburger 1 Large Patty With Condiments On Bun From Fast Food / Restaurant ☞ serving size: 1 (1/3 lb) cheeseburger = 335 g; Calories = 794

Bacon Cheeseburger 1 Medium Patty Plain On Bun From Fast Food / Restaurant ☞ serving size: 1 (1/4 lb) bacon cheeseburger = 170 g; Calories = 553

Bacon Cheeseburger 1 Medium Patty Plain On White Bun ☞ serving size: 1 (1/4 lb) bacon cheeseburger = 180 g; Calories = 544

Bacon Cheeseburger 1 Medium Patty With Condiments On Bun From Fast Food / Restaurant ☛ serving size: 1 (1/4 lb) bacon cheeseburger = 240 g; Calories = 677

Bacon Cheeseburger 1 Medium Patty With Condiments On Wheat Bun ☛ serving size: 1 (1/4 lb) bacon cheeseburger = 240 g; Calories = 586

Bacon Cheeseburger 1 Medium Patty With Condiments On White Bun ☛ serving size: 1 (1/4 lb) bacon cheeseburger = 240 g; Calories = 595

Bacon Cheeseburger 1 Medium Patty With Condiments On Whole Wheat Bun ☛ serving size: 1 (1/4 lb) bacon cheeseburger = 240 g; Calories = 586

Bacon Cheeseburger 1 Small Patty With Condiments On Bun From Fast Food / Restaurant ☛ serving size: 1 bacon cheeseburger = 160 g; Calories = 459

Bacon Cheeseburger 1 Small Patty With Condiments On Bun From Fast Food / Restaurant (Wendy's Jr. Bacon Cheeseburger) ☛ serving size: 1 wendy's jr. bacon cheeseburger = 150 g; Calories = 408

Bacon Chicken And Tomato Club Sandwich On Multigrain Roll With Lettuce And Spread ☛ serving size: 1 sandwich = 194 g; Calories = 433

Bacon Lettuce And Tomato Sandwich With Spread ☛ serving size: 1 sandwich = 164 g; Calories = 340

Bacon Lettuce Tomato And Cheese Submarine Sandwich With Spread ☛ serving size: 1 submarine = 260 g; Calories = 606

Bacon On Biscuit ☛ serving size: 1 sandwich = 93 g; Calories = 330

Bacon Sandwich With Spread ☛ serving size: 1 sandwich = 91 g; Calories = 324

Bagel With Breakfast Steak Egg Cheese And Condiments ☛ serving size: 1 item = 254 g; Calories = 716

Bagel With Egg Sausage Patty Cheese And Condiments ☛ serving size: 1 item = 219 g; Calories = 646

Beef Barbecue Sandwich Or Sloppy Joe On Bun ☛ serving size: 1 barbecue sandwich = 186 g; Calories = 433

Beef Barbecue Submarine Sandwich On Bun ☛ serving size: 1 sandwich = 192 g; Calories = 424

Beef Sandwich Nfs ☛ serving size: 1 sandwich = 133 g; Calories = 253

Biscuit With Crispy Chicken Fillet ☛ serving size: 1 item = 132 g; Calories = 396

Biscuit With Egg And Bacon ☛ serving size: 1 biscuit = 150 g; Calories = 458

Biscuit With Egg And Ham ☛ serving size: 1 biscuit = 182 g; Calories = 424

Biscuit With Egg Cheese And Bacon ☛ serving size: 1 item = 145 g; Calories = 437

Biscuit With Gravy ☛ serving size: 1 biscuit with gravy = 221 g; Calories = 475

Biscuit With Ham ☛ serving size: 1 biscuit = 162 g; Calories = 554

Biscuit With Sausage ☛ serving size: 1 item = 111 g; Calories = 412

Blended Soft Serve Ice Cream With Cookies ☛ serving size: 12 fl oz cup = 337 g; Calories = 570

Blintz Cheese-Filled ☛ serving size: 1 blintz = 70 g; Calories = 130

Blintz Fruit-Filled ☛ serving size: 1 blintz = 70 g; Calories = 123

Bologna And Cheese Sandwich With Spread ☞ serving size: 1 sandwich = 111 g; Calories = 335

Bologna Sandwich With Spread ☞ serving size: 1 sandwich = 83 g; Calories = 250

Breadstick Soft Prepared With Garlic And Parmesan Cheese ☞ serving size: 1 breadstick = 43 g; Calories = 148

Breakfast Burrito With Egg Cheese And Sausage ☞ serving size: 1 burrito = 109 g; Calories = 302

Breakfast Pizza With Egg ☞ serving size: 1 piece, nfs = 144 g; Calories = 428

Bruschetta ☞ serving size: 1 slice = 43 g; Calories = 74

Buffalo Chicken Submarine Sandwich ☞ serving size: 1 submarine = 240 g; Calories = 446

Buffalo Chicken Submarine Sandwich With Cheese ☞ serving size: 1 submarine = 260 g; Calories = 528

Burger King Cheeseburger ☞ serving size: 1 item = 133 g; Calories = 380

Burger King Chicken Strips ☞ serving size: 1 strip = 36 g; Calories = 105

Burger King Croissanwich With Egg And Cheese ☞ serving size: 1 item = 110 g; Calories = 311

Burger King Croissanwich With Sausage And Cheese ☞ serving size: 1 item = 131 g; Calories = 493

Burger King Croissanwich With Sausage Egg And Cheese ☞ serving size: 1 sandwich = 171 g; Calories = 527

Burger King Double Cheeseburger ☞ serving size: 1 sandwich = 162 g; Calories = 457

Burger King Double Whopper No Cheese ☛ serving size: 1 item = 374 g; Calories = 943

Burger King Double Whopper With Cheese ☛ serving size: 1 item = 399 g; Calories = 1061

Burger King French Fries ☛ serving size: 1 small serving = 74 g; Calories = 207

Burger King French Toast Sticks ☛ serving size: 1 stick = 21 g; Calories = 73

Burger King Hamburger ☛ serving size: 1 sandwich = 99 g; Calories = 258

Burger King Hash Brown Rounds ☛ serving size: 1 piece = 5.6 g; Calories = 17

Burger King Onion Rings ☛ serving size: 1 small = 91 g; Calories = 380

Burger King Original Chicken Sandwich ☛ serving size: 1 sandwich = 199 g; Calories = 569

Burger King Premium Fish Sandwich ☛ serving size: 1 sandwich = 220 g; Calories = 572

Burger King Vanilla Shake ☛ serving size: 1 fl oz = 24.8 g; Calories = 42

Burger King Whopper No Cheese ☛ serving size: 1 item = 291 g; Calories = 678

Burger King Whopper With Cheese ☛ serving size: 1 item = 316 g; Calories = 790

Burrito Taco Or Quesadilla With Egg ☛ serving size: 1 small = 110 g; Calories = 252

Burrito Taco Or Quesadilla With Egg And Breakfast Meat ☛ serving size: 1 small = 123 g; Calories = 298

Burrito Taco Or Quesadilla With Egg And Potato ☞ serving size: 1 small = 127 g; Calories = 299

Burrito Taco Or Quesadilla With Egg Beans And Breakfast Meat ☞ serving size: 1 small = 150 g; Calories = 336

Burrito Taco Or Quesadilla With Egg Potato And Breakfast Meat ☞ serving size: 1 small = 144 g; Calories = 354

Burrito Taco Or Quesadilla With Egg Potato And Breakfast Meat From Fast Food ☞ serving size: 1 small = 144 g; Calories = 349

Burrito With Beans ☞ serving size: 2 pieces = 217 g; Calories = 447

Burrito With Beans And Beef ☞ serving size: 1 item = 241 g; Calories = 460

Burrito With Beans And Cheese ☞ serving size: 1 each burrito = 185 g; Calories = 379

Burrito With Beans Cheese And Beef ☞ serving size: 1 burrito = 241 g; Calories = 434

Cheese Pizza ☞ serving size: 1 slice = 107 g; Calories = 285

Cheeseburger 1 Large Patty Plain On Bun From Fast Food / Restaurant ☞ serving size: 1 (1/3 lb) cheeseburger = 200 g; Calories = 600

Cheeseburger 1 Large Patty With Condiments On Bun From Fast Food / Restaurant ☞ serving size: 1 (1/3 lb) cheeseburger = 315 g; Calories = 690

Cheeseburger 1 Medium Patty Plain On Wheat Bun ☞ serving size: 1 (1/4 lb) cheeseburger = 165 g; Calories = 462

Cheeseburger 1 Medium Patty Plain On White Bun ☞ serving size: 1 (1/4 lb) cheeseburger = 165 g; Calories = 472

Cheeseburger 1 Medium Patty Plain On Whole Wheat Bun ☞ serving size: 1 cheeseburger = 165 g; Calories = 462

🍔 Cheeseburger 1 Medium Patty With Condiments On Wheat Bun ☛ serving size: 1 (1/4 lb) cheeseburger = 225 g; Calories = 513

🍔 Cheeseburger 1 Medium Patty With Condiments On White Bun ☛ serving size: 1 (1/4 lb) cheeseburger = 225 g; Calories = 524

🍔 Cheeseburger 1 Medium Patty With Condiments On Whole Wheat Bun ☛ serving size: 1 (1/4 lb) cheeseburger = 225 g; Calories = 513

🍔 Cheeseburger 1 Miniature Patty On Miniature Bun From School ☛ serving size: 1 miniature = 60 g; Calories = 150

🍔 Cheeseburger 1 Miniature Patty Plain On Miniature Bun From Fast Food / Restaurant ☛ serving size: 1 miniature = 60 g; Calories = 179

🍔 Cheeseburger 1 Miniature Patty With Condiments On Miniature Bun From Fast Food / Restaurant ☛ serving size: 1 miniature = 75 g; Calories = 198

🍔 Cheeseburger 1 Small Patty Plain On Wheat Bun ☛ serving size: 1 cheeseburger = 140 g; Calories = 395

🍔 Cheeseburger 1 Small Patty Plain On White Bun ☛ serving size: 1 cheeseburger = 140 g; Calories = 403

🍔 Cheeseburger 1 Small Patty With Condiments On Bun From Fast Food / Restaurant (Burger King Whopper Jr. With Cheese) ☛ serving size: 1 burger king whopper jr = 170 g; Calories = 383

🍔 Cheeseburger 1 Small Patty With Condiments On Bun From Fast Food / Restaurant (Wendy's Jr. Cheeseburger Deluxe) ☛ serving size: 1 wendy's jr. cheeseburger deluxe = 160 g; Calories = 360

🍔 Cheeseburger 1 Small Patty With Condiments On Wheat Bun ☛ serving size: 1 cheeseburger = 195 g; Calories = 435

🍔 Cheeseburger 1 Small Patty With Condiments On White Bun ☛ serving size: 1 cheeseburger = 195 g; Calories = 443

Cheeseburger 1 Small Patty With Condiments On Whole Wheat Bun ☛ serving size: 1 cheeseburger = 195 g; Calories = 435

Cheeseburger Double Regular Patty And Bun With Condiments ☛ serving size: 1 sandwich = 155 g; Calories = 437

Cheeseburger Nfs ☛ serving size: 1 cheeseburger = 225 g; Calories = 524

Cheeseburger On Bun From School ☛ serving size: 1 cheeseburger = 115 g; Calories = 281

Cheeseburger; Double Large Patty; With Condiments ☛ serving size: 1 item = 280 g; Calories = 762

Cheeseburger; Double Regular Patty; Double Decker Bun With Condiments And Special Sauce ☛ serving size: 1 item = 219 g; Calories = 572

Cheeseburger; Double Regular Patty; With Condiments ☛ serving size: 1 sandwich = 155 g; Calories = 437

Cheeseburger; Single Large Patty; Plain ☛ serving size: 1 sandwich = 182 g; Calories = 564

Cheeseburger; Single Large Patty; With Condiments ☛ serving size: 1 item = 199 g; Calories = 535

Cheeseburger; Single Large Patty; With Condiments Vegetables And Mayonnaise ☛ serving size: 1 sandwich = 215 g; Calories = 576

Cheeseburger; Single Regular Patty With Condiments ☛ serving size: 1 item = 127 g; Calories = 343

Cheeseburger; Single Regular Patty With Condiments And Vegetables ☛ serving size: 1 sandwich = 115 g; Calories = 292

Cheeseburger; Single Regular Patty; Plain ☛ serving size: 1 sandwich = 91 g; Calories = 280

Chick-Fil-A Chick-N-Strips ☛ serving size: 1 strip = 50 g; Calories = 114

Chick-Fil-A Chicken Sandwich ☛ serving size: 1 sandwich = 187 g; Calories = 466

Chick-Fil-A Hash Browns ☛ serving size: 1 piece = 5.5 g; Calories = 17

Chicken Barbecue Sandwich ☛ serving size: 1 sandwich = 239 g; Calories = 531

Chicken Breaded And Fried Boneless Pieces Plain ☛ serving size: 6 pieces = 96 g; Calories = 295

Chicken Fillet Breaded Fried Sandwich With Cheese Lettuce Tomato And Spread ☛ serving size: 1 sandwich = 241 g; Calories = 689

Chicken Fillet Broiled Sandwich On Oat Bran Bun With Lettuce Tomato Spread ☛ serving size: 1 burger king sandwich = 155 g; Calories = 312

Chicken Fillet Broiled Sandwich On Whole Wheat Roll With Lettuce Tomato And Spread ☛ serving size: 1 sandwich = 173 g; Calories = 353

Chicken Fillet Broiled Sandwich With Cheese On Whole Wheat Roll With Lettuce Tomato And Non-Mayonnaise Type Spread ☛ serving size: 1 wendy's sandwich = 242 g; Calories = 479

Chicken Fillet Sandwich Plain With Pickles ☛ serving size: 1 sandwich = 187 g; Calories = 468

Chicken Patty Sandwich Miniature With Spread ☛ serving size: 1 miniature sandwich = 31 g; Calories = 94

Chicken Patty Sandwich Or Biscuit ☛ serving size: 1 sandwich = 173 g; Calories = 533

Chicken Patty Sandwich With Cheese On Wheat Bun With

Lettuce Tomato And Spread ☛ serving size: 1 sandwich = 227 g; Calories = 577

Chicken Salad Or Chicken Spread Sandwich ☛ serving size: 1 sandwich = 141 g; Calories = 324

Chicken Sandwich With Cheese And Spread ☛ serving size: 1 sandwich = 136 g; Calories = 321

Chicken Sandwich With Spread ☛ serving size: 1 sandwich = 112 g; Calories = 250

Chicken Tenders ☛ serving size: 1 strip = 30 g; Calories = 81

Chiliburger With Or Without Cheese On Bun ☛ serving size: 1 chiliburger = 160 g; Calories = 403

Chinese Pancake ☛ serving size: 1 pancake = 28 g; Calories = 58

Coleslaw (Fast Food) ☛ serving size: 1 cup = 191 g; Calories = 292

Corned Beef Sandwich ☛ serving size: 1 sandwich = 130 g; Calories = 268

Crab Cake Sandwich On Bun ☛ serving size: 1 sandwich = 140 g; Calories = 328

Crepe Chocolate Filled ☛ serving size: 1 crepe with filling, any size = 80 g; Calories = 125

Crepe Fruit Filled ☛ serving size: 1 crepe with filling, any size = 80 g; Calories = 147

Crepe Nfs ☛ serving size: 1 crepe, any size = 80 g; Calories = 178

Crepe Ns As To Filling ☛ serving size: 1 crepe with filling, any size = 80 g; Calories = 147

Crepe Plain ☛ serving size: 1 crepe, any size = 65 g; Calories = 145

Crispy Chicken Bacon And Tomato Club Sandwich With Cheese

Lettuce And Mayonnaise 🐄 serving size: 1 sandwich = 271 g; Calories = 697

🍔 Crispy Chicken In Tortilla With Lettuce Cheese And Ranch Sauce 🐄 serving size: 1 item = 133 g; Calories = 366

🍔 Croissant Sandwich Filled With Broccoli And Cheese 🐄 serving size: 1 croissant = 113 g; Calories = 303

🍔 Croissant Sandwich Filled With Chicken Broccoli And Cheese Sauce 🐄 serving size: 1 croissant = 128 g; Calories = 347

🍔 Croissant Sandwich Filled With Ham And Cheese 🐄 serving size: 1 croissant = 113 g; Calories = 338

🍔 Croissant Sandwich With Bacon And Egg 🐄 serving size: 1 croissant = 113 g; Calories = 372

🍔 Croissant Sandwich With Bacon Egg And Cheese 🐄 serving size: 1 croissant = 131 g; Calories = 409

🍔 Croissant Sandwich With Sausage And Egg 🐄 serving size: 1 croissant = 142 g; Calories = 497

🍔 Croissant With Egg Cheese And Bacon 🐄 serving size: 1 item = 128 g; Calories = 370

🍔 Croissant With Egg Cheese And Ham 🐄 serving size: 1 item = 155 g; Calories = 405

🍔 Croissant With Egg Cheese And Sausage 🐄 serving size: 1 sandwich = 171 g; Calories = 527

🍔 Cuban Sandwich With Spread 🐄 serving size: 1 sandwich (6" long) = 255 g; Calories = 699

🍔 Digiorno Pizza Cheese Topping Cheese Stuffed Crust Frozen Baked 🐄 serving size: 1 slice 1/4 of pie = 164 g; Calories = 458

🍔 Digiorno Pizza Cheese Topping Rising Crust Frozen Baked 🐄 serving size: 1 slice 1/4 of pie = 183 g; Calories = 469

Digiorno Pizza Cheese Topping Thin Crispy Crust Frozen Baked ☛ serving size: 1 slice 1/4 of pie = 161 g; Calories = 398

Digiorno Pizza Pepperoni Topping Cheese Stuffed Crust Frozen Baked ☛ serving size: 1 slice 1/4 of pie = 179 g; Calories = 499

Digiorno Pizza Pepperoni Topping Rising Crust Frozen Baked ☛ serving size: 1 slice 1/4 of pie = 207 g; Calories = 549

Digiorno Pizza Pepperoni Topping Thin Crispy Crust Frozen Baked ☛ serving size: 1 slice 1/4 of pie = 145 g; Calories = 410

Digiorno Pizza Supreme Topping Rising Crust Frozen Baked ☛ serving size: 1 slice 1/4 of pie = 227 g; Calories = 579

Digiorno Pizza Supreme Topping Thin Crispy Crust Frozen Baked ☛ serving size: 1 slice 1/4 of pie = 155 g; Calories = 395

Dominos 14 Inch Cheese Pizza Classic Hand-Tossed Crust ☛ serving size: 1 slice = 108 g; Calories = 278

Dominos 14 Inch Cheese Pizza Crunchy Thin Crust ☛ serving size: 1 slice = 70 g; Calories = 209

Dominos 14 Inch Cheese Pizza Ultimate Deep Dish Crust ☛ serving size: 1 slice = 118 g; Calories = 313

Dominos 14 Inch Extravaganzza Feast Pizza Classic Hand-Tossed Crust ☛ serving size: 1 slice = 151 g; Calories = 368

Dominos 14 Inch Pepperoni Pizza Classic Hand-Tossed Crust ☛ serving size: 1 slice = 113 g; Calories = 309

Dominos 14 Inch Pepperoni Pizza Crunchy Thin Crust ☛ serving size: 1 slice = 79 g; Calories = 259

Dominos 14 Inch Pepperoni Pizza Ultimate Deep Dish Crust ☛ serving size: 1 slice = 123 g; Calories = 348

Dominos 14 Inch Sausage Pizza Classic Hand-Tossed Crust ☛ serving size: 1 slice = 114 g; Calories = 311

Dominos 14 Inch Sausage Pizza Crunchy Thin Crust ☞ serving size: 1 slice = 78 g; Calories = 249

Dominos 14 Inch Sausage Pizza Ultimate Deep Dish Crust ☞ serving size: 1 slice = 129 g; Calories = 357

Dosa (Indian) Plain ☞ serving size: 1 small = 35 g; Calories = 73

Double Bacon Cheeseburger 2 Large Patties With Condiments On Bun From Fast Food / Restaurant ☞ serving size: 1 sandwich = 400 g; Calories = 1172

Double Bacon Cheeseburger 2 Medium Patties Plain On Bun From Fast Food / Restaurant ☞ serving size: 1 double bacon cheeseburger = 275 g; Calories = 855

Double Bacon Cheeseburger 2 Medium Patties With Condiments On Bun From Fast Food / Restaurant ☞ serving size: 1 double bacon cheeseburger = 335 g; Calories = 908

Double Bacon Cheeseburger 2 Medium Patties With Condiments On Bun From Fast Food / Restaurant (Wendy's Baconator) ☞ serving size: 1 wendy's baconator = 335 g; Calories = 908

Double Bacon Cheeseburger 2 Small Patties With Condiments On Bun From Fast Food / Restaurant (Burger King Bacon Double Cheeseburger) ☞ serving size: 1 burger king double bacon cheeseburger = 200 g; Calories = 510

Double Cheeseburger 2 Medium Patties Plain On Bun From Fast Food / Restaurant ☞ serving size: 1 double cheeseburger = 235 g; Calories = 717

Double Cheeseburger 2 Small Patties Plain On Bun From Fast Food / Restaurant ☞ serving size: 1 double cheeseburger = 155 g; Calories = 473

Double Hamburger 2 Medium Patties Plain On Bun From Fast Food / Restaurant ☞ serving size: 1 double hamburger = 220 g; Calories = 638

Double Hamburger 2 Small Patties Plain On Bun From Fast Food / Restaurant ☛ serving size: 1 double hamburger = 135 g; Calories = 389

Double Hamburger 2 Small Patties With Condiments On Bun From Fast Food / Restaurant ☛ serving size: 1 double hamburger = 190 g; Calories = 428

Egg And Cheese On Biscuit ☛ serving size: 1 sandwich = 140 g; Calories = 378

Egg And Steak On Biscuit ☛ serving size: 1 sandwich = 179 g; Calories = 508

Egg Cheese And Bacon On Bagel ☛ serving size: 1 sandwich = 246 g; Calories = 590

Egg Cheese And Beef On English Muffin ☛ serving size: 1 great starts sandwich (5.2 oz) = 147 g; Calories = 403

Egg Cheese And Ham On Bagel ☛ serving size: 1 mcdonald's sandwich = 218 g; Calories = 569

Egg Cheese And Ham On Biscuit ☛ serving size: 1 sandwich = 174 g; Calories = 440

Egg Cheese And Sausage On Bun ☛ serving size: 1 sandwich = 148 g; Calories = 401

Egg Cheese Ham And Bacon On Bun ☛ serving size: 1 jack-in-the-box sandwich = 226 g; Calories = 590

Egg Extra Cheese And Extra Sausage On Bun ☛ serving size: 1 jack-in-the-box sandwich = 213 g; Calories = 584

Egg Salad Sandwich ☛ serving size: 1 sandwich = 159 g; Calories = 471

Egg Scrambled ☛ serving size: 2 eggs = 96 g; Calories = 204

English Muffin With Cheese And Sausage ☛ serving size: 1 item = 108 g; Calories = 365

English Muffin With Egg Cheese And Canadian Bacon ☞ serving size: 1 sandwich = 126 g; Calories = 287

English Muffin With Egg Cheese And Sausage ☞ serving size: 1 item = 165 g; Calories = 472

Fajita-Style Beef Sandwich With Cheese On Pita Bread With Lettuce And Tomato ☞ serving size: 1 pita sandwich = 175 g; Calories = 280

Fajita-Style Chicken Sandwich With Cheese On Pita Bread With Lettuce And Tomato ☞ serving size: 1 pita sandwich = 207 g; Calories = 323

Fast Food Biscuit ☞ serving size: 1 biscuit = 55 g; Calories = 204

Fast Food Pizza Chain 14 Inch Pizza Cheese Topping Stuffed Crust ☞ serving size: 1 slice 1/8 pizza = 117 g; Calories = 321

Fast Food Pizza Chain 14 Inch Pizza Cheese Topping Thick Crust ☞ serving size: 1 slice = 115 g; Calories = 312

Fast Food Pizza Chain 14 Inch Pizza Cheese Topping Thin Crust ☞ serving size: 1 slice = 76 g; Calories = 230

Fast Food Pizza Chain 14 Inch Pizza Meat And Vegetable Topping Regular Crust ☞ serving size: 1 slice = 136 g; Calories = 332

Fast Food Pizza Chain 14 Inch Pizza Pepperoni Topping Thick Crust ☞ serving size: 1 slice = 118 g; Calories = 339

Fast Food Pizza Chain 14 Inch Pizza Pepperoni Topping Thin Crust ☞ serving size: 1 slice = 79 g; Calories = 262

Fast Food Pizza Chain 14 Inch Pizza Sausage Topping Thick Crust ☞ serving size: 1 slice = 127 g; Calories = 358

Fast Food Pizza Chain 14 Inch Pizza Sausage Topping Thin Crust ☞ serving size: 1 slice = 88 g; Calories = 283

Fast Foods Biscuit With Egg And Sausage ☛ serving size: 1 item = 162 g; Calories = 505

Fast Foods Cheeseburger; Double Large Patty; With Condiments Vegetables And Mayonnaise ☛ serving size: 1 item = 355 g; Calories = 898

Fast Foods Crispy Chicken Filet Sandwich With Lettuce And Mayonnaise ☛ serving size: 1 sandwich = 152 g; Calories = 420

Fast Foods Fried Chicken Breast Meat And Skin And Breading ☛ serving size: 1 breast, with skin = 203 g; Calories = 467

Fast Foods Fried Chicken Breast Meat Only Skin And Breading Removed ☛ serving size: 1 breast without skin = 142 g; Calories = 217

Fast Foods Fried Chicken Drumstick Meat And Skin With Breading ☛ serving size: 1 drumstick, with skin = 75 g; Calories = 200

Fast Foods Fried Chicken Drumstick Meat Only Skin And Breading Removed ☛ serving size: 1 drumstick, bone, and skin removed = 40 g; Calories = 69

Fast Foods Fried Chicken Thigh Meat And Skin And Breading ☛ serving size: 1 thigh with skin = 136 g; Calories = 373

Fast Foods Fried Chicken Thigh Meat Only Skin And Breading Removed ☛ serving size: 1 thigh without skin = 84 g; Calories = 150

Fast Foods Fried Chicken Wing Meat And Skin And Breading ☛ serving size: 1 wing, with skin = 58 g; Calories = 180

Fast Foods Fried Chicken Wing Meat Only Skin And Breading Removed ☛ serving size: 1 wing without skin = 37 g; Calories = 80

Fast Foods Grilled Chicken Filet Sandwich With Lettuce Tomato And Spread ☛ serving size: 1 sandwich = 230 g; Calories = 419

Fish Sandwich With Tartar Sauce ☛ serving size: 1 sandwich = 220 g; Calories = 565

🍔 Fish Sandwich With Tartar Sauce And Cheese 🐂 serving size: 1 sandwich = 134 g; Calories = 374

🍔 Frankfurter Or Hot Dog Sandwich Beef And Pork Plain On Multigrain Bread 🐂 serving size: 1 frankfurter on bread = 93 g; Calories = 267

🍔 Frankfurter Or Hot Dog Sandwich Beef And Pork Plain On Multigrain Bun 🐂 serving size: 1 frankfurter on bun = 102 g; Calories = 291

🍔 Frankfurter Or Hot Dog Sandwich Beef And Pork Plain On Wheat Bread 🐂 serving size: 1 frankfurter on bread = 85 g; Calories = 247

🍔 Frankfurter Or Hot Dog Sandwich Beef And Pork Plain On Wheat Bun 🐂 serving size: 1 frankfurter on bun = 102 g; Calories = 294

🍔 Frankfurter Or Hot Dog Sandwich Beef And Pork Plain On White Bread 🐂 serving size: 1 frankfurter on bread = 85 g; Calories = 245

🍔 Frankfurter Or Hot Dog Sandwich Beef And Pork Plain On White Bun 🐂 serving size: 1 frankfurter on bun = 102 g; Calories = 299

🍔 Frankfurter Or Hot Dog Sandwich Beef And Pork Plain On Whole Grain White Bread 🐂 serving size: 1 frankfurter on bread = 93 g; Calories = 257

🍔 Frankfurter Or Hot Dog Sandwich Beef And Pork Plain On Whole Grain White Bun 🐂 serving size: 1 frankfurter on bun = 102 g; Calories = 287

🍔 Frankfurter Or Hot Dog Sandwich Beef And Pork Plain On Whole Wheat Bread 🐂 serving size: 1 frankfurter on bread = 93 g; Calories = 261

🍔 Frankfurter Or Hot Dog Sandwich Beef And Pork Plain On Whole Wheat Bun 🐂 serving size: 1 frankfurter on bun = 102 g; Calories = 294

🍔 Frankfurter Or Hot Dog Sandwich Beef Plain On Multigrain Bread 🐂 serving size: 1 frankfurter on bread = 93 g; Calories = 285

Frankfurter Or Hot Dog Sandwich Beef Plain On Multigrain Bun serving size: 1 frankfurter on bun = 102 g; Calories = 307

Frankfurter Or Hot Dog Sandwich Beef Plain On Wheat Bread serving size: 1 frankfurter on bread = 85 g; Calories = 266

Frankfurter Or Hot Dog Sandwich Beef Plain On Wheat Bun serving size: 1 frankfurter on bun = 102 g; Calories = 310

Frankfurter Or Hot Dog Sandwich Beef Plain On White Bread serving size: 1 frankfurter on bread = 85 g; Calories = 264

Frankfurter Or Hot Dog Sandwich Beef Plain On White Bun serving size: 1 frankfurter on bun = 102 g; Calories = 314

Frankfurter Or Hot Dog Sandwich Beef Plain On Whole Grain White Bread serving size: 1 frankfurter on bread = 93 g; Calories = 274

Frankfurter Or Hot Dog Sandwich Beef Plain On Whole Grain White Bun serving size: 1 frankfurter on bun = 102 g; Calories = 304

Frankfurter Or Hot Dog Sandwich Beef Plain On Whole Wheat Bread serving size: 1 frankfurter on bread = 93 g; Calories = 280

Frankfurter Or Hot Dog Sandwich Beef Plain On Whole Wheat Bun serving size: 1 frankfurter on bun = 102 g; Calories = 310

Frankfurter Or Hot Dog Sandwich Chicken And/or Turkey Plain On Multigrain Bread serving size: 1 frankfurter on bread = 93 g; Calories = 229

Frankfurter Or Hot Dog Sandwich Chicken And/or Turkey Plain On Multigrain Bun serving size: 1 frankfurter on bun = 102 g; Calories = 252

Frankfurter Or Hot Dog Sandwich Chicken And/or Turkey Plain On Wheat Bread serving size: 1 frankfurter on bread = 85 g; Calories = 211

Frankfurter Or Hot Dog Sandwich Chicken And/or Turkey Plain

On Wheat Bun ☞ serving size: 1 frankfurter on bun = 102 g; Calories = 255

Frankfurter Or Hot Dog Sandwich Chicken And/or Turkey Plain On White Bread ☞ serving size: 1 frankfurter on bread = 85 g; Calories = 208

Frankfurter Or Hot Dog Sandwich Chicken And/or Turkey Plain On White Bun ☞ serving size: 1 frankfurter on bun = 102 g; Calories = 259

Frankfurter Or Hot Dog Sandwich Chicken And/or Turkey Plain On Whole Grain White Bread ☞ serving size: 1 frankfurter on bread = 93 g; Calories = 220

Frankfurter Or Hot Dog Sandwich Chicken And/or Turkey Plain On Whole Grain White Bun ☞ serving size: 1 frankfurter on bun = 102 g; Calories = 249

Frankfurter Or Hot Dog Sandwich Chicken And/or Turkey Plain On Whole Wheat Bread ☞ serving size: 1 frankfurter on bread = 93 g; Calories = 224

Frankfurter Or Hot Dog Sandwich Chicken And/or Turkey Plain On Whole Wheat Bun ☞ serving size: 1 frankfurter on bun = 102 g; Calories = 255

Frankfurter Or Hot Dog Sandwich Fat Free Plain On Multigrain Bread ☞ serving size: 1 frankfurter on bread = 93 g; Calories = 161

Frankfurter Or Hot Dog Sandwich Fat Free Plain On Multigrain Bun ☞ serving size: 1 frankfurter on bun = 102 g; Calories = 184

Frankfurter Or Hot Dog Sandwich Fat Free Plain On Wheat Bread ☞ serving size: 1 frankfurter on bread = 85 g; Calories = 142

Frankfurter Or Hot Dog Sandwich Fat Free Plain On Wheat Bun ☞ serving size: 1 frankfurter on bun = 102 g; Calories = 187

Frankfurter Or Hot Dog Sandwich Fat Free Plain On White Bread serving size: 1 frankfurter on bread = 85 g; Calories = 140

Frankfurter Or Hot Dog Sandwich Fat Free Plain On White Bun serving size: 1 frankfurter on bun = 102 g; Calories = 191

Frankfurter Or Hot Dog Sandwich Fat Free Plain On Whole Grain White Bread serving size: 1 frankfurter on bread = 93 g; Calories = 151

Frankfurter Or Hot Dog Sandwich Fat Free Plain On Whole Grain White Bun serving size: 1 frankfurter on bun = 102 g; Calories = 181

Frankfurter Or Hot Dog Sandwich Fat Free Plain On Whole Wheat Bread serving size: 1 frankfurter on bread = 93 g; Calories = 156

Frankfurter Or Hot Dog Sandwich Fat Free Plain On Whole Wheat Bun serving size: 1 frankfurter on bun = 102 g; Calories = 187

Frankfurter Or Hot Dog Sandwich Meat And Poultry Plain On Multigrain Bread serving size: 1 frankfurter on bread = 93 g; Calories = 261

Frankfurter Or Hot Dog Sandwich Meat And Poultry Plain On Multigrain Bun serving size: 1 frankfurter on bun = 102 g; Calories = 285

Frankfurter Or Hot Dog Sandwich Meat And Poultry Plain On Wheat Bread serving size: 1 frankfurter on bread = 85 g; Calories = 243

Frankfurter Or Hot Dog Sandwich Meat And Poultry Plain On Wheat Bun serving size: 1 frankfurter on bun = 102 g; Calories = 288

Frankfurter Or Hot Dog Sandwich Meat And Poultry Plain On White Bread serving size: 1 frankfurter on bread = 85 g; Calories = 241

🍔 Frankfurter Or Hot Dog Sandwich Meat And Poultry Plain On White Bun ☛ serving size: 1 frankfurter on bun = 102 g; Calories = 292

🍔 Frankfurter Or Hot Dog Sandwich Meat And Poultry Plain On Whole Grain White Bread ☛ serving size: 1 frankfurter on bread = 93 g; Calories = 252

🍔 Frankfurter Or Hot Dog Sandwich Meat And Poultry Plain On Whole Grain White Bun ☛ serving size: 1 frankfurter on bun = 102 g; Calories = 281

🍔 Frankfurter Or Hot Dog Sandwich Meat And Poultry Plain On Whole Wheat Bread ☛ serving size: 1 frankfurter on bread = 93 g; Calories = 257

🍔 Frankfurter Or Hot Dog Sandwich Meat And Poultry Plain On Whole Wheat Bun ☛ serving size: 1 frankfurter on bun = 102 g; Calories = 288

🍔 Frankfurter Or Hot Dog Sandwich Meatless On Bread With Meatless Chili ☛ serving size: 1 frankfurter on bread = 162 g; Calories = 303

🍔 Frankfurter Or Hot Dog Sandwich Meatless On Bun With Meatless Chili ☛ serving size: 1 frankfurter on bun = 179 g; Calories = 354

🍔 Frankfurter Or Hot Dog Sandwich Meatless Plain On Bread ☛ serving size: 1 frankfurter on bread = 98 g; Calories = 237

🍔 Frankfurter Or Hot Dog Sandwich Meatless Plain On Bun ☛ serving size: 1 frankfurter on bun = 115 g; Calories = 289

🍔 Frankfurter Or Hot Dog Sandwich NFS Plain On Multigrain Bread ☛ serving size: 1 frankfurter on bread = 93 g; Calories = 285

🍔 Frankfurter Or Hot Dog Sandwich NFS Plain On Multigrain Bun ☛ serving size: 1 frankfurter on bun = 102 g; Calories = 307

🍔 Frankfurter Or Hot Dog Sandwich NFS Plain On Wheat Bread ☛ serving size: 1 frankfurter on bread = 85 g; Calories = 266

Frankfurter Or Hot Dog Sandwich NFS Plain On Wheat Bun ☞ serving size: 1 frankfurter on bun = 102 g; Calories = 310

Frankfurter Or Hot Dog Sandwich NFS Plain On White Bread ☞ serving size: 1 frankfurter on bread = 85 g; Calories = 264

Frankfurter Or Hot Dog Sandwich NFS Plain On White Bun ☞ serving size: 1 frankfurter on bun = 102 g; Calories = 314

Frankfurter Or Hot Dog Sandwich NFS Plain On Whole Grain White Bread ☞ serving size: 1 frankfurter on bread = 93 g; Calories = 274

Frankfurter Or Hot Dog Sandwich NFS Plain On Whole Grain White Bun ☞ serving size: 1 frankfurter on bun = 102 g; Calories = 304

Frankfurter Or Hot Dog Sandwich NFS Plain On Whole Wheat Bread ☞ serving size: 1 frankfurter on bread = 93 g; Calories = 280

Frankfurter Or Hot Dog Sandwich NFS Plain On Whole Wheat Bun ☞ serving size: 1 frankfurter on bun = 102 g; Calories = 310

Frankfurter Or Hot Dog Sandwich Reduced Fat Or Light Plain On Multigrain Bread ☞ serving size: 1 frankfurter on bread = 93 g; Calories = 168

Frankfurter Or Hot Dog Sandwich Reduced Fat Or Light Plain On Multigrain Bun ☞ serving size: 1 frankfurter on bun = 102 g; Calories = 191

Frankfurter Or Hot Dog Sandwich Reduced Fat Or Light Plain On Wheat Bread ☞ serving size: 1 frankfurter on bread = 85 g; Calories = 150

Frankfurter Or Hot Dog Sandwich Reduced Fat Or Light Plain On Wheat Bun ☞ serving size: 1 frankfurter on bun = 102 g; Calories = 194

Frankfurter Or Hot Dog Sandwich Reduced Fat Or Light Plain On White Bread ☞ serving size: 1 frankfurter on bread = 85 g; Calories = 147

🍔 Frankfurter Or Hot Dog Sandwich Reduced Fat Or Light Plain On White Bun ☛ serving size: 1 frankfurter on bun = 102 g; Calories = 198

🍔 Frankfurter Or Hot Dog Sandwich Reduced Fat Or Light Plain On Whole Grain White Bread ☛ serving size: 1 frankfurter on bread = 93 g; Calories = 158

🍔 Frankfurter Or Hot Dog Sandwich Reduced Fat Or Light Plain On Whole Grain White Bun ☛ serving size: 1 frankfurter on bun = 102 g; Calories = 188

🍔 Frankfurter Or Hot Dog Sandwich Reduced Fat Or Light Plain On Whole Wheat Bread ☛ serving size: 1 frankfurter on bread = 93 g; Calories = 164

🍔 Frankfurter Or Hot Dog Sandwich Reduced Fat Or Light Plain On Whole Wheat Bun ☛ serving size: 1 frankfurter on bun = 102 g; Calories = 194

🍔 Frankfurter Or Hot Dog Sandwich With Chili On Multigrain Bread ☛ serving size: 1 frankfurter on bread = 157 g; Calories = 353

🍔 Frankfurter Or Hot Dog Sandwich With Chili On Multigrain Bun ☛ serving size: 1 frankfurter on bun = 166 g; Calories = 375

🍔 Frankfurter Or Hot Dog Sandwich With Chili On Wheat Bread ☛ serving size: 1 frankfurter on bread = 149 g; Calories = 334

🍔 Frankfurter Or Hot Dog Sandwich With Chili On Wheat Bun ☛ serving size: 1 frankfurter on bun = 166 g; Calories = 379

🍔 Frankfurter Or Hot Dog Sandwich With Chili On White Bread ☛ serving size: 1 frankfurter on bread = 149 g; Calories = 332

🍔 Frankfurter Or Hot Dog Sandwich With Chili On White Bun ☛ serving size: 1 frankfurter on bun = 166 g; Calories = 384

🍔 Frankfurter Or Hot Dog Sandwich With Chili On Whole Grain White Bread ☛ serving size: 1 frankfurter on bread = 157 g; Calories = 344

Frankfurter Or Hot Dog Sandwich With Chili On Whole Grain White Bun ☛ serving size: 1 frankfurter on bun = 166 g; Calories = 372

Frankfurter Or Hot Dog Sandwich With Chili On Whole Wheat Bread ☛ serving size: 1 frankfurter on bread = 157 g; Calories = 349

Frankfurter Or Hot Dog Sandwich With Chili On Whole Wheat Bun ☛ serving size: 1 frankfurter on bun = 166 g; Calories = 379

Frankfurter Or Hot Dog Sandwich With Meatless Chili On Multi-grain Bread ☛ serving size: 1 frankfurter on bread = 157 g; Calories = 350

Frankfurter Or Hot Dog Sandwich With Meatless Chili On Multi-grain Bun ☛ serving size: 1 frankfurter on bun = 166 g; Calories = 374

Frankfurter Or Hot Dog Sandwich With Meatless Chili On Wheat Bread ☛ serving size: 1 frankfurter on bread = 149 g; Calories = 332

Frankfurter Or Hot Dog Sandwich With Meatless Chili On Wheat Bun ☛ serving size: 1 frankfurter on bun = 166 g; Calories = 375

Frankfurter Or Hot Dog Sandwich With Meatless Chili On White Bread ☛ serving size: 1 frankfurter on bread = 149 g; Calories = 329

Frankfurter Or Hot Dog Sandwich With Meatless Chili On White Bun ☛ serving size: 1 frankfurter on bun = 166 g; Calories = 380

Frankfurter Or Hot Dog Sandwich With Meatless Chili On Whole Grain White Bread ☛ serving size: 1 frankfurter on bread = 157 g; Calories = 341

Frankfurter Or Hot Dog Sandwich With Meatless Chili On Whole Grain White Bun ☛ serving size: 1 frankfurter on bun = 166 g; Calories = 370

Frankfurter Or Hot Dog Sandwich With Meatless Chili On Whole Wheat Bread ☛ serving size: 1 frankfurter on bread = 157 g; Calories = 349

Frankfurter Or Hot Dog Sandwich With Meatless Chili On Whole Wheat Bun ☛ serving size: 1 frankfurter on bun = 166 g; Calories = 375

French Toast From School Nfs ☛ serving size: 1 bite size = 10 g; Calories = 16

French Toast Gluten Free ☛ serving size: 1 slice, any size = 65 g; Calories = 170

French Toast Gluten Free From Frozen ☛ serving size: 1 bite size = 10 g; Calories = 17

French Toast Nfs ☛ serving size: 1 slice, any size = 65 g; Calories = 176

French Toast Plain ☛ serving size: 1 slice, any size = 65 g; Calories = 176

French Toast Plain From Fast Food / Restaurant ☛ serving size: 1 slice, any size = 85 g; Calories = 260

French Toast Plain From Frozen ☛ serving size: 1 bite size = 10 g; Calories = 18

French Toast Plain Reduced Fat ☛ serving size: 1 slice, any size = 65 g; Calories = 154

French Toast Sticks ☛ serving size: 3 pieces = 65 g; Calories = 221

French Toast Sticks From School Nfs ☛ serving size: 1 stick = 25 g; Calories = 40

French Toast Sticks Nfs ☛ serving size: 1 stick = 25 g; Calories = 71

French Toast Sticks Plain From Fast Food / Restaurant ☛ serving size: 1 stick = 25 g; Calories = 100

French Toast Sticks Plain From Frozen ☛ serving size: 1 stick = 45 g; Calories = 127

French Toast Sticks Whole Grain ☛ serving size: 1 stick = 45 g; Calories = 121

French Toast Whole Grain ☛ serving size: 1 slice, any size = 65 g; Calories = 175

French Toast Whole Grain From Fast Food / Restaurant ☛ serving size: 1 slice, any size = 85 g; Calories = 258

French Toast Whole Grain From Frozen ☛ serving size: 1 bite size = 10 g; Calories = 18

French Toast Whole Grain Reduced Fat ☛ serving size: 1 slice, any size = 65 g; Calories = 153

Fried Bread Puerto Rican Style ☛ serving size: 2 fritters with syrup (4" x 2-1/2" x 3-1/4") = 110 g; Calories = 283

Fried Egg Sandwich ☛ serving size: 1 sandwich = 96 g; Calories = 225

Griddle Cake Sandwich Egg Cheese And Bacon ☛ serving size: 1 item 6.1 oz = 174 g; Calories = 473

Griddle Cake Sandwich Egg Cheese And Sausage ☛ serving size: 1 item = 199 g; Calories = 579

Griddle Cake Sandwich Sausage ☛ serving size: 1 item = 135 g; Calories = 429

Grilled Chicken Bacon And Tomato Club Sandwich With Cheese Lettuce And Mayonnaise ☛ serving size: 1 sandwich = 268 g; Calories = 590

Grilled Chicken In Tortilla With Lettuce Cheese And Ranch Sauce ☛ serving size: 1 item = 123 g; Calories = 273

Gyro Sandwich (Pita Bread Beef Lamb Onion Condiments) With Tomato And Spread ☛ serving size: 1 gyro = 390 g; Calories = 651

Ham And Cheese On English Muffin ☛ serving size: 1 jimmy dean sandwich = 57 g; Calories = 145

Ham And Cheese Sandwich On Bun With Lettuce And Spread ☞ serving size: 1 sandwich = 154 g; Calories = 328

Ham And Cheese Sandwich With Lettuce And Spread ☞ serving size: 1 sandwich = 155 g; Calories = 360

Ham And Cheese Sandwich With Spread Grilled ☞ serving size: 1 sandwich = 141 g; Calories = 360

Ham And Egg Sandwich ☞ serving size: 1 sandwich = 124 g; Calories = 272

Ham And Tomato Club Sandwich With Lettuce And Spread ☞ serving size: 1 sandwich = 254 g; Calories = 602

Ham Salad Sandwich ☞ serving size: 1 sandwich = 141 g; Calories = 312

Ham Sandwich With Lettuce And Spread ☞ serving size: 1 sandwich = 127 g; Calories = 273

Ham Sandwich With Spread ☞ serving size: 1 sandwich = 112 g; Calories = 270

Hamburger 1 Medium Patty Plain On Wheat Bun ☞ serving size: 1 hamburger = 145 g; Calories = 389

Hamburger 1 Medium Patty Plain On White Bun ☞ serving size: 1 hamburger = 145 g; Calories = 399

Hamburger 1 Medium Patty Plain On Whole Wheat Bun ☞ serving size: 1 hamburger = 145 g; Calories = 389

Hamburger 1 Medium Patty With Condiments On Wheat Bun ☞ serving size: 1 hamburger = 200 g; Calories = 430

Hamburger 1 Medium Patty With Condiments On White Bun ☞ serving size: 1 hamburger = 200 g; Calories = 440

Hamburger 1 Medium Patty With Condiments On Whole Wheat Bun ☞ serving size: 1 hamburger = 200 g; Calories = 430

Hamburger 1 Miniature Patty On Miniature Bun From School ☞ serving size: 1 miniature hamburger = 50 g; Calories = 119

Hamburger 1 Miniature Patty Plain On Miniature Bun From Fast Food / Restaurant ☞ serving size: 1 miniature hamburger = 50 g; Calories = 143

Hamburger 1 Miniature Patty With Condiments On Miniature Bun From Fast Food / Restaurant ☞ serving size: 1 miniature hamburger = 65 g; Calories = 163

Hamburger 1 Small Patty Plain On Wheat Bun ☞ serving size: 1 hamburger = 115 g; Calories = 308

Hamburger 1 Small Patty Plain On White Bun ☞ serving size: 1 hamburger = 115 g; Calories = 316

Hamburger 1 Small Patty Plain On Whole Wheat Bun ☞ serving size: 1 hamburger = 115 g; Calories = 308

Hamburger 1 Small Patty With Condiments On Bun From Fast Food / Restaurant (Burger King Whopper Jr.) ☞ serving size: 1 burger king whopper jr = 150 g; Calories = 311

Hamburger 1 Small Patty With Condiments On White Bun ☞ serving size: 1 hamburger = 175 g; Calories = 369

Hamburger 1 Small Patty With Condiments On Whole Wheat Bun ☞ serving size: 1 hamburger = 175 g; Calories = 361

Hamburger Large Single Patty With Condiments ☞ serving size: 1 item = 171 g; Calories = 438

Hamburger Nfs ☞ serving size: 1 hamburger = 200 g; Calories = 440

Hamburger On Bun From School ☞ serving size: 1 hamburger = 95 g; Calories = 225

Hamburger; Double Large Patty; With Condiments Vegetables And Mayonnaise ☞ serving size: 1 item = 374 g; Calories = 943

Hamburger; Single Large Patty; With Condiments Vegetables And Mayonnaise ☛ serving size: 1 item = 247 g; Calories = 558

Hamburger; Single Regular Patty; Double Decker Bun With Condiments And Special Sauce ☛ serving size: 1 item = 205 g; Calories = 531

Hamburger; Single Regular Patty; Plain ☛ serving size: 1 sandwich = 78 g; Calories = 232

Hamburger; Single Regular Patty; With Condiments ☛ serving size: 1 sandwich = 97 g; Calories = 255

Hors D'oeuvres With Spread ☛ serving size: 1 hors d'oeuvre = 23 g; Calories = 47

Hot Ham And Cheese Sandwich On Bun ☛ serving size: 1 sandwich = 162 g; Calories = 345

Hush Puppies ☛ serving size: 1 piece = 22 g; Calories = 65

Kfc Biscuit ☛ serving size: 1 biscuit = 49 g; Calories = 175

Kfc Coleslaw ☛ serving size: 1 package = 112 g; Calories = 161

Kfc Crispy Chicken Strips ☛ serving size: 1 strip = 47 g; Calories = 129

Kfc Fried Chicken Breast ☛ serving size: 1 breast, with skin = 212 g; Calories = 568

Kfc Fried Chicken Extra Crispy Breast Meat Only Skin And Breading Removed ☛ serving size: 1 breast, without skin = 140 g; Calories = 214

Kfc Fried Chicken Extra Crispy Drumstick Meat And Skin With Breading ☛ serving size: 1 drumstick, with skin = 81 g; Calories = 222

Kfc Fried Chicken Extra Crispy Drumstick Meat Only Skin And Breading Removed ☛ serving size: 1 drumstick, bone and skin removed = 41 g; Calories = 70

Kfc Fried Chicken Extra Crispy Thigh Meat And Skin With Breading ☛ serving size: 1 thigh, with skin = 152 g; Calories = 470

Kfc Fried Chicken Extra Crispy Thigh Meat Only Skin And Breading Removed ☛ serving size: 1 thigh, without skin = 91 g; Calories = 163

Kfc Fried Chicken Extra Crispy Wing Meat And Skin With Breading ☛ serving size: 1 wing, with skin = 68 g; Calories = 229

Kfc Fried Chicken Extra Crispy Wing Meat Only Skin And Breading Removed ☛ serving size: 1 wing, without skin = 44 g; Calories = 104

Kfc Fried Chicken Original Recipe Breast Meat And Skin With Breading ☛ serving size: 1 breast, with skin = 212 g; Calories = 490

Kfc Fried Chicken Original Recipe Breast Meat Only Skin And Breading Removed ☛ serving size: 1 breast without skin = 152 g; Calories = 227

Kfc Fried Chicken Original Recipe Drumstick Meat And Skin With Breading ☛ serving size: 1 drumstick, with skin = 75 g; Calories = 179

Kfc Fried Chicken Original Recipe Drumstick Meat Only Skin And Breading Removed ☛ serving size: 1 drumstick, bone and skin removed = 40 g; Calories = 70

Kfc Fried Chicken Original Recipe Thigh Meat And Skin With Breading ☛ serving size: 1 thigh, with skin = 135 g; Calories = 363

Kfc Fried Chicken Original Recipe Thigh Meat Only Skin And Breading Removed ☛ serving size: 1 thigh without skin = 86 g; Calories = 151

Kfc Fried Chicken Original Recipe Wing Meat And Skin With Breading ☛ serving size: 1 wing, with skin = 60 g; Calories = 178

Kfc Fried Chicken Original Recipe Wing Meat Only Skin And

Breading Removed ☛ serving size: 1 wing wing without skin = 39 g; Calories = 84

🍔 Kfc Popcorn Chicken ☛ serving size: 1 piece = 6.4 g; Calories = 23

🍔 Little Caesars 14 Inch Cheese Pizza Large Deep Dish Crust ☛ serving size: 1 slice = 102 g; Calories = 268

🍔 Little Caesars 14 Inch Cheese Pizza Thin Crust ☛ serving size: 1 slice = 48 g; Calories = 148

🍔 Little Caesars 14 Inch Original Round Cheese Pizza Regular Crust ☛ serving size: 1 slice = 89 g; Calories = 236

🍔 Little Caesars 14 Inch Original Round Meat And Vegetable Pizza Regular Crust ☛ serving size: 1 slice = 115 g; Calories = 280

🍔 Little Caesars 14 Inch Original Round Pepperoni Pizza Regular Crust ☛ serving size: 1 slice = 90 g; Calories = 246

🍔 Little Caesars 14 Inch Pepperoni Pizza Large Deep Dish Crust ☛ serving size: 1 slice = 104 g; Calories = 276

🍔 McDonalds Bacon Egg & Cheese Biscuit ☛ serving size: 1 item 4.9 oz = 142 g; Calories = 432

🍔 McDonalds Bacon Egg & Cheese Mcgriddles ☛ serving size: 1 item 5.8 oz = 165 g; Calories = 449

🍔 McDonalds Bacon Ranch Salad With Crispy Chicken ☛ serving size: 1 item 11.3 oz = 319 g; Calories = 389

🍔 McDonalds Bacon Ranch Salad With Grilled Chicken ☛ serving size: 1 item 10.8 oz = 305 g; Calories = 247

🍔 McDonalds Bacon Ranch Salad Without Chicken ☛ serving size: 1 item 7.8 oz = 223 g; Calories = 136

🍔 McDonalds Big Breakfast ☛ serving size: 1 item 9.5 oz = 269 g; Calories = 767

McDonalds Big Mac ☛ serving size: 1 item 7.6 oz = 219 g; Calories = 563

McDonalds Big Mac (Without Big Mac Sauce) ☛ serving size: 1 item = 200 g; Calories = 468

McDonalds Cheeseburger ☛ serving size: 1 item 4 oz = 119 g; Calories = 313

McDonalds Chicken Mcnuggets ☛ serving size: 4 pieces = 64 g; Calories = 193

McDonalds Deluxe Breakfast With Syrup And Margarine ☛ serving size: 1 item 14.8 oz = 420 g; Calories = 1197

McDonalds Double Cheeseburger ☛ serving size: 1 sandwich = 155 g; Calories = 437

McDonalds Double Quarter Pounder With Cheese ☛ serving size: 1 item = 280 g; Calories = 734

McDonalds Egg Mcmuffin ☛ serving size: 1 sandwich = 126 g; Calories = 287

McDonalds Filet-O-Fish ☛ serving size: 1 sandwich = 134 g; Calories = 378

McDonalds Filet-O-Fish (Without Tartar Sauce) ☛ serving size: 1 item = 124 g; Calories = 301

McDonalds French Fries ☛ serving size: 1 small serving = 71 g; Calories = 229

McDonalds Fruit N Yogurt Parfait ☛ serving size: 1 item 5.2 oz = 149 g; Calories = 157

McDonalds Fruit N Yogurt Parfait (Without Granola) ☛ serving size: 1 item = 142 g; Calories = 128

McDonalds Hamburger ☛ serving size: 1 sandwich = 95 g; Calories = 251

McDonalds Hash Brown ☛ serving size: 1 serving 1 patty = 53 g; Calories = 144

McDonalds Hot Caramel Sundae ☛ serving size: 1 item (6.4 oz) = 182 g; Calories = 342

McDonalds Hot Fudge Sundae ☛ serving size: 1 item (6.3 oz) = 179 g; Calories = 333

McDonalds Hotcakes (Plain) ☛ serving size: 3 hotcakes 5.3 oz = 149 g; Calories = 340

McDonalds Hotcakes And Sausage ☛ serving size: 1 item = 192 g; Calories = 565

McDonalds Mcchicken Sandwich ☛ serving size: 1 sandwich = 131 g; Calories = 358

McDonalds Mcchicken Sandwich (Without Mayonnaise) ☛ serving size: 1 item = 138 g; Calories = 331

McDonalds Mcflurry With M&Ms ☛ serving size: 1 regular (12 fl oz) = 348 g; Calories = 616

McDonalds Mcflurry With Oreo Cookies ☛ serving size: 1 regular (12 fl oz) = 337 g; Calories = 556

McDonalds Pancakes ☛ serving size: 1 item = 221 g; Calories = 601

McDonalds Quarter Pounder ☛ serving size: 1 item = 171 g; Calories = 417

McDonalds Quarter Pounder With Cheese ☛ serving size: 1 item 7.1 oz = 199 g; Calories = 513

McDonalds Ranch Snack Wrap Crispy ☛ serving size: 1 wrap = 133 g; Calories = 366

McDonalds Ranch Snack Wrap Grilled ☛ serving size: 1 wrap = 123 g; Calories = 273

McDonalds Sausage Biscuit ☛ serving size: 1 item 4.1 oz = 117 g; Calories = 440

McDonalds Sausage Biscuit With Egg ☛ serving size: 1 item 5.7 oz = 163 g; Calories = 507

McDonalds Sausage Burrito ☛ serving size: 1 burrito = 109 g; Calories = 302

McDonalds Sausage Egg & Cheese Mcgriddles ☛ serving size: 1 item 7 oz = 199 g; Calories = 563

McDonalds Sausage Mcgriddles ☛ serving size: 1 item = 135 g; Calories = 421

McDonalds Sausage Mcmuffin ☛ serving size: 1 item 4 oz = 115 g; Calories = 383

McDonalds Sausage Mcmuffin With Egg ☛ serving size: 1 item 5.8 oz = 165 g; Calories = 452

McDonalds Side Salad ☛ serving size: 1 item 3.1 oz = 87 g; Calories = 17

McDonalds Southern Style Chicken Biscuit ☛ serving size: 1 biscuit regular size biscuit = 132 g; Calories = 401

McDonalds Strawberry Sundae ☛ serving size: 1 item (6.3 oz) = 178 g; Calories = 281

McDonalds Vanilla Reduced Fat Ice Cream Cone ☛ serving size: 1 item (3.2 oz) = 90 g; Calories = 146

Meat Sandwich Nfs ☛ serving size: 1 sandwich = 83 g; Calories = 250

Meat Spread Or Potted Meat Sandwich ☛ serving size: 1 sandwich = 107 g; Calories = 268

Midnight Sandwich With Spread ☛ serving size: 1 sandwich = 201 g; Calories = 472

Miniature Cinnamon Rolls ☛ serving size: 1 each = 25 g; Calories = 101

Nachos With Cheese ☛ serving size: 1 serving = 80 g; Calories = 274

Nachos With Cheese Beans Ground Beef And Tomatoes ☛ serving size: 1 serving = 222 g; Calories = 486

Onion Rings Breaded And Fried ☛ serving size: 1 package (18 onion rings) = 117 g; Calories = 481

Pancakes Buckwheat ☛ serving size: 1 miniature/bite size pancake = 10 g; Calories = 27

Pancakes Cornmeal ☛ serving size: 1 miniature/bite size pancake = 10 g; Calories = 20

Pancakes From School Nfs ☛ serving size: 1 miniature/bite size pancake = 10 g; Calories = 23

Pancakes Nfs ☛ serving size: 1 miniature/bite size pancake = 10 g; Calories = 28

Pancakes Plain ☛ serving size: 1 miniature/bite size pancake = 10 g; Calories = 28

Pancakes Plain From Fast Food / Restaurant ☛ serving size: 1 miniature/bite size pancake = 10 g; Calories = 30

Pancakes Plain Reduced Fat From Fozen ☛ serving size: 1 miniature/bite size pancake = 10 g; Calories = 26

Pancakes Pumpkin ☛ serving size: 1 miniature/bite size pancake = 10 g; Calories = 24

Pancakes Whole Grain ☛ serving size: 1 miniature/bite size pancake = 10 g; Calories = 27

Pancakes Whole Grain And Nuts From Fast Food / Restaurant ☛ serving size: 1 miniature/bite size pancake = 10 g; Calories = 35

🍔 Pancakes Whole Grain From Fast Food / Restaurant ☞ serving size: 1 miniature/bite size pancake = 10 g; Calories = 30

🍔 Pancakes Whole Grain From Frozen ☞ serving size: 1 miniature/bite size pancake = 10 g; Calories = 23

🍔 Pancakes Whole Grain Reduced Fat ☞ serving size: 1 miniature/bite size pancake = 10 g; Calories = 25

🍔 Pancakes Whole Grain Reduced Fat From Frozen ☞ serving size: 1 miniature/bite size pancake = 10 g; Calories = 23

🍔 Pancakes With Chocolate ☞ serving size: 1 miniature/bite size pancake = 10 g; Calories = 34

🍔 Pancakes With Chocolate From Fast Food / Restaurant ☞ serving size: 1 miniature/bite size pancake = 10 g; Calories = 36

🍔 Pancakes With Chocolate From Frozen ☞ serving size: 1 miniature/bite size pancake = 10 g; Calories = 25

🍔 Pancakes With Fruit ☞ serving size: 1 miniature/bite size pancake = 10 g; Calories = 23

🍔 Pancakes With Fruit From Fast Food / Restaurant ☞ serving size: 1 miniature/bite size pancake = 10 g; Calories = 25

🍔 Pancakes With Fruit From Frozen ☞ serving size: 1 miniature/bite size pancake = 10 g; Calories = 22

🍔 Papa Johns 14 Inch Cheese Pizza Original Crust ☞ serving size: 1 slice = 117 g; Calories = 304

🍔 Papa Johns 14 Inch Cheese Pizza Thin Crust ☞ serving size: 1 slice = 87 g; Calories = 257

🍔 Papa Johns 14 Inch Pepperoni Pizza Original Crust ☞ serving size: 1 slice = 123 g; Calories = 338

🍔 Papa Johns 14 Inch The Works Pizza Original Crust ☞ serving size: 1 slice = 153 g; Calories = 367

🍔 Pastrami Sandwich 🖝 serving size: 1 sandwich = 134 g; Calories = 221

🍔 Pepperoni And Salami Submarine Sandwich With Lettuce Tomato And Spread 🖝 serving size: 1 submarine = 240 g; Calories = 540

🍔 Pepperoni Pizza 🖝 serving size: 1 slice = 111 g; Calories = 313

🍔 Pig In A Blanket Frankfurter Or Hot Dog Wrapped In Dough 🖝 serving size: 1 pig in blanket = 85 g; Calories = 275

🍔 Pizza Cheese Topping Regular Crust Frozen Cooked 🖝 serving size: 1 serving 9 servings per 24 oz package = 81 g; Calories = 217

🍔 Pizza Cheese Topping Rising Crust Frozen Cooked 🖝 serving size: 1 serving 6 servings per 29.25 oz package = 139 g; Calories = 361

🍔 Pizza Cheese Topping Thin Crust Frozen Cooked 🖝 serving size: 1 slice = 69 g; Calories = 182

🍔 Pizza Hut 12 Inch Cheese Pizza Hand-Tossed Crust 🖝 serving size: 1 slice = 96 g; Calories = 260

🍔 Pizza Hut 12 Inch Cheese Pizza Pan Crust 🖝 serving size: 1 slice = 100 g; Calories = 280

🍔 Pizza Hut 12 Inch Cheese Pizza Thin N Crispy Crust 🖝 serving size: 1 slice = 69 g; Calories = 209

🍔 Pizza Hut 12 Inch Pepperoni Pizza Hand-Tossed Crust 🖝 serving size: 1 slice = 96 g; Calories = 269

🍔 Pizza Hut 12 Inch Pepperoni Pizza Pan Crust 🖝 serving size: 1 slice = 96 g; Calories = 286

🍔 Pizza Hut 12 Inch Super Supreme Pizza Hand-Tossed Crust 🖝 serving size: 1 slice = 127 g; Calories = 309

🍔 Pizza Hut 14 Inch Cheese Pizza Hand-Tossed Crust 🖝 serving size: 1 slice = 105 g; Calories = 289

Pizza Hut 14 Inch Cheese Pizza Pan Crust ☛ serving size: 1 slice = 112 g; Calories = 309

Pizza Hut 14 Inch Cheese Pizza Stuffed Crust ☛ serving size: 1 slice = 117 g; Calories = 321

Pizza Hut 14 Inch Cheese Pizza Thin N Crispy Crust ☛ serving size: 1 slice = 79 g; Calories = 242

Pizza Hut 14 Inch Pepperoni Pizza Hand-Tossed Crust ☛ serving size: 1 slice = 110 g; Calories = 320

Pizza Hut 14 Inch Pepperoni Pizza Pan Crust ☛ serving size: 1 slice = 113 g; Calories = 329

Pizza Hut 14 Inch Pepperoni Pizza Thin N Crispy Crust ☛ serving size: 1 slice = 80 g; Calories = 266

Pizza Hut 14 Inch Sausage Pizza Hand-Tossed Crust ☛ serving size: 1 slice = 119 g; Calories = 342

Pizza Hut 14 Inch Sausage Pizza Pan Crust ☛ serving size: 1 slice = 125 g; Calories = 359

Pizza Hut 14 Inch Sausage Pizza Thin N Crispy Crust ☛ serving size: 1 slice = 92 g; Calories = 297

Pizza Hut 14 Inch Super Supreme Pizza Hand-Tossed Crust ☛ serving size: 1 slice = 123 g; Calories = 305

Pizza Hut Breadstick Parmesan Garlic ☛ serving size: 1 breadstick = 43 g; Calories = 148

Pizza Meat And Vegetable Topping Regular Crust Frozen Cooked ☛ serving size: 1 serving 5 servings per 24.2 oz package = 143 g; Calories = 395

Pizza Meat And Vegetable Topping Rising Crust Frozen Cooked ☛ serving size: 1 serving 6 servings per 34.98 oz package = 170 g; Calories = 461

Pizza Meat Topping Thick Crust Frozen Cooked ☛ serving size: 1 slice 1/8 of 12 inch pizza = 103 g; Calories = 282

Pizza Pepperoni Topping Regular Crust Frozen Cooked ☛ serving size: 1/4 pizza 12 inch diameter = 127 g; Calories = 348

Popeyes Biscuit ☛ serving size: 1 biscuit = 60 g; Calories = 241

Popeyes Coleslaw ☛ serving size: 1 package = 120 g; Calories = 193

Popeyes Fried Chicken Mild Breast Meat And Skin With Breading ☛ serving size: 1 breast, with skin = 194 g; Calories = 532

Popeyes Fried Chicken Mild Breast Meat Only Skin And Breading Removed ☛ serving size: 1 breast without skin = 132 g; Calories = 207

Popeyes Fried Chicken Mild Drumstick Meat And Skin With Breading ☛ serving size: 1 drumstick, with skin = 76 g; Calories = 223

Popeyes Fried Chicken Mild Drumstick Meat Only Skin And Breading Removed ☛ serving size: 1 drumstick, bone and skin removed = 44 g; Calories = 75

Popeyes Fried Chicken Mild Thigh Meat And Skin With Breading ☛ serving size: 1 thigh with skin = 138 g; Calories = 428

Popeyes Fried Chicken Mild Thigh Meat Only Skin And Breading Removed ☛ serving size: 1 thigh thigh without skin = 83 g; Calories = 156

Popeyes Fried Chicken Mild Wing Meat And Skin With Breading ☛ serving size: 1 wing, with skin = 57 g; Calories = 193

Popeyes Fried Chicken Mild Wing Meat Only Skin And Breading Removed ☛ serving size: 1 wing without skin, bone and breading = 16 g; Calories = 34

Popeyes Mild Chicken Strips Analyzed 2006 ☛ serving size: 1 strip = 54 g; Calories = 146

Popeyes Spicy Chicken Strips Analyzed 2006 ☞ serving size: 1 strip = 53 g; Calories = 134

Pork Barbecue Sandwich Or Sloppy Joe On Bun ☞ serving size: 1 barbecue sandwich = 186 g; Calories = 389

Pork Sandwich ☞ serving size: 1 sandwich = 136 g; Calories = 316

Pork Sandwich On White Roll With Onions Dill Pickles And Barbecue Sauce ☞ serving size: 1 sandwich = 189 g; Calories = 422

Pork Sandwich With Gravy ☞ serving size: 1 sandwich = 218 g; Calories = 325

Potato French Fried In Vegetable Oil ☞ serving size: 1 serving small = 71 g; Calories = 222

Potato French Fries From Fresh Baked ☞ serving size: 1 shoestring = 2 g; Calories = 3

Potato French Fries From Fresh Fried ☞ serving size: 1 shoestring = 2 g; Calories = 4

Potato French Fries From Frozen Fried ☞ serving size: 1 shoestring = 2 g; Calories = 5

Potato French Fries Nfs ☞ serving size: 1 shoestring = 2 g; Calories = 5

Potato French Fries Ns As To Fresh Or Frozen ☞ serving size: 1 shoestring = 2 g; Calories = 5

Potato French Fries School ☞ serving size: 1 shoestring = 2 g; Calories = 3

Potato French Fries With Cheese ☞ serving size: 1 fry, any cut = 8 g; Calories = 21

Potato French Fries With Cheese Fast Food / Restaurant ☞ serving size: 1 kids meal order = 107 g; Calories = 277

Potato French Fries With Cheese School 🐀 serving size: 1 fry, any cut = 11 g; Calories = 20

Potato French Fries With Chili 🐀 serving size: 1 fry, any cut = 8 g; Calories = 19

Potato French Fries With Chili And Cheese 🐀 serving size: 1 fry, any cut = 10 g; Calories = 22

Potato French Fries With Chili And Cheese Fast Food / Restaurant 🐀 serving size: 1 fry, any cut = 10 g; Calories = 22

Potato French Fries With Chili Fast Food / Restaurant 🐀 serving size: 1 fry, any cut = 8 g; Calories = 19

Potato Hash Brown From Dry Mix 🐀 serving size: 1 cup = 160 g; Calories = 347

Potato Hash Brown From Fast Food With Cheese 🐀 serving size: 1 patty = 55 g; Calories = 162

Potato Hash Brown From Fresh 🐀 serving size: 1 cup = 160 g; Calories = 302

Potato Hash Brown From Fresh With Cheese 🐀 serving size: 1 cup = 160 g; Calories = 354

Potato Hash Brown From Restaurant With Cheese 🐀 serving size: 1 patty = 55 g; Calories = 162

Potato Hash Brown From School Lunch 🐀 serving size: 1 patty = 55 g; Calories = 120

Potato Hash Brown Nfs 🐀 serving size: 1 patty = 55 g; Calories = 119

Potato Hash Brown Ready-To-Heat 🐀 serving size: 1 patty = 55 g; Calories = 119

Potato Hash Brown Ready-To-Heat With Cheese 🐀 serving size: 1 patty = 55 g; Calories = 136

Potato Home Fries From Fresh ☞ serving size: 1 cup = 200 g; Calories = 366

Potato Home Fries From Restaurant / Fast Food ☞ serving size: 1 cup = 200 g; Calories = 426

Potato Home Fries Nfs ☞ serving size: 1 cup = 200 g; Calories = 390

Potato Home Fries Ready-To-Heat ☞ serving size: 1 cup = 200 g; Calories = 390

Potato Home Fries With Vegetables ☞ serving size: 1 cup = 200 g; Calories = 342

Potato Mashed ☞ serving size: 1 cup = 242 g; Calories = 215

Potato Patty ☞ serving size: 1 patty = 55 g; Calories = 94

Potato Skins Nfs ☞ serving size: skin from 1 small = 25 g; Calories = 50

Potato Skins With Cheese ☞ serving size: skin from 1 small = 35 g; Calories = 69

Potato Skins With Cheese And Bacon ☞ serving size: skin from 1 small = 35 g; Calories = 75

Potato Skins Without Topping ☞ serving size: skin from 1 small = 25 g; Calories = 38

Potato Tots Fast Food / Restaurant ☞ serving size: 1 cup = 130 g; Calories = 307

Potato Tots From Fresh Fried Or Baked ☞ serving size: 1 cup = 130 g; Calories = 307

Potato Tots Frozen Baked ☞ serving size: 1 cup = 130 g; Calories = 243

Potato Tots Frozen Fried ☞ serving size: 1 cup = 130 g; Calories = 307

Potato Tots Frozen Ns As To Fried Or Baked 🖝 serving size: 1 cup = 130 g; Calories = 307

Potato Tots Nfs 🖝 scrving size: 1 cup = 130 g; Calories = 307

Potato Tots School 🖝 serving size: 1 cup = 130 g; Calories = 213

Potatoes Hash Browns Round Pieces Or Patty 🖝 serving size: 1 round piece = 5.5 g; Calories = 15

Puerto Rican Sandwich 🖝 serving size: 1 sandwich = 160 g; Calories = 534

Quesadilla With Chicken 🖝 serving size: 1 each quesadilla = 180 g; Calories = 529

Reuben Sandwich Corned Beef Sandwich With Sauerkraut And Cheese With Spread 🖝 serving size: 1 sandwich = 181 g; Calories = 516

Roast Beef Sandwich Plain 🖝 serving size: 1 sandwich = 149 g; Calories = 364

Roast Beef Sandwich With Bacon And Cheese Sauce 🖝 serving size: 1 sandwich = 218 g; Calories = 754

Roast Beef Sandwich With Cheese 🖝 serving size: 1 sandwich = 190 g; Calories = 619

Roast Beef Sandwich With Gravy 🖝 serving size: 1 sandwich = 222 g; Calories = 491

Roast Beef Submarine Sandwich On Roll Au Jus 🖝 serving size: 1 sandwich = 193 g; Calories = 461

Roast Beef Submarine Sandwich With Cheese Lettuce Tomato And Spread 🖝 serving size: 1 submarine = 260 g; Calories = 494

Roast Beef Submarine Sandwich With Lettuce Tomato And Spread 🖝 serving size: 1 submarine = 240 g; Calories = 434

Salami Sandwich With Spread 🖝 serving size: 1 sandwich = 82 g; Calories = 254

Sandwich Nfs ☛ serving size: 1 sandwich = 83 g; Calories = 250

Sardine Sandwich With Lettuce And Spread ☛ serving size: 1 sandwich = 214 g; Calories = 484

Sausage And Spaghetti Sauce Sandwich ☛ serving size: 1 sandwich = 189 g; Calories = 480

Sausage Pizza ☛ serving size: 1 slice = 116 g; Calories = 325

Sausage Sandwich ☛ serving size: 1 sandwich = 107 g; Calories = 317

School Lunch Chicken Nuggets Whole Grain Breaded ☛ serving size: 5 pieces = 88 g; Calories = 238

School Lunch Chicken Patty Whole Grain Breaded ☛ serving size: 1 patty = 86 g; Calories = 212

School Lunch Pizza Big Daddys Ls 16 Inch 51% Whole Grain Rolled Edge Cheese Pizza Frozen ☛ serving size: 1 slice 1/8 per pizza = 155 g; Calories = 377

School Lunch Pizza Big Daddys Ls 16 Inch 51% Whole Grain Rolled Edge Turkey Pepperoni Pizza Frozen ☛ serving size: 1 slice 1/8 per pizza = 156 g; Calories = 387

School Lunch Pizza Cheese Topping Thick Crust Whole Grain Frozen Cooked ☛ serving size: 1 slice per 1/10 pizza = 124 g; Calories = 315

School Lunch Pizza Cheese Topping Thin Crust Whole Grain Frozen Cooked ☛ serving size: 1 piece 4 inchx6 inch = 130 g; Calories = 321

School Lunch Pizza Pepperoni Topping Thick Crust Whole Grain Frozen Cooked ☛ serving size: 1 slice per 1/10 pizza = 124 g; Calories = 321

School Lunch Pizza Pepperoni Topping Thin Crust Whole Grain

Frozen Cooked 🖝 serving size: 1 piece 4 inchx6 inch = 127 g; Calories = 323

School Lunch Pizza Sausage Topping Thick Crust Whole Grain Frozen Cooked 🖝 serving size: 1 slice per 1/10 pizza = 129 g; Calories = 332

School Lunch Pizza Sausage Topping Thin Crust Whole Grain Frozen Cooked 🖝 serving size: 1 piece 4 inch x 6 inch = 133 g; Calories = 333

School Lunch Pizza Tonys Breakfast Pizza Sausage Frozen 🖝 serving size: 1 piece 3.2 oz = 91 g; Calories = 218

School Lunch Pizza Tonys Smartpizza Whole Grain 4x6 Cheese Pizza 50/50 Cheese Frozen 🖝 serving size: 1 piece 4 inch x 6 inch = 130 g; Calories = 303

School Lunch Pizza Tonys Smartpizza Whole Grain 4x6 Pepperoni Pizza 50/50 Cheese Frozen 🖝 serving size: 1 piece 4 inchx6 inch = 127 g; Calories = 302

Scrambled Egg Sandwich 🖝 serving size: 1 sandwich = 112 g; Calories = 230

Shrimp Breaded And Fried 🖝 serving size: 3 pieces shrimp = 39 g; Calories = 120

Soft Serve Blended With Chocolate Candy 🖝 serving size: 12 fl oz cup = 348 g; Calories = 633

Steak And Cheese Sandwich Plain On Roll 🖝 serving size: 1 sandwich = 170 g; Calories = 422

Steak And Cheese Submarine Sandwich Plain On Roll 🖝 serving size: 1 submarine = 197 g; Calories = 496

Steak And Cheese Submarine Sandwich With Fried Peppers And Onions On Roll 🖝 serving size: 1 submarine = 260 g; Calories = 603

Steak Sandwich Plain On Biscuit ☛ serving size: 1 sandwich = 142 g; Calories = 408

Steak Sandwich Plain On Roll ☛ serving size: 1 sandwich = 142 g; Calories = 329

Steak Submarine Sandwich With Lettuce And Tomato ☛ serving size: 1 sandwich = 186 g; Calories = 376

Strawberry Banana Smoothie Made With Ice And Low-Fat Yogurt ☛ serving size: 12 fl oz = 347 g; Calories = 226

Submarine Sandwich Bacon Lettuce And Tomato On White Bread ☛ serving size: 6 inch sub = 148 g; Calories = 303

Submarine Sandwich Cold Cut On White Bread With Lettuce And Tomato ☛ serving size: 6 inch sub = 196 g; Calories = 418

Submarine Sandwich Ham On White Bread With Lettuce And Tomato ☛ serving size: 6 inch sub = 184 g; Calories = 278

Submarine Sandwich Meatball Marinara On White Bread ☛ serving size: 6 inch sub = 209 g; Calories = 458

Submarine Sandwich Oven Roasted Chicken On White Bread With Lettuce And Tomato ☛ serving size: 6 inch sub = 198 g; Calories = 311

Submarine Sandwich Roast Beef On White Bread With Lettuce And Tomato ☛ serving size: 6 inch sub = 190 g; Calories = 296

Submarine Sandwich Steak And Cheese On White Bread With Cheese Lettuce And Tomato ☛ serving size: 6 inch sub = 201 g; Calories = 368

Submarine Sandwich Sweet Onion Chicken Teriyaki On White Bread With Lettuce Tomato And Sweet Onion Sauce ☛ serving size: 6 inch sub = 228 g; Calories = 353

Submarine Sandwich Tuna On White Bread With Lettuce And Tomato ☛ serving size: 6 inch sub = 237 g; Calories = 517

Submarine Sandwich Turkey Breast On White Bread With Lettuce And Tomato ☛ serving size: 6 inch sub = 184 g; Calories = 271

Submarine Sandwich Turkey Roast Beef And Ham On White Bread With Lettuce And Tomato ☛ serving size: 12 inch sub = 413 g; Calories = 603

Subway B.l.t. Sub On White Bread With Bacon Lettuce And Tomato ☛ serving size: 6 inch sub = 148 g; Calories = 303

Subway Black Forest Ham Sub On White Bread With Lettuce And Tomato ☛ serving size: 6 inch sub = 184 g; Calories = 278

Subway Cold Cut Sub On White Bread With Lettuce And Tomato ☛ serving size: 6 inch sub = 196 g; Calories = 419

Subway Meatball Marinara Sub On White Bread (No Toppings) ☛ serving size: 6 inch sub = 209 g; Calories = 458

Subway Oven Roasted Chicken Sub On White Bread With Lettuce And Tomato ☛ serving size: 6 inch sub = 198 g; Calories = 311

Subway Roast Beef Sub On White Bread With Lettuce And Tomato ☛ serving size: 6 inch sub = 190 g; Calories = 295

Subway Steak & Cheese Sub On White Bread With American Cheese Lettuce And Tomato ☛ serving size: 6 inch sub = 201 g; Calories = 368

Subway Subway Club Sub On White Bread With Lettuce And Tomato ☛ serving size: 6 inch sub = 207 g; Calories = 302

Subway Sweet Onion Chicken Teriyaki Sub On White Bread With Lettuce Tomato And Sweet Onion Sauce ☛ serving size: 6 inch sub = 228 g; Calories = 353

Subway Tuna Sub ☛ serving size: 6 inch sub = 237 g; Calories = 524

Subway Turkey Breast Sub On White Bread With Lettuce And Tomato ☛ serving size: 6 inch sub = 184 g; Calories = 271

Sundae Caramel ☛ serving size: 1 sundae = 155 g; Calories = 304

Sundae Hot Fudge ☛ serving size: 1 sundae = 158 g; Calories = 284

Sundae Strawberry ☛ serving size: 1 sundae = 153 g; Calories = 268

Taco Bell Bean Burrito ☛ serving size: 1 each burrito = 185 g; Calories = 387

Taco Bell Burrito Supreme With Beef ☛ serving size: 1 burrito = 241 g; Calories = 441

Taco Bell Burrito Supreme With Chicken ☛ serving size: 1 item = 248 g; Calories = 444

Taco Bell Burrito Supreme With Steak ☛ serving size: 1 item = 248 g; Calories = 454

Taco Bell Nachos ☛ serving size: 1 serving = 80 g; Calories = 280

Taco Bell Nachos Supreme ☛ serving size: 1 serving = 222 g; Calories = 495

Taco Bell Original Taco With Beef Cheese And Lettuce ☛ serving size: 1 each taco = 69 g; Calories = 158

Taco Bell Soft Taco With Beef Cheese And Lettuce ☛ serving size: 1 each taco = 102 g; Calories = 210

Taco Bell Soft Taco With Chicken Cheese And Lettuce ☛ serving size: 1 each taco = 98 g; Calories = 185

Taco Bell Soft Taco With Steak ☛ serving size: 1 item = 127 g; Calories = 286

Taco Bell Taco Salad ☛ serving size: 1 item = 533 g; Calories = 906

Taco With Beef Cheese And Lettuce Hard Shell ☛ serving size: 1 each taco = 69 g; Calories = 156

Taco With Beef Cheese And Lettuce Soft ☛ serving size: 1 each taco = 102 g; Calories = 210

Taco With Chicken Lettuce And Cheese Soft ☞ serving size: 1 each taco = 98 g; Calories = 185

Taquito Or Flauta With Egg ☞ serving size: 1 small taquito = 36 g; Calories = 92

Taquito Or Flauta With Egg And Breakfast Meat ☞ serving size: 1 small taquito = 36 g; Calories = 96

Tomato Sandwich ☞ serving size: 1 sandwich = 134 g; Calories = 235

Triple Cheeseburger 3 Medium Patties With Condiments On Bun From Fast Food / Restaurant ☞ serving size: 1 triple cheeseburger = 420 g; Calories = 1193

Tuna Melt Sandwich ☞ serving size: 1 sandwich = 150 g; Calories = 348

Tuna Salad Sandwich ☞ serving size: 1 sandwich = 157 g; Calories = 254

Tuna Salad Sandwich With Lettuce ☞ serving size: 1 sandwich = 167 g; Calories = 256

Turkey And Bacon Submarine Sandwich With Cheese Lettuce Tomato And Spread ☞ serving size: 1 submarine = 260 g; Calories = 577

Turkey And Bacon Submarine Sandwich With Lettuce Tomato And Spread ☞ serving size: 1 submarine = 240 g; Calories = 494

Turkey Ham And Roast Beef Club Sandwich With Lettuce Tomato And Spread ☞ serving size: 1 sandwich = 240 g; Calories = 398

Turkey Or Chicken Burger Plain On Bun From Fast Food / Restaurant ☞ serving size: 1 sandwich = 145 g; Calories = 338

Turkey Or Chicken Burger Plain On Wheat Bun ☞ serving size: 1 sandwich = 145 g; Calories = 329

Turkey Or Chicken Burger Plain On White Bun ☛ serving size: 1 sandwich = 145 g; Calories = 338

Turkey Or Chicken Burger With Condiments On Bun From Fast Food / Restaurant ☛ serving size: 1 sandwich = 200 g; Calories = 380

Turkey Or Chicken Burger With Condiments On Wheat Bun ☛ serving size: 1 sandwich = 200 g; Calories = 370

Turkey Or Chicken Burger With Condiments On White Bun ☛ serving size: 1 sandwich = 200 g; Calories = 380

Turkey Or Chicken Burger With Condiments On Whole Wheat Bun ☛ serving size: 1 sandwich = 200 g; Calories = 370

Turkey Salad Or Turkey Spread Sandwich ☛ serving size: 1 sandwich = 141 g; Calories = 322

Turkey Sandwich With Gravy ☛ serving size: 1 sandwich = 284 g; Calories = 383

Turkey Sandwich With Spread ☛ serving size: 1 sandwich = 143 g; Calories = 319

Vanilla Light Soft-Serve Ice Cream With Cone ☛ serving size: 1 item = 120 g; Calories = 196

Vegetable Submarine Sandwich With Fat Free Spread ☛ serving size: 1 submarine = 240 g; Calories = 300

Vegetable Submarine Sandwich With Spread ☛ serving size: 1 submarine = 167 g; Calories = 311

Waffle Chocolate ☛ serving size: 1 miniature/bite size waffle = 10 g; Calories = 43

Waffle Chocolate From Fast Food / Restaurant ☛ serving size: 1 miniature/bite size waffle = 10 g; Calories = 48

Waffle Chocolate From Frozen ☛ serving size: 1 miniature/bite size waffle = 10 g; Calories = 32

🍔 Waffle Cinnamon 🠒 serving size: 1 miniature/bite size waffle = 10 g; Calories = 37

🍔 Waffle Cornmeal 🠒 serving size: 1 miniature/bite size waffle = 10 g; Calories = 26

🍔 Waffle Fruit 🠒 serving size: 1 miniature/bite size waffle = 10 g; Calories = 30

🍔 Waffle Fruit From Fast Food / Restaurant 🠒 serving size: 1 miniature/bite size waffle = 10 g; Calories = 35

🍔 Waffle Fruit From Frozen 🠒 serving size: 1 miniature/bite size waffle = 10 g; Calories = 30

🍔 Waffle Plain 🠒 serving size: 1 miniature/bite size waffle = 10 g; Calories = 37

🍔 Waffle Plain From Fast Food / Restaurant 🠒 serving size: 1 miniature/bite size waffle = 10 g; Calories = 42

🍔 Waffle Plain Reduced Fat 🠒 serving size: 1 miniature/bite size waffle = 10 g; Calories = 34

🍔 Waffle Plain Reduced Fat From Frozen 🠒 serving size: 1 miniature/bite size waffle = 10 g; Calories = 29

🍔 Waffle Whole Grain 🠒 serving size: 1 miniature/bite size waffle = 10 g; Calories = 36

🍔 Waffle Whole Grain From Fast Food / Restaurant 🠒 serving size: 1 miniature/bite size waffle = 10 g; Calories = 42

🍔 Waffle Whole Grain From Frozen 🠒 serving size: 1 miniature/bite size waffle = 10 g; Calories = 29

🍔 Waffle Whole Grain Fruit From Frozen 🠒 serving size: 1 miniature/bite size waffle = 10 g; Calories = 28

🍔 Waffle Whole Grain Reduced Fat 🠒 serving size: 1 miniature/bite size waffle = 10 g; Calories = 33

Wendys Chicken Nuggets ☛ serving size: 5 pieces = 68 g; Calories = 222

Wendys Classic Double With Cheese ☛ serving size: 1 item = 310 g; Calories = 747

Wendys Classic Single Hamburger No Cheese ☛ serving size: 1 item = 218 g; Calories = 464

Wendys Classic Single Hamburger With Cheese ☛ serving size: 1 item = 236 g; Calories = 522

Wendys Crispy Chicken Sandwich ☛ serving size: 1 sandwich = 126 g; Calories = 350

Wendys Daves Hot N Juicy 1/4 Lb Single ☛ serving size: 1 sandwich = 215 g; Calories = 576

Wendys Double Stack With Cheese ☛ serving size: 1 sandwich = 146 g; Calories = 416

Wendys French Fries ☛ serving size: 1 kid's meal serving = 71 g; Calories = 214

Wendys Frosty Dairy Dessert ☛ serving size: 1 junior 6 oz. cup = 113 g; Calories = 149

Wendys Homestyle Chicken Fillet Sandwich ☛ serving size: 1 item = 230 g; Calories = 492

Wendys Jr. Hamburger With Cheese ☛ serving size: 1 item = 129 g; Calories = 330

Wendys Jr. Hamburger Without Cheese ☛ serving size: 1 item = 117 g; Calories = 284

Wendys Ultimate Chicken Grill Sandwich ☛ serving size: 1 item = 225 g; Calories = 403

Wrap Sandwich Filled With Beef Patty Cheese And Spread And/or Sauce ☛ serving size: 1 snack wrap sandwich = 126 g; Calories

= 340

🍔 Wrap Sandwich Filled With Meat Poultry Or Fish And Vegetables 🖝 serving size: 1 sandwich = 240 g; Calories = 449

🍔 Wrap Sandwich Filled With Meat Poultry Or Fish Vegetables And Cheese 🖝 serving size: 1 sandwich = 280 g; Calories = 574

🍔 Wrap Sandwich Filled With Meat Poultry Or Fish Vegetables And Rice 🖝 serving size: 1 sandwich = 433 g; Calories = 680

🍔 Wrap Sandwich Filled With Meat Poultry Or Fish Vegetables Rice And Cheese 🖝 serving size: 1 sandwich = 467 g; Calories = 761

🍔 Wrap Sandwich Filled With Vegetables 🖝 serving size: 1 sandwich = 273 g; Calories = 333

🍔 Wrap Sandwich Filled With Vegetables And Rice 🖝 serving size: 1 sandwich = 404 g; Calories = 549

🍔 Yogurt Parfait Lowfat With Fruit And Granola 🖝 serving size: 1 item = 149 g; Calories = 125

14

FATS AND OILS

🍪 Almond Oil ☛ serving size: 1 tablespoon = 13.6 g; Calories = 120

🍪 Animal Fat Or Drippings ☛ serving size: 1 cup = 205 g; Calories = 1724

🍪 Apricot Kernel Oil ☛ serving size: 1 tablespoon = 13.6 g; Calories = 120

🍪 Avocado Oil ☛ serving size: 1 tbsp = 14 g; Calories = 124

🍪 Bacon Grease ☛ serving size: 1 tsp = 4.3 g; Calories = 39

🍪 Beef Tallow ☛ serving size: 1 tbsp = 12.8 g; Calories = 116

🍪 Butter Light Stick With Salt ☛ serving size: 1 tablespoon = 14 g; Calories = 70

🍪 Butter Light Stick Without Salt ☛ serving size: 1 tablespoon = 14 g; Calories = 70

🍪 Butter Replacement Without Fat Powder ☛ serving size: 1 cup = 80 g; Calories = 298

🍪 Butter Whipped Tub Salted ☛ serving size: 1 cup = 151 g; Calories = 1084

🍪 Butter-Margarine Blend Stick Salted ☛ serving size: 1 cup = 227 g; Calories = 1628

🍪 Canola Oil ☛ serving size: 1 tbsp = 14 g; Calories = 124

🍪 Cheese Cream Light Or Lite ☛ serving size: 1 cup = 240 g; Calories = 482

🍪 Cheese Spread Cream Cheese Light Or Lite ☛ serving size: 1 cup = 240 g; Calories = 482

🍪 Cocoa Butter ☛ serving size: 1 tablespoon = 13.6 g; Calories = 120

🍪 Coconut Oil ☛ serving size: 1 tbsp = 13.6 g; Calories = 121

🍪 Cod Liver Oil ☛ serving size: 1 tsp = 4.5 g; Calories = 41

🍪 Coffee Creamer Liquid Fat Free Flavored ☛ serving size: 1 cup = 240 g; Calories = 360

🍪 Coleslaw Dressing ☛ serving size: 1 cup = 250 g; Calories = 975

🍪 Coleslaw Salad Dressing ☛ serving size: 1 tbsp = 16 g; Calories = 65

🍪 Corn Oil ☛ serving size: 1 tbsp = 13.6 g; Calories = 122

🍪 Cottonseed Oil ☛ serving size: 1 tablespoon = 13.6 g; Calories = 120

🍪 Cream Half And Half ☛ serving size: 1 cup = 240 g; Calories = 295

🍪 Cream Half And Half Flavored ☛ serving size: 1 cup = 240 g; Calories = 293

🍪 Cream Heavy ☛ serving size: 1 cup = 240 g; Calories = 816

🍪 Cream Light ☛ serving size: 1 cup = 240 g; Calories = 458

🍪 Cream Ns As To Light Heavy Or Half And Half ☛ serving size: 1 cup = 240 g; Calories = 295

🍪 Cream Whipped ☛ serving size: 1 cup = 120 g; Calories = 412

Creamy Dressing Made With Sour Cream And/or Buttermilk And Oil Reduced Calorie ☞ serving size: 1 tbsp = 15 g; Calories = 24

Creamy Dressing Made With Sour Cream And/or Buttermilk And Oil Reduced Calorie Cholesterol-Free ☞ serving size: 1 tbsp = 15 g; Calories = 21

Creamy Dressing Made With Sour Cream And/or Buttermilk And Oil Reduced Calorie Fat-Free ☞ serving size: 1 tbsp = 17 g; Calories = 18

Creamy Poppyseed Salad Dressing ☞ serving size: 2 tbsp = 33 g; Calories = 132

Dressing Honey Mustard Fat-Free ☞ serving size: 2 tbsp (1 nlea serving) = 30 g; Calories = 51

Fat Back Cooked ☞ serving size: 1 slice (2-1/4" x 1-3/4" x 1/4") = 26 g; Calories = 195

Fat Goose ☞ serving size: 1 tbsp = 12.8 g; Calories = 115

Fat Turkey ☞ serving size: 1 tbsp = 12.8 g; Calories = 115

Fish Oil Menhaden Fully Hydrogenated ☞ serving size: 1 tbsp = 12.5 g; Calories = 113

Flaxseed Oil ☞ serving size: 1 tbsp = 13.6 g; Calories = 120

French Or Catalina Dressing ☞ serving size: 1 cup = 250 g; Calories = 1143

Grapeseed Oil ☞ serving size: 1 tablespoon = 13.6 g; Calories = 120

Hazelnut Oil ☞ serving size: 1 tablespoon = 13.6 g; Calories = 120

Herring Oil ☞ serving size: 1 tbsp = 13.6 g; Calories = 123

Honey Butter ☞ serving size: 1 cup = 288 g; Calories = 1354

Honey Mustard Salad Dressing ☞ serving size: 2 tbsp = 30 g; Calories = 139

◉ Hydrogenated Soybean And Palm Oil ☛ serving size: 1 tbsp = 12.8 g; Calories = 113

◉ Italian Salad Dressing ☛ serving size: 1 tablespoon = 15 g; Calories = 15

◉ Korean Dressing Or Marinade ☛ serving size: 1 cup = 246 g; Calories = 832

◉ Lard ☛ serving size: 1 tbsp = 12.8 g; Calories = 116

◉ Lowfat French Salad Dressing ☛ serving size: 1 tablespoon = 16 g; Calories = 37

◉ Margarine ☛ serving size: 1 tsp = 4.7 g; Calories = 34

◉ Margarine (Unsalted) ☛ serving size: 1 tbsp = 14.2 g; Calories = 102

◉ Margarine 80% Fat Stick Includes Regular And Hydrogenated Corn And Soybean Oils ☛ serving size: 1 tbsp = 14 g; Calories = 100

◉ Margarine 80% Fat Tub Canola Harvest Soft Spread (Canola Palm And Palm Kernel Oils) ☛ serving size: 1 tablespoon (1 nlea serving) = 14 g; Calories = 102

◉ Margarine Industrial Non-Dairy Cottonseed Soy Oil (Partially Hydrogenated) For Flaky Pastries ☛ serving size: 1 tbsp = 14 g; Calories = 100

◉ Margarine Industrial Soy And Partially Hydrogenated Soy Oil Use For Baking Sauces And Candy ☛ serving size: 1 tbsp = 14 g; Calories = 100

◉ Margarine Like Spread Whipped Tub Salted ☛ serving size: 1 tablespoon = 10 g; Calories = 53

◉ Margarine Margarine-Like Vegetable Oil Spread 67-70% Fat Tub ☛ serving size: 1 tbsp (1 nlea serving) = 14 g; Calories = 85

◉ Margarine Margarine-Type Vegetable Oil Spread 70% Fat

Soybean And Partially Hydrogenated Soybean Stick ☞ serving size: 1 tbsp (1 nlea serving) = 14 g; Calories = 88

☕ Margarine Regular 80% Fat Composite Stick With Salt ☞ serving size: 1 tbsp = 14 g; Calories = 100

☕ Margarine Regular 80% Fat Composite Stick With Salt With Added Vitamin D ☞ serving size: 1 tablespoon = 14 g; Calories = 100

☕ Margarine Regular 80% Fat Composite Stick Without Salt With Added Vitamin D ☞ serving size: 1 tbsp = 14 g; Calories = 100

☕ Margarine Regular 80% Fat Composite Tub With Salt ☞ serving size: 1 tbsp = 14.2 g; Calories = 101

☕ Margarine Regular 80% Fat Composite Tub With Salt With Added Vitamin D ☞ serving size: 1 tbsp = 14 g; Calories = 100

☕ Margarine Regular 80% Fat Composite Tub Without Salt ☞ serving size: 1 tbsp = 14.2 g; Calories = 101

☕ Margarine Spread Approximately 48% Fat Tub ☞ serving size: 1 tbsp = 14 g; Calories = 56

☕ Margarine-Like Butter-Margarine Blend 80% Fat Stick Without Salt ☞ serving size: 1 tablespoon = 14 g; Calories = 101

☕ Margarine-Like Margarine-Butter Blend Soybean Oil And Butter ☞ serving size: 1 tbsp = 14.1 g; Calories = 103

☕ Margarine-Like Shortening Industrial Soy (Partially Hydrogenated) Cottonseed And Soy Principal Use Flaky Pastries ☞ serving size: 1 tbsp = 14 g; Calories = 88

☕ Margarine-Like Spread Benecol Light Spread ☞ serving size: 1 tablespoon (1 nlea serving) = 14 g; Calories = 50

☕ Margarine-Like Spread Liquid Salted ☞ serving size: 1 cup = 227 g; Calories = 1196

⚘ Margarine-Like Spread Smart Balance Light Buttery Spread ☛ serving size: 1 tbsp = 14 g; Calories = 47

⚘ Margarine-Like Spread Smart Balance Omega Plus Spread (With Plant Sterols & Fish Oil) ☛ serving size: 1 tablespoon = 14 g; Calories = 85

⚘ Margarine-Like Spread Smart Balance Regular Buttery Spread With Flax Oil ☛ serving size: 1 tablespoon = 14 g; Calories = 82

⚘ Margarine-Like Spread Smart Beat Smart Squeeze ☛ serving size: 1 tablespoon = 14 g; Calories = 7

⚘ Margarine-Like Spread Smart Beat Super Light Without Saturated Fat ☛ serving size: 1 tablespoon = 14 g; Calories = 22

⚘ Margarine-Like Spread With Yogurt 70% Fat Stick With Salt ☛ serving size: 1 tablespoon = 14 g; Calories = 88

⚘ Margarine-Like Spread With Yogurt Approximately 40% Fat Tub With Salt ☛ serving size: 1 tablespoon = 14 g; Calories = 46

⚘ Margarine-Like Vegetable Oil Spread 20% Fat With Salt ☛ serving size: 1 tbsp = 15 g; Calories = 26

⚘ Margarine-Like Vegetable Oil Spread 20% Fat Without Salt ☛ serving size: 1 tbsp = 12.8 g; Calories = 22

⚘ Margarine-Like Vegetable Oil Spread 60% Fat Stick With Salt ☛ serving size: 1 tbsp = 14.3 g; Calories = 77

⚘ Margarine-Like Vegetable Oil Spread 60% Fat Stick With Salt With Added Vitamin D ☛ serving size: 1 tbsp = 14 g; Calories = 75

⚘ Margarine-Like Vegetable Oil Spread 60% Fat Stick/tub/bottle With Salt ☛ serving size: 1 tbsp = 14.3 g; Calories = 75

⚘ Margarine-Like Vegetable Oil Spread 60% Fat Stick/tub/bottle Without Salt ☛ serving size: 1 tbsp = 14 g; Calories = 75

⚘ Margarine-Like Vegetable Oil Spread 60% Fat Stick/tub/bottle

Without Salt With Added Vitamin D ☛ serving size: 1 tbsp = 14 g; Calories = 76

☙ Margarine-Like Vegetable Oil Spread 60% Fat Tub With Salt ☛ serving size: 1 tbsp = 14 g; Calories = 75

☙ Margarine-Like Vegetable Oil Spread 60% Fat Tub With Salt With Added Vitamin D ☛ serving size: 1 tbsp = 14 g; Calories = 75

☙ Margarine-Like Vegetable Oil Spread Approximately 37% Fat Unspecified Oils With Salt With Added Vitamin D ☛ serving size: 1 tbsp = 14.9 g; Calories = 51

☙ Margarine-Like Vegetable Oil Spread Fat Free Liquid With Salt ☛ serving size: 1 tbsp = 15 g; Calories = 7

☙ Margarine-Like Vegetable Oil Spread Fat-Free Tub ☛ serving size: 1 tbsp = 14.6 g; Calories = 6

☙ Margarine-Like Vegetable Oil Spread Stick Or Tub Sweetened ☛ serving size: 1 tablespoon = 14 g; Calories = 75

☙ Margarine-Like Vegetable Oil Spread Unspecified Oils Approximately 37% Fat With Salt ☛ serving size: 1 tbsp = 14.9 g; Calories = 52

☙ Margarine-Like Vegetable Oil-Butter Spread Reduced Calorie Tub With Salt ☛ serving size: 1 tablespoon = 14 g; Calories = 63

☙ Margarine-Like Vegetable Oil-Butter Spread Tub With Salt ☛ serving size: 1 tablespoon = 14 g; Calories = 51

☙ Margarine-Like Vegetable-Oil Spread Stick/tub/bottle 60% Fat With Added Vitamin D ☛ serving size: 1 tbsp = 14 g; Calories = 75

☙ Mayonnaise Dressing No Cholesterol ☛ serving size: 1 tbsp = 15 g; Calories = 103

☙ Mayonnaise Low Sodium Low Calorie Or Diet ☛ serving size: 1 tbsp = 14 g; Calories = 32

☕ Mayonnaise Made With Tofu ☛ serving size: 1 tbsp = 15 g; Calories = 48

☕ Mayonnaise Reduced Fat With Olive Oil ☛ serving size: 1 tbsp = 15 g; Calories = 54

☕ Mayonnaise Reduced-Calorie Or Diet Cholesterol-Free ☛ serving size: 1 tbsp = 14.6 g; Calories = 49

☕ Mayonnaise Salad Dressing ☛ serving size: 1 tbsp = 14.7 g; Calories = 37

☕ Menhaden Oil ☛ serving size: 1 tbsp = 13.6 g; Calories = 123

☕ Mustard Oil ☛ serving size: 1 tbsp = 14 g; Calories = 124

☕ Oil Babassu ☛ serving size: 1 tbsp = 13.6 g; Calories = 120

☕ Oil Cooking And Salad Enova 80% Diglycerides ☛ serving size: 1 tbsp (1 nlea serving) = 14 g; Calories = 124

☕ Oil Corn And Canola ☛ serving size: 1 tbsp = 14 g; Calories = 124

☕ Oil Corn Peanut And Olive ☛ serving size: 1 tablespoon = 14 g; Calories = 124

☕ Oil Cupu Assu ☛ serving size: 1 tablespoon = 13.6 g; Calories = 120

☕ Oil Flaxseed Contains Added Sliced Flaxseed ☛ serving size: 1 tablespoon = 13.7 g; Calories = 120

☕ Oil Industrial Canola (Partially Hydrogenated) Oil For Deep Fat Frying ☛ serving size: 1 tablespoon = 13.6 g; Calories = 120

☕ Oil Industrial Canola For Salads Woks And Light Frying ☛ serving size: 1 tablespoon = 13.6 g; Calories = 120

☕ Oil Industrial Canola High Oleic ☛ serving size: 1 tablespoon = 14 g; Calories = 126

☕ Oil Industrial Canola With Antifoaming Agent Principal Uses

Salads Woks And Light Frying ☛ serving size: 1 tablespoon = 13.6 g; Calories = 120

☟ Oil Industrial Coconut (Hydrogenated) Used For Whipped Toppings And Coffee Whiteners ☛ serving size: 1 tbsp = 13.6 g; Calories = 120

☟ Oil Industrial Coconut Confection Fat Typical Basis For Ice Cream Coatings ☛ serving size: 1 tbsp = 13.6 g; Calories = 120

☟ Oil Industrial Coconut Principal Uses Candy Coatings Oil Sprays Roasting Nuts ☛ serving size: 1 tbsp = 13.6 g; Calories = 120

☟ Oil Industrial Cottonseed Fully Hydrogenated ☛ serving size: 1 tablespoon = 13.6 g; Calories = 120

☟ Oil Industrial Mid-Oleic Sunflower ☛ serving size: 1 tablespoon = 13.6 g; Calories = 120

☟ Oil Industrial Palm And Palm Kernel Filling Fat (Non-Hydrogenated) ☛ serving size: 1 tbsp = 13.6 g; Calories = 120

☟ Oil Industrial Palm Kernel (Hydrogenated) Used For Whipped Toppings Non-Dairy ☛ serving size: 1 tbsp = 13.6 g; Calories = 120

☟ Oil Industrial Palm Kernel (Hydrogenated) Confection Fat Intermediate Grade Product ☛ serving size: 1 tbsp = 13.6 g; Calories = 120

☟ Oil Industrial Palm Kernel (Hydrogenated) Confection Fat Uses Similar To 95 Degree Hard Butter ☛ serving size: 1 tbsp = 13.6 g; Calories = 120

☟ Oil Industrial Palm Kernel (Hydrogenated) Filling Fat ☛ serving size: 1 tbsp = 13.6 g; Calories = 120

☟ Oil Industrial Palm Kernel Confection Fat Uses Similar To High Quality Cocoa Butter ☛ serving size: 1 tbsp = 13.6 g; Calories = 120

☟ Oil Industrial Soy (Partially Hydrogenated) All Purpose ☛ serving size: 1 tbsp = 13.6 g; Calories = 120

Oil Industrial Soy (Partially Hydrogenated) And Soy (Winterized) Pourable Clear Fry ☛ serving size: 1 tbsp = 13.6 g; Calories = 120

Oil Industrial Soy (Partially Hydrogenated) Palm Principal Uses Icings And Fillings ☛ serving size: 1 tbsp = 13.6 g; Calories = 120

Oil Industrial Soy (Partially Hydrogenated) And Cottonseed Principal Use As A Tortilla Shortening ☛ serving size: 1 tbsp = 13.6 g; Calories = 120

Oil Industrial Soy (Partially Hydrogenated) Multiuse For Non-Dairy Butter Flavor ☛ serving size: 1 tbsp = 13.6 g; Calories = 120

Oil Industrial Soy (Partially Hydrogenated) Principal Uses Popcorn And Flavoring Vegetables ☛ serving size: 1 tbsp = 13.6 g; Calories = 120

Oil Industrial Soy Fully Hydrogenated ☛ serving size: 1 tablespoon = 13.6 g; Calories = 120

Oil Industrial Soy Low Linolenic ☛ serving size: 1 tablespoon = 14 g; Calories = 126

Oil Industrial Soy Refined For Woks And Light Frying ☛ serving size: 1 tbsp = 13.6 g; Calories = 120

Oil Industrial Soy Ultra Low Linolenic ☛ serving size: 1 tablespoon = 13.6 g; Calories = 120

Oil Nutmeg Butter ☛ serving size: 1 tbsp = 13.6 g; Calories = 120

Oil Oat ☛ serving size: 1 tbsp = 13.6 g; Calories = 120

Oil Or Table Fat Nfs ☛ serving size: 1 cup = 224 g; Calories = 1711

Oil Pam Cooking Spray Original ☛ serving size: 1 spray , about 1/3 second (1 nlea serving) = 0.3 g; Calories = 2

Oil Safflower Salad Or Cooking High Oleic (Primary Safflower Oil Of Commerce) ☛ serving size: 1 tablespoon = 13.6 g; Calories = 120

Oil Safflower Salad Or Cooking Linoleic (Over 70%) ☛ serving size: 1 tbsp = 13.6 g; Calories = 120

Oil Sheanut ☛ serving size: 1 tablespoon = 13.6 g; Calories = 120

Oil Soybean Salad Or Cooking (Partially Hydrogenated) ☛ serving size: 1 tbsp = 13.6 g; Calories = 120

Oil Soybean Salad Or Cooking (Partially Hydrogenated) And Cottonseed ☛ serving size: 1 tablespoon = 13.6 g; Calories = 120

Oil Sunflower High Oleic (70% And Over) ☛ serving size: 1 tbsp = 14 g; Calories = 124

Oil Sunflower Linoleic (Approx. 65%) ☛ serving size: 1 tbsp = 13.6 g; Calories = 120

Oil Sunflower Linoleic (Less Than 60%) ☛ serving size: 1 tbsp = 13.6 g; Calories = 120

Oil Sunflower Linoleic (Partially Hydrogenated) ☛ serving size: 1 tbsp = 13.6 g; Calories = 120

Oil Ucuhuba Butter ☛ serving size: 1 tbsp = 13.6 g; Calories = 120

Oil Vegetable Natreon Canola High Stability Non Trans High Oleic (70%) ☛ serving size: 1 tbsp = 14 g; Calories = 124

Olive Oil ☛ serving size: 1 tablespoon = 13.5 g; Calories = 119

Palm Kernel Oil ☛ serving size: 1 tablespoon = 13.6 g; Calories = 117

Palm Oil ☛ serving size: 1 tbsp = 13.6 g; Calories = 120

Peanut Oil ☛ serving size: 1 tbsp = 13.5 g; Calories = 119

Poppyseed Oil ☛ serving size: 1 tablespoon = 13.6 g; Calories = 120

Rendered Chicken Fat ☛ serving size: 1 tbsp = 12.8 g; Calories = 115

Rice Bran Oil ☛ serving size: 1 tablespoon = 13.6 g; Calories = 120

Russian Dressing ☛ serving size: 1 tbsp = 15 g; Calories = 53

⊌ Salad Dressing Bacon And Tomato ☛ serving size: 1 tbsp = 15 g;
Calories = 49

⊌ Salad Dressing Blue Or Roquefort Cheese Dressing Commercial
Regular ☛ serving size: 1 tbsp = 15 g; Calories = 73

⊌ Salad Dressing Blue Or Roquefort Cheese Dressing Fat-Free ☛
serving size: 1 tbsp = 17 g; Calories = 20

⊌ Salad Dressing Blue Or Roquefort Cheese Dressing Light ☛
serving size: 1 tbsp = 16 g; Calories = 14

⊌ Salad Dressing Blue Or Roquefort Cheese Low Calorie ☛ serving
size: 1 tbsp = 15 g; Calories = 15

⊌ Salad Dressing Buttermilk Lite ☛ serving size: 1 tablespoon = 15 g;
Calories = 30

⊌ Salad Dressing Caesar Dressing Regular ☛ serving size: 1 tbsp =
14.7 g; Calories = 80

⊌ Salad Dressing Caesar Fat-Free ☛ serving size: 2 tbsp (1 nlea serving) = 34 g; Calories = 45

⊌ Salad Dressing Caesar Low Calorie ☛ serving size: 1 tbsp = 15 g;
Calories = 17

⊌ Salad Dressing Coleslaw Dressing Reduced Fat ☛ serving size: 1
tbsp = 17 g; Calories = 56

⊌ Salad Dressing French Cottonseed Oil Home Recipe ☛ serving
size: 1 tablespoon = 14 g; Calories = 88

⊌ Salad Dressing French Dressing Commercial Regular ☛ serving
size: 1 tbsp = 16 g; Calories = 67

⊌ Salad Dressing French Dressing Commercial Regular Without
Salt ☛ serving size: 1 tablespoon = 15 g; Calories = 69

⊌ Salad Dressing French Dressing Fat-Free ☛ serving size: 1 tablespoon = 16 g; Calories = 21

✅ Salad Dressing French Dressing Reduced Calorie ☛ serving size: 1 tbsp = 16 g; Calories = 36

✅ Salad Dressing French Dressing Reduced Fat ☛ serving size: 1 tablespoon = 16 g; Calories = 36

✅ Salad Dressing French Home Recipe ☛ serving size: 1 tablespoon = 14 g; Calories = 88

✅ Salad Dressing Green Goddess Regular ☛ serving size: 1 tbsp = 15 g; Calories = 64

✅ Salad Dressing Home Recipe Vinegar And Oil ☛ serving size: 1 tablespoon = 16 g; Calories = 72

✅ Salad Dressing Honey Mustard Dressing Reduced Calorie ☛ serving size: 2 tbsp (1 serving) = 30 g; Calories = 62

✅ Salad Dressing Italian Dressing Commercial Regular ☛ serving size: 1 tbsp = 14.7 g; Calories = 35

✅ Salad Dressing Italian Dressing Commercial Regular Without Salt ☛ serving size: 1 tablespoon = 14.7 g; Calories = 43

✅ Salad Dressing Italian Dressing Fat-Free ☛ serving size: 1 tbsp = 14 g; Calories = 7

✅ Salad Dressing Italian Dressing Reduced Calorie ☛ serving size: 1 tbsp = 14 g; Calories = 28

✅ Salad Dressing Italian Dressing Reduced Fat Without Salt ☛ serving size: 1 tablespoon = 15 g; Calories = 11

✅ Salad Dressing Kraft Mayo Fat Free Mayonnaise Dressing ☛ serving size: 1 tbsp = 16 g; Calories = 10

✅ Salad Dressing Kraft Mayo Light Mayonnaise ☛ serving size: 1 tbsp = 15 g; Calories = 50

✅ Salad Dressing Kraft Miracle Whip Free Nonfat Dressing ☛ serving size: 1 tbsp = 16 g; Calories = 13

💿 Salad Dressing Mayonnaise And Mayonnaise-Type Low Calorie ☞ serving size: 1 tbsp = 14.5 g; Calories = 38

💿 Salad Dressing Mayonnaise Imitation Milk Cream ☞ serving size: 1 tablespoon = 15 g; Calories = 15

💿 Salad Dressing Mayonnaise Imitation Soybean ☞ serving size: 1 tbsp = 15 g; Calories = 35

💿 Salad Dressing Mayonnaise Imitation Soybean Without Cholesterol ☞ serving size: 1 tablespoon = 14.1 g; Calories = 68

💿 Salad Dressing Mayonnaise Light ☞ serving size: 1 tablespoon = 15 g; Calories = 36

💿 Salad Dressing Mayonnaise Light Smart Balance Omega Plus Light ☞ serving size: 1 tbsp (1 nlea serving) = 14 g; Calories = 47

💿 Salad Dressing Mayonnaise Regular ☞ serving size: 1 tbsp = 13.8 g; Calories = 94

💿 Salad Dressing Mayonnaise Soybean And Safflower Oil With Salt ☞ serving size: 1 tablespoon = 13.8 g; Calories = 99

💿 Salad Dressing Mayonnaise Soybean Oil Without Salt ☞ serving size: 1 tablespoon = 13.8 g; Calories = 99

💿 Salad Dressing Mayonnaise-Like Fat-Free ☞ serving size: 1 tbsp = 16 g; Calories = 13

💿 Salad Dressing NFS For Sandwiches ☞ serving size: 1 cup = 237 g; Calories = 1408

💿 Salad Dressing Peppercorn Dressing Commercial Regular ☞ serving size: 1 tbsp = 13.4 g; Calories = 76

💿 Salad Dressing Ranch Dressing Fat-Free ☞ serving size: 1 tablespoon = 14 g; Calories = 17

💿 Salad Dressing Ranch Dressing Reduced Fat ☞ serving size: 1 tablespoon = 15 g; Calories = 29

Salad Dressing Ranch Dressing Regular ☛ serving size: 1 tablespoon = 15 g; Calories = 65

Salad Dressing Russian Dressing Low Calorie ☛ serving size: 1 tablespoon = 16 g; Calories = 23

Salad Dressing Spray-Style Dressing Assorted Flavors ☛ serving size: 1 serving (approximately 10 sprays) = 8 g; Calories = 13

Salad Dressing Sweet And Sour ☛ serving size: 1 tbsp = 16 g; Calories = 2

Salad Dressing Thousand Island Dressing Fat-Free ☛ serving size: 1 tbsp = 16 g; Calories = 21

Salad Dressing Thousand Island Dressing Reduced Fat ☛ serving size: 1 tablespoon = 15 g; Calories = 29

Salmon Oil ☛ serving size: 1 tbsp = 13.6 g; Calories = 123

Sandwich Spread With Chopped Pickle Regular Unspecified Oils ☛ serving size: 1 tablespoon = 15 g; Calories = 58

Sardine Oil ☛ serving size: 1 tbsp = 13.6 g; Calories = 123

Sesame Oil ☛ serving size: 1 tablespoon = 13.6 g; Calories = 120

Sesame Seed Dressing ☛ serving size: 1 tablespoon = 15 g; Calories = 67

Shortening ☛ serving size: 1 tbsp = 12.8 g; Calories = 115

Shortening Bread Soybean (Hydrogenated) And Cottonseed ☛ serving size: 1 tablespoon = 12.8 g; Calories = 113

Shortening Cake Mix Soybean (Hydrogenated) And Cottonseed (Hydrogenated) ☛ serving size: 1 tbsp = 12.8 g; Calories = 113

Shortening Confectionery Coconut (Hydrogenated) And Or Palm Kernel (Hydrogenated) ☛ serving size: 1 tbsp = 12.8 g; Calories = 113

☺ Shortening Confectionery Fractionated Palm ☞ serving size: 1 tbsp = 13.6 g; Calories = 120

☺ Shortening Frying (Heavy Duty) Beef Tallow And Cottonseed ☞ serving size: 1 tbsp = 12.8 g; Calories = 115

☺ Shortening Frying (Heavy Duty) Palm (Hydrogenated) ☞ serving size: 1 tbsp = 12.8 g; Calories = 113

☺ Shortening Frying (Heavy Duty) Soybean (Hydrogenated) Linoleic (Less Than 1%) ☞ serving size: 1 tbsp = 12.8 g; Calories = 113

☺ Shortening Household Lard And Vegetable Oil ☞ serving size: 1 tablespoon = 12.8 g; Calories = 115

☺ Shortening Household Soybean (Hydrogenated) And Palm ☞ serving size: 1 tbsp = 12.8 g; Calories = 113

☺ Shortening Household Soybean (Partially Hydrogenated)-Cottonseed (Partially Hydrogenated) ☞ serving size: 1 tbsp = 12.8 g; Calories = 113

☺ Shortening Industrial Soy (Partially Hydrogenated) And Corn For Frying ☞ serving size: 1 tbsp = 12.8 g; Calories = 113

☺ Shortening Industrial Soy (Partially Hydrogenated) For Baking And Confections ☞ serving size: 1 tbsp = 12.8 g; Calories = 113

☺ Shortening Industrial Soy (Partially Hydrogenated) Pourable Liquid Fry Shortening ☞ serving size: 1 tbsp = 13.6 g; Calories = 120

☺ Shortening Industrial Soybean (Hydrogenated) And Cottonseed ☞ serving size: 1 tbsp = 12.8 g; Calories = 113

☺ Shortening Special Purpose For Baking Soybean (Hydrogenated) Palm And Cottonseed ☞ serving size: 1 tbsp = 12.8 g; Calories = 113

☺ Shortening Special Purpose For Cakes And Frostings Soybean (Hydrogenated) ☞ serving size: 1 tbsp = 12.8 g; Calories = 113

Soybean Lecithin ☛ serving size: 1 tablespoon = 13.6 g; Calories = 104

Soybean Oil ☛ serving size: 1 tbsp = 13.6 g; Calories = 120

Table Fat Nfs ☛ serving size: 1 cup = 227 g; Calories = 1460

Tartar Sauce Reduced Fat/calorie ☛ serving size: 1 cup = 224 g; Calories = 193

Teaseed Oil ☛ serving size: 1 tablespoon = 13.6 g; Calories = 120

Thousand Island ☛ serving size: 1 tbsp = 16 g; Calories = 61

Tomatoseed Oil ☛ serving size: 1 tablespoon = 13.6 g; Calories = 120

USDA Commodity Food Oil Vegetable Soybean Refined ☛ serving size: 1 tablespoon = 13.6 g; Calories = 120

Vegetable Oil Nfs ☛ serving size: 1 cup = 218 g; Calories = 1932

Vegetable Oil-Butter Spread Reduced Calorie ☛ serving size: 1 tbsp = 13 g; Calories = 61

Vegetable Oil-Butter Spread Stick Salted ☛ serving size: 1 cup = 227 g; Calories = 1210

Vegetable Shortening ☛ serving size: 1 tbsp = 12.8 g; Calories = 113

Walnut Oil ☛ serving size: 1 tbsp = 13.6 g; Calories = 120

Wheat Germ Oil ☛ serving size: 1 tsp = 4.5 g; Calories = 40

Yogurt Dressing ☛ serving size: 1 cup = 246 g; Calories = 541

15

FISH AND SEAFOOD

🐟 Abalone (Cooked) ☛ serving size: 3 oz = 85 g; Calories = 161

🐟 Abalone Cooked Ns As To Cooking Method ☛ serving size: 1 oz, boneless, cooked = 28 g; Calories = 44

🐟 Abalone Floured Or Breaded Fried ☛ serving size: 1 oz, cooked = 28 g; Calories = 68

🐟 Abalone Steamed Or Poached ☛ serving size: 1 oz, cooked = 28 g; Calories = 59

🐟 Alaskan King Crab ☛ serving size: 1 leg = 134 g; Calories = 130

🐟 Anchovies (Raw) ☛ serving size: 3 oz = 85 g; Calories = 111

🐟 Atlantic Herring ☛ serving size: 1 fillet = 143 g; Calories = 290

🐟 Atlantic Mackerel (Cooked) ☛ serving size: 1 fillet = 88 g; Calories = 231

🐟 Atlantic Mackerel (Raw) ☛ serving size: 1 fillet = 112 g; Calories = 230

🐟 Baked Conch ☛ serving size: 1 cup, sliced = 127 g; Calories = 165

🦞 Barracuda Baked Or Broiled Fat Added In Cooking ☞ serving size: 1 small fillet = 113 g; Calories = 255

🦞 Barracuda Baked Or Broiled Fat Not Added In Cooking ☞ serving size: 1 small fillet = 113 g; Calories = 225

🦞 Barracuda Coated Baked Or Broiled Fat Added In Cooking ☞ serving size: 1 small fillet = 113 g; Calories = 298

🦞 Barracuda Coated Baked Or Broiled Fat Not Added In Cooking ☞ serving size: 1 small fillet = 113 g; Calories = 253

🦞 Barracuda Coated Fried ☞ serving size: 1 small fillet = 113 g; Calories = 315

🦞 Barracuda Cooked Ns As To Cooking Method ☞ serving size: 1 small fillet = 113 g; Calories = 255

🦞 Barracuda Steamed Or Poached ☞ serving size: 1 small fillet = 113 g; Calories = 225

🦞 Bass Freshwater Mixed Species Cooked Dry Heat ☞ serving size: 1 fillet = 62 g; Calories = 91

🦞 Biscayne Codfish Puerto Rican Style ☞ serving size: 1 cup = 175 g; Calories = 324

🦞 Blue Crab ☞ serving size: 1 cup, flaked and pieces = 118 g; Calories = 98

🦞 Blue Crab Cakes ☞ serving size: 1 cake = 60 g; Calories = 93

🦞 Bluefin Tuna (Cooked) ☞ serving size: 3 oz = 85 g; Calories = 156

🦞 Bluefin Tuna (Raw) ☞ serving size: 3 oz = 85 g; Calories = 122

🦞 Bluefish Cooked Dry Heat ☞ serving size: 1 fillet = 117 g; Calories = 186

🦞 Bluefish Raw ☞ serving size: 1 fillet = 150 g; Calories = 186

🦞 Bouillabaisse ☞ serving size: 1 cup = 227 g; Calories = 223

🐙 Burbot Cooked Dry Heat ☛ serving size: 1 fillet = 90 g; Calories = 104

🐙 Burbot Raw ☛ serving size: 1 fillet = 116 g; Calories = 104

🐙 Butterfish Cooked Dry Heat ☛ serving size: 1 fillet = 25 g; Calories = 47

🐙 Butterfish Raw ☛ serving size: 1 fillet = 32 g; Calories = 47

🐙 Cake Or Patty Ns As To Fish ☛ serving size: 1 cake or patty = 120 g; Calories = 245

🐙 Canned Anchovies ☛ serving size: 1 oz, boneless = 28.4 g; Calories = 60

🐙 Canned Atlantic Cod ☛ serving size: 3 oz = 85 g; Calories = 89

🐙 Canned Blue Crab ☛ serving size: 1 cup = 135 g; Calories = 112

🐙 Canned Clams ☛ serving size: 3 oz = 85 g; Calories = 121

🐙 Canned Eastern Oysters ☛ serving size: 3 oz = 85 g; Calories = 58

🐙 Canned Pink Salmon ☛ serving size: 3 oz = 85 g; Calories = 116

🐙 Canned Pink Salmon (With Skin And Bones) ☛ serving size: 3 oz = 85 g; Calories = 117

🐙 Canned Salmon ☛ serving size: 3 oz = 85 g; Calories = 142

🐙 Canned Sardines ☛ serving size: 1 cup, drained = 149 g; Calories = 310

🐙 Canned Shrimp ☛ serving size: 1 cup = 128 g; Calories = 128

🐙 Canned Sockeye Salmon ☛ serving size: 3 oz = 85 g; Calories = 134

🐙 Canned Sockeye Salmon (With Bones) ☛ serving size: 3 oz = 85 g; Calories = 130

🐙 Canned Sockeye Salmon (With Skin And Bones) ☛ serving size: 3 oz = 85 g; Calories = 130

🦐 Canned White Tuna (Oil Packed) ☛ serving size: 3 oz = 85 g; Calories = 158

🦐 Canned White Tuna (Water Packed) ☛ serving size: 3 oz = 85 g; Calories = 109

🦐 Carp Baked Or Broiled Fat Added In Cooking ☛ serving size: 1 small fillet = 170 g; Calories = 320

🦐 Carp Baked Or Broiled Fat Not Added In Cooking ☛ serving size: 1 small fillet = 170 g; Calories = 272

🦐 Carp Coated Baked Or Broiled Fat Added In Cooking ☛ serving size: 1 small fillet = 170 g; Calories = 400

🦐 Carp Coated Baked Or Broiled Fat Not Added In Cooking ☛ serving size: 1 small fillet = 170 g; Calories = 330

🦐 Carp Coated Fried ☛ serving size: 1 small fillet = 170 g; Calories = 430

🦐 Carp Cooked Dry Heat ☛ serving size: 3 oz = 85 g; Calories = 138

🦐 Carp Cooked Ns As To Cooking Method ☛ serving size: 1 small fillet = 170 g; Calories = 430

🦐 Carp Raw ☛ serving size: 3 oz = 85 g; Calories = 108

🦐 Carp Smoked ☛ serving size: 1 oz = 28 g; Calories = 55

🦐 Carp Steamed Or Poached ☛ serving size: 1 small fillet = 170 g; Calories = 272

🦐 Cassava Fritter Stuffed With Crab Meat Puerto Rican Style ☛ serving size: 1 empanada (5" x 2-1/2" x 1/2") = 126 g; Calories = 335

🦐 Catfish Baked Or Broiled Made With Butter ☛ serving size: 1 small fillet = 113 g; Calories = 196

🦐 Catfish Baked Or Broiled Made With Cooking Spray ☛ serving size: 1 small fillet = 113 g; Calories = 174

Catfish Baked Or Broiled Made With Margarine ☞ serving size: 1 small fillet = 113 g; Calories = 188

Catfish Baked Or Broiled Made With Oil ☞ serving size: 1 small fillet = 113 g; Calories = 201

Catfish Baked Or Broiled Made Without Fat ☞ serving size: 1 small fillet = 113 g; Calories = 170

Catfish Channel Cooked Breaded And Fried ☞ serving size: 1 fillet = 87 g; Calories = 199

Catfish Channel Farmed Cooked Dry Heat ☞ serving size: 1 fillet = 143 g; Calories = 206

Catfish Channel Farmed Raw ☞ serving size: 3 oz = 85 g; Calories = 101

Catfish Channel Wild Raw ☞ serving size: 3 oz = 85 g; Calories = 81

Catfish Coated Baked Or Broiled Made With Butter ☞ serving size: 1 small fillet = 113 g; Calories = 249

Catfish Coated Baked Or Broiled Made With Cooking Spray ☞ serving size: 1 small fillet = 113 g; Calories = 214

Catfish Coated Baked Or Broiled Made With Margarine ☞ serving size: 1 small fillet = 113 g; Calories = 236

Catfish Coated Baked Or Broiled Made With Oil ☞ serving size: 1 small fillet = 113 g; Calories = 258

Catfish Coated Baked Or Broiled Made Without Fat ☞ serving size: 1 small fillet = 113 g; Calories = 210

Catfish Coated Fried Made With Butter ☞ serving size: 1 small fillet = 113 g; Calories = 261

Catfish Coated Fried Made With Cooking Spray ☞ serving size: 1 small fillet = 113 g; Calories = 227

Catfish Coated Fried Made With Margarine ☞ serving size: 1 small fillet = 113 g; Calories = 243

Catfish Coated Fried Made With Oil ☞ serving size: 1 small fillet = 113 g; Calories = 278

Catfish Coated Fried Made Without Fat ☞ serving size: 1 small fillet = 113 g; Calories = 225

Catfish Cooked Ns As To Cooking Method ☞ serving size: 1 small fillet = 113 g; Calories = 278

Catfish Steamed Or Poached ☞ serving size: 1 small fillet = 113 g; Calories = 170

Caviar Black And Red Granular ☞ serving size: 1 tbsp = 16 g; Calories = 42

Ceviche ☞ serving size: 1 cup = 250 g; Calories = 155

Cisco Raw ☞ serving size: 1 fillet = 79 g; Calories = 77

Cisco Smoked ☞ serving size: 1 oz = 28.4 g; Calories = 50

Clam Cake Or Patty ☞ serving size: 1 cake or patty = 120 g; Calories = 295

Clam Sauce White ☞ serving size: 1 cup = 240 g; Calories = 470

Clams (Raw) ☞ serving size: 3 oz = 85 g; Calories = 73

Clams Baked Or Broiled Fat Added In Cooking ☞ serving size: 1 oz, without shell, cooked = 28 g; Calories = 38

Clams Baked Or Broiled Fat Not Added In Cooking ☞ serving size: 1 oz, without shell, cooked = 28 g; Calories = 30

Clams Canned ☞ serving size: 1 oz = 28 g; Calories = 30

Cod Atlantic Raw ☞ serving size: 3 oz = 85 g; Calories = 70

Cod Cooked Ns As To Cooking Method ☞ serving size: 1 small fillet = 170 g; Calories = 199

🐟 Cod Pacific Raw (May Have Been Previously Frozen) ☛ serving size: 1 fillet = 116 g; Calories = 80

🐟 Cod Smoked ☛ serving size: 1 oz, boneless = 28 g; Calories = 30

🐟 Cod Steamed Or Poached ☛ serving size: 1 small fillet = 170 g; Calories = 148

🐟 Codfish Ball Or Cake ☛ serving size: 1 ball = 63 g; Calories = 112

🐟 Codfish Fritter Puerto Rican Style ☛ serving size: 1 fritter (3-1/2" x 3-1/2") = 34 g; Calories = 95

🐟 Cooked Alaska Pollock ☛ serving size: 1 fillet = 60 g; Calories = 67

🐟 Cooked Atlantic Cod ☛ serving size: 3 oz = 85 g; Calories = 89

🐟 Cooked Atlantic Perch ☛ serving size: 1 fillet = 50 g; Calories = 48

🐟 Cooked Blue Mussels ☛ serving size: 3 oz = 85 g; Calories = 146

🐟 Cooked Catfish ☛ serving size: 1 fillet = 143 g; Calories = 150

🐟 Cooked Clams ☛ serving size: 3 oz = 85 g; Calories = 126

🐟 Cooked Cod ☛ serving size: 3 oz = 85 g; Calories = 71

🐟 Cooked Coho Salmon (Farmed) ☛ serving size: 1 fillet = 143 g; Calories = 255

🐟 Cooked Coho Salmon (Wild Moist Heat) ☛ serving size: 3 oz = 85 g; Calories = 156

🐟 Cooked Coho Salmon (Wild) ☛ serving size: 3 oz = 85 g; Calories = 118

🐟 Cooked Crayfish ☛ serving size: 3 oz = 85 g; Calories = 74

🐟 Cooked Cuttlefish ☛ serving size: 3 oz = 85 g; Calories = 134

🐟 Cooked Dry Heat ☛ serving size: 1 fillet = 95 g; Calories = 106

🐟 Cooked Dungeness Crab ☛ serving size: 3 oz = 85 g; Calories = 94

🐟 Cooked Eastern Oysters (Farmed) ☛ serving size: 3 oz = 85 g; Calories = 67

🐟 Cooked Eastern Oysters (Wild) ☛ serving size: 3 oz = 85 g; Calories = 67

🐟 Cooked Eel ☛ serving size: 1 oz, boneless = 28.4 g; Calories = 67

🐟 Cooked Grouper ☛ serving size: 3 oz = 85 g; Calories = 100

🐟 Cooked Haddock ☛ serving size: 1 fillet = 150 g; Calories = 135

🐟 Cooked Halibut ☛ serving size: 3 oz = 85 g; Calories = 94

🐟 Cooked King Mackerel ☛ serving size: 3 oz = 85 g; Calories = 114

🐟 Cooked Lingcod ☛ serving size: 3 oz = 85 g; Calories = 93

🐟 Cooked Mahimahi ☛ serving size: 3 oz = 85 g; Calories = 93

🐟 Cooked Northern Pike ☛ serving size: 3 oz = 85 g; Calories = 96

🐟 Cooked Orange Roughy ☛ serving size: 3 oz = 85 g; Calories = 89

🐟 Cooked Pacific Cod ☛ serving size: 1 fillet = 90 g; Calories = 77

🐟 Cooked Pacific Herring ☛ serving size: 1 fillet = 144 g; Calories = 360

🐟 Cooked Pacific Oysters ☛ serving size: 1 medium = 25 g; Calories = 41

🐟 Cooked Pollock ☛ serving size: 3 oz = 85 g; Calories = 100

🐟 Cooked Pompano ☛ serving size: 1 fillet = 88 g; Calories = 186

🐟 Cooked Rainbow Trout ☛ serving size: 1 fillet = 71 g; Calories = 119

🐟 Cooked Sablefish ☛ serving size: 3 oz = 85 g; Calories = 213

🐟 Cooked Sea Bass ☛ serving size: 1 fillet = 101 g; Calories = 125

🐟 Cooked Shrimp ☛ serving size: 3 oz = 85 g; Calories = 101

🐟 Cooked Skipjack ☛ serving size: 3 oz = 85 g; Calories = 112

🦐 Cooked Smelt ☛ serving size: 3 oz = 85 g; Calories = 105

🦐 Cooked Snapper ☛ serving size: 3 oz = 85 g; Calories = 109

🦐 Cooked Sockeye Salmon ☛ serving size: 3 oz = 85 g; Calories = 133

🦐 Cooked Spiny Lobster ☛ serving size: 3 oz = 85 g; Calories = 122

🦐 Cooked Striped Bass ☛ serving size: 1 fillet = 124 g; Calories = 154

🦐 Cooked Sturgeon ☛ serving size: 3 oz = 85 g; Calories = 115

🦐 Cooked Swordfish ☛ serving size: 3 oz = 85 g; Calories = 146

🦐 Cooked Tilapia ☛ serving size: 1 fillet = 87 g; Calories = 111

🦐 Cooked Tilefish ☛ serving size: 1/2 fillet = 150 g; Calories = 221

🦐 Cooked Trout ☛ serving size: 1 fillet = 143 g; Calories = 215

🦐 Cooked Turbot ☛ serving size: 3 oz = 85 g; Calories = 104

🦐 Cooked Walleye Pike ☛ serving size: 1 fillet = 124 g; Calories = 148

🦐 Cooked Whitefish ☛ serving size: 3 oz = 85 g; Calories = 146

🦐 Cooked Whiting ☛ serving size: 1 fillet = 72 g; Calories = 84

🦐 Cooked Wild Eastern Oysters ☛ serving size: 3 oz = 85 g; Calories = 87

🦐 Cooked Yellowfin Tuna ☛ serving size: 3 oz = 85 g; Calories = 111

🦐 Cooked Yellowtail ☛ serving size: 1/2 fillet = 146 g; Calories = 273

🦐 Crab Cooked Ns As To Cooking Method ☛ serving size: 1 oz, without shell, cooked = 28 g; Calories = 23

🦐 Crab Deviled ☛ serving size: 1 cup = 175 g; Calories = 327

🦐 Crab Hard Shell Steamed ☛ serving size: 1 cup, cooked, flaked and pieces = 118 g; Calories = 97

🦐 Crab Imperial ☛ serving size: 1 cup = 259 g; Calories = 355

🦐 Crayfish ☛ serving size: 3 oz = 85 g; Calories = 70

🦐 Crayfish Boiled Or Steamed ☛ serving size: 1 oz, without shell, cooked = 28 g; Calories = 23

🦐 Crayfish Coated Fried ☛ serving size: 1 oz, without shell, cooked = 28 g; Calories = 61

🦐 Croaker Atlantic Cooked Breaded And Fried ☛ serving size: 1 fillet = 87 g; Calories = 192

🦐 Croaker Atlantic Raw ☛ serving size: 1 fillet = 79 g; Calories = 82

🦐 Croaker Baked Or Broiled Fat Added In Cooking ☛ serving size: 1 small fillet = 113 g; Calories = 181

🦐 Croaker Steamed Or Poached ☛ serving size: 1 small fillet = 113 g; Calories = 148

🦐 Crustaceans Crab Alaska King Raw ☛ serving size: 3 oz = 85 g; Calories = 71

🦐 Crustaceans Crab Blue Raw ☛ serving size: 3 oz = 85 g; Calories = 74

🦐 Crustaceans Crayfish Mixed Species Farmed Raw ☛ serving size: 3 oz = 85 g; Calories = 61

🦐 Crustaceans Crayfish Mixed Species Wild Raw ☛ serving size: 3 oz = 85 g; Calories = 66

🦐 Crustaceans Lobster Northern Raw ☛ serving size: 1 lobster = 150 g; Calories = 116

🦐 Crustaceans Shrimp Cooked (Not Previously Frozen) ☛ serving size: 3 oz = 85 g; Calories = 84

🦐 Crustaceans Shrimp Mixed Species Cooked Breaded And Fried ☛ serving size: 3 oz = 85 g; Calories = 206

🦐 Crustaceans Shrimp Mixed Species Imitation Made From Surimi ☛ serving size: 3 oz = 85 g; Calories = 86

🦐 Crustaceans Shrimp Mixed Species Raw (May Have Been Previously Frozen) ☛ serving size: 1 medium = 6 g; Calories = 4

🦐 Crustaceans Shrimp Raw (Not Previously Frozen) ☛ serving size: 3 oz = 85 g; Calories = 72

🦐 Crustaceans Spiny Lobster Mixed Species Raw ☛ serving size: 3 oz = 85 g; Calories = 95

🦐 Curry ☛ serving size: 1 cup = 236 g; Calories = 165

🦐 Cusk Raw ☛ serving size: 1 fillet = 122 g; Calories = 106

🦐 Dried Salted Atlantic Cod ☛ serving size: 1 oz = 28.4 g; Calories = 82

🦐 Drum Freshwater Cooked Dry Heat ☛ serving size: 3 oz = 85 g; Calories = 130

🦐 Drum Freshwater Raw ☛ serving size: 3 oz = 85 g; Calories = 101

🦐 Dungeness Crab (Raw) ☛ serving size: 3 oz = 85 g; Calories = 73

🦐 Eel Cooked Ns As To Cooking Method ☛ serving size: 1 oz, boneless, cooked = 28 g; Calories = 83

🦐 Farmed Atlantic Salmon ☛ serving size: 3 oz = 85 g; Calories = 175

🦐 Farmed Atlantic Salmon (Raw) ☛ serving size: 3 oz = 85 g; Calories = 177

🦐 Flat Fish (Flounder Or Sole) ☛ serving size: 1 fillet = 127 g; Calories = 109

🦐 Flatfish (Flounder And Sole Species) Raw ☛ serving size: 1 oz, boneless = 28.4 g; Calories = 20

🦐 Flounder Cooked Ns As To Cooking Method ☛ serving size: 1 small fillet = 113 g; Calories = 231

🦐 Flounder Smoked ☛ serving size: 1 oz, boneless = 28 g; Calories = 47

🦞 Flounder Steamed Or Poached ☛ serving size: 1 small fillet = 113 g; Calories = 99

🦞 Fresh Water Bass (Raw) ☛ serving size: 1 fillet = 79 g; Calories = 90

🦞 Fried Calamari ☛ serving size: 3 oz = 85 g; Calories = 149

🦞 Frog Legs Ns As To Cooking Method ☛ serving size: 1 oz, boneless, cooked = 28 g; Calories = 60

🦞 Frog Legs Raw ☛ serving size: 1 leg = 45 g; Calories = 33

🦞 Frog Legs Steamed ☛ serving size: 1 oz, boneless, cooked = 28 g; Calories = 26

🦞 Gefilte Fish ☛ serving size: 1 cup = 227 g; Calories = 257

🦞 Gefiltefish Commercial Sweet Recipe ☛ serving size: 1 piece = 42 g; Calories = 35

🦞 Grouper Mixed Species Raw ☛ serving size: 3 oz = 85 g; Calories = 78

🦞 Gumbo No Rice ☛ serving size: 1 cup = 244 g; Calories = 200

🦞 Gumbo With Rice ☛ serving size: 1 cup = 244 g; Calories = 215

🦞 Haddock Baked Or Broiled Fat Added In Cooking ☛ serving size: 1 small fillet = 170 g; Calories = 209

🦞 Haddock Baked Or Broiled Fat Not Added In Cooking ☛ serving size: 1 small fillet = 170 g; Calories = 160

🦞 Haddock Cake Or Patty ☛ serving size: 1 cake or patty = 120 g; Calories = 245

🦞 Haddock Raw ☛ serving size: 3 oz = 85 g; Calories = 63

🦞 Haddock Steamed Or Poached ☛ serving size: 1 small fillet = 170 g; Calories = 158

🦞 Halibut Atlantic And Pacific Raw ☛ serving size: 3 oz = 85 g; Calories = 77

Halibut Cooked Ns As To Cooking Method ☛ serving size: 1 small fillet = 170 g; Calories = 245

Halibut Greenland Cooked Dry Heat ☛ serving size: 3 oz = 85 g; Calories = 203

Halibut Greenland Raw ☛ serving size: 3 oz = 85 g; Calories = 158

Halibut Smoked ☛ serving size: 1 oz, boneless = 28 g; Calories = 61

Halibut Steamed Or Poached ☛ serving size: 1 small fillet = 170 g; Calories = 194

Herring Atlantic Raw ☛ serving size: 1 oz, boneless = 28.4 g; Calories = 45

Herring Coated Fried ☛ serving size: 1 oz, boneless, raw (yield after cooking) = 27 g; Calories = 75

Herring Cooked Ns As To Cooking Method ☛ serving size: 1 oz, boneless, raw (yield after cooking) = 23 g; Calories = 52

Herring Dried Salted ☛ serving size: 1 oz, boneless = 28 g; Calories = 137

Herring Pacific Raw ☛ serving size: 3 oz = 85 g; Calories = 166

Herring Pickled In Cream Sauce ☛ serving size: 1 oz, boneless = 28 g; Calories = 70

Imitation Crab Meat ☛ serving size: 3 oz = 85 g; Calories = 81

Jellyfish Dried Salted ☛ serving size: 1 cup = 58 g; Calories = 21

Kippered Herring ☛ serving size: 1 oz, boneless = 28.4 g; Calories = 62

Lau Lau ☛ serving size: 1 lau lau = 214 g; Calories = 300

Ling Cooked Dry Heat ☛ serving size: 3 oz = 85 g; Calories = 94

Ling Raw ☛ serving size: 3 oz = 85 g; Calories = 74

🦞 Lingcod Raw ☛ serving size: 3 oz = 85 g; Calories = 72

🦞 Lobster (Cooked) ☛ serving size: 1 cup = 145 g; Calories = 129

🦞 Lobster Cooked Ns As To Cooking Method ☛ serving size: 1 small lobster (1 lb live weight) (yield after cooking, shell removed) = 118 g; Calories = 104

🦞 Lobster Gumbo ☛ serving size: 1 cup = 244 g; Calories = 144

🦞 Lobster Newburg ☛ serving size: 1 cup = 244 g; Calories = 588

🦞 Lomi Salmon ☛ serving size: 1 cup = 234 g; Calories = 140

🦞 Mackerel Cake Or Patty ☛ serving size: 1 cake or patty = 120 g; Calories = 310

🦞 Mackerel Cooked Ns As To Cooking Method ☛ serving size: 1 small fillet = 170 g; Calories = 449

🦞 Mackerel Jack Canned Drained Solids ☛ serving size: 1 oz, boneless = 28.4 g; Calories = 44

🦞 Mackerel King Raw ☛ serving size: 3 oz = 85 g; Calories = 89

🦞 Mackerel Pacific And Jack Mixed Species Cooked Dry Heat ☛ serving size: 1 oz, boneless = 28.4 g; Calories = 57

🦞 Mackerel Pacific And Jack Mixed Species Raw ☛ serving size: 3 oz = 85 g; Calories = 134

🦞 Mackerel Pickled ☛ serving size: 1 oz, boneless = 28 g; Calories = 61

🦞 Mackerel Raw ☛ serving size: 1 oz, boneless, raw = 28 g; Calories = 53

🦞 Mackerel Salted ☛ serving size: 1 piece (5-1/2 inch x 1-1/2 inch x 1/2 inch) = 80 g; Calories = 244

🦞 Mackerel Smoked ☛ serving size: 1 oz, boneless = 28 g; Calories = 56

Mackerel Spanish Cooked Dry Heat ☛ serving size: 1 fillet = 146 g; Calories = 231

Mackerel Spanish Raw ☛ serving size: 3 oz = 85 g; Calories = 118

Mahimahi Raw ☛ serving size: 3 oz = 85 g; Calories = 72

Milkfish Cooked Dry Heat ☛ serving size: 3 oz = 85 g; Calories = 162

Milkfish Raw ☛ serving size: 3 oz = 85 g; Calories = 126

Mollusks Abalone Mixed Species Raw ☛ serving size: 3 oz = 85 g; Calories = 89

Mollusks Clam Mixed Species Canned Liquid ☛ serving size: 3 oz = 85 g; Calories = 2

Mollusks Clam Mixed Species Cooked Breaded And Fried ☛ serving size: 3 oz = 85 g; Calories = 172

Mollusks Cuttlefish Mixed Species Raw ☛ serving size: 3 oz = 85 g; Calories = 67

Mollusks Mussel Blue Raw ☛ serving size: 1 cup = 150 g; Calories = 129

Mollusks Octopus Common Raw ☛ serving size: 3 oz = 85 g; Calories = 70

Mollusks Oyster Eastern Cooked Breaded And Fried ☛ serving size: 3 oz = 85 g; Calories = 169

Mollusks Oyster Eastern Wild Raw ☛ serving size: 6 medium = 84 g; Calories = 43

Mollusks Scallop Mixed Species Cooked Breaded And Fried ☛ serving size: 2 large = 31 g; Calories = 67

Mollusks Scallop Mixed Species Imitation Made From Surimi ☛ serving size: 3 oz = 85 g; Calories = 84

🐚 Mollusks Snail Raw ☛ serving size: 3 oz = 85 g; Calories = 77

🐚 Mollusks Whelk Unspecified Raw ☛ serving size: 3 oz = 85 g; Calories = 117

🐚 Monkfish Cooked Dry Heat ☛ serving size: 3 oz = 85 g; Calories = 83

🐚 Monkfish Raw ☛ serving size: 3 oz = 85 g; Calories = 65

🐚 Moochim ☛ serving size: 1 tablespoon = 5 g; Calories = 17

🐚 Mullet Cooked Ns As To Cooking Method ☛ serving size: 1 small fillet = 113 g; Calories = 276

🐚 Mullet Steamed Or Poached ☛ serving size: 1 small fillet = 113 g; Calories = 166

🐚 Mullet Striped Raw ☛ serving size: 1 oz = 28.4 g; Calories = 33

🐚 Mussels Cooked Ns As To Cooking Method ☛ serving size: 1 oz, cooked = 28 g; Calories = 48

🐚 Mussels Steamed Or Poached ☛ serving size: 1 oz, cooked = 28 g; Calories = 48

🐚 Ocean Perch Atlantic Raw ☛ serving size: 1 oz, boneless = 28.4 g; Calories = 22

🐚 Ocean Perch Cooked Ns As To Cooking Method ☛ serving size: 1 small fillet = 113 g; Calories = 146

🐚 Ocean Perch Steamed Or Poached ☛ serving size: 1 small fillet = 113 g; Calories = 112

🐚 Octopus (Cooked) ☛ serving size: 3 oz = 85 g; Calories = 139

🐚 Octopus Cooked Ns As To Cooking Method ☛ serving size: 1 oz, boneless, cooked = 28 g; Calories = 62

🐚 Octopus Dried ☛ serving size: 1 oz = 28 g; Calories = 87

🦑 Octopus Dried Boiled ☛ serving size: 1 cup, cooked = 106 g; Calories = 173

🦑 Octopus Smoked ☛ serving size: 1 oz, boneless, cooked = 28 g; Calories = 46

🦑 Octopus Steamed ☛ serving size: 1 oz, boneless, cooked = 28 g; Calories = 46

🦑 Oyster Fritter ☛ serving size: 1 fritter = 40 g; Calories = 78

🦑 Oyster Pie ☛ serving size: 1 pie = 656 g; Calories = 1607

🦑 Oysters Baked Or Broiled Fat Added In Cooking ☛ serving size: 1 oz, without shell, cooked = 28 g; Calories = 26

🦑 Oysters Cooked Ns As To Cooking Method ☛ serving size: 1 oz, without shell, cooked = 28 g; Calories = 55

🦑 Oysters Rockefeller ☛ serving size: 1 oyster, no shell = 24 g; Calories = 31

🦑 Oysters Smoked ☛ serving size: 1 oz = 28 g; Calories = 23

🦑 Oysters Steamed ☛ serving size: 1 oz, without shell, cooked = 28 g; Calories = 29

🦑 Perch Cooked Ns As To Cooking Method ☛ serving size: 1 small fillet = 113 g; Calories = 251

🦑 Perch Mixed Species Cooked Dry Heat ☛ serving size: 1 fillet = 46 g; Calories = 54

🦑 Perch Mixed Species Raw ☛ serving size: 1 fillet = 60 g; Calories = 55

🦑 Perch Steamed Or Poached ☛ serving size: 1 small fillet = 113 g; Calories = 129

🦑 Pickled Herring ☛ serving size: 1 cup = 140 g; Calories = 367

🦑 Pike Cooked Ns As To Cooking Method ☛ serving size: 1 small fillet = 170 g; Calories = 401

🦑 Pike Northern Raw ☛ serving size: 3 oz = 85 g; Calories = 75

🦑 Pike Steamed Or Poached ☛ serving size: 1 small fillet = 170 g; Calories = 189

🦑 Pike Walleye Raw ☛ serving size: 3 oz = 85 g; Calories = 79

🦑 Pink Salmon (Raw) ☛ serving size: 3 oz = 85 g; Calories = 108

🦑 Pollock Alaska Cooked (Not Previously Frozen) ☛ serving size: 3 oz = 85 g; Calories = 74

🦑 Pollock Alaska Raw (May Have Been Previously Frozen) ☛ serving size: 1 fillet = 77 g; Calories = 43

🦑 Pollock Alaska Raw (Not Previously Frozen) ☛ serving size: 3 oz = 85 g; Calories = 65

🦑 Pollock Atlantic Raw ☛ serving size: 3 oz = 85 g; Calories = 78

🦑 Pompano Cooked Ns As To Cooking Method ☛ serving size: 1 small fillet = 113 g; Calories = 263

🦑 Pompano Florida Raw ☛ serving size: 1 oz, boneless = 28.4 g; Calories = 47

🦑 Pompano Smoked ☛ serving size: 1 oz, boneless = 28 g; Calories = 54

🦑 Pompano Steamed Or Poached ☛ serving size: 1 small fillet = 113 g; Calories = 233

🦑 Porgy Cooked Ns As To Cooking Method ☛ serving size: 1 small fillet = 113 g; Calories = 182

🦑 Porgy Steamed Or Poached ☛ serving size: 1 small fillet = 113 g; Calories = 149

🐟 Pout Ocean Cooked Dry Heat ☛ serving size: 1/2 fillet = 137 g; Calories = 140

🐟 Pout Ocean Raw ☛ serving size: 3 oz = 85 g; Calories = 67

🐟 Queen Crab (Cooked) ☛ serving size: 3 oz = 85 g; Calories = 98

🐟 Queen Crab (Raw) ☛ serving size: 3 oz = 85 g; Calories = 77

🐟 Rainbow Trout (Raw) ☛ serving size: 1 fillet = 79 g; Calories = 111

🐟 Raw Coho Salmon ☛ serving size: 3 oz = 85 g; Calories = 136

🐟 Raw Eastern Oysters ☛ serving size: 3 oz = 85 g; Calories = 50

🐟 Raw Pacific Oysters ☛ serving size: 1 medium = 50 g; Calories = 41

🐟 Raw Scallops ☛ serving size: 1 unit 2 large or 5 small = 30 g; Calories = 21

🐟 Raw Tilapia ☛ serving size: 1 fillet = 116 g; Calories = 111

🐟 Raw Whiting ☛ serving size: 1 fillet = 92 g; Calories = 83

🐟 Ray Cooked Ns As To Cooking Method ☛ serving size: 1 oz, boneless, raw (yield after cooking) = 23 g; Calories = 44

🐟 Ray Steamed Or Poached ☛ serving size: 1 oz, boneless, raw (yield after cooking) = 23 g; Calories = 38

🐟 Rockfish Pacific Mixed Species Cooked Dry Heat ☛ serving size: 1 fillet = 149 g; Calories = 162

🐟 Rockfish Pacific Mixed Species Raw ☛ serving size: 3 oz = 85 g; Calories = 77

🐟 Roe ☛ serving size: 1 tbsp = 14 g; Calories = 20

🐟 Roe (Cooked) ☛ serving size: 1 oz = 28.4 g; Calories = 58

🐟 Roe Shad Cooked ☛ serving size: 1 oz = 28 g; Calories = 58

🐟 Roughy Orange Raw ☛ serving size: 3 oz = 85 g; Calories = 65

Sablefish Raw ☛ serving size: 3 oz = 85 g; Calories = 166

Sablefish Smoked ☛ serving size: 1 oz = 28.4 g; Calories = 73

Salmon Cake Or Patty ☛ serving size: 1 ball = 63 g; Calories = 155

Salmon Canned ☛ serving size: 1 oz = 28 g; Calories = 38

Salmon Chinook Cooked Dry Heat ☛ serving size: 3 oz = 85 g; Calories = 196

Salmon Chinook Raw ☛ serving size: 3 oz = 85 g; Calories = 152

Salmon Chinook Smoked (Lox) Regular ☛ serving size: 1 oz = 28.4 g; Calories = 33

Salmon Chum Canned Drained Solids With Bone ☛ serving size: 3 oz = 85 g; Calories = 120

Salmon Chum Canned Without Salt Drained Solids With Bone ☛ serving size: 3 oz = 85 g; Calories = 120

Salmon Chum Cooked Dry Heat ☛ serving size: 3 oz = 85 g; Calories = 131

Salmon Chum Raw ☛ serving size: 3 oz = 85 g; Calories = 102

Salmon Coated Baked Or Broiled Made With Butter ☛ serving size: 1 small fillet = 170 g; Calories = 386

Salmon Coated Baked Or Broiled Made With Cooking Spray ☛ serving size: 1 small fillet = 170 g; Calories = 335

Salmon Cooked Ns As To Cooking Method ☛ serving size: 1 small fillet = 170 g; Calories = 320

Salmon Dried ☛ serving size: 1 oz, boneless = 28 g; Calories = 111

Salmon Loaf ☛ serving size: 1 slice = 105 g; Calories = 202

Salmon Pink Canned Total Can Contents ☛ serving size: 3 oz = 85 g; Calories = 110

🦞 Salmon Pink Canned Without Salt Solids With Bone And Liquid ☛ serving size: 3 oz = 85 g; Calories = 118

🦞 Salmon Pink Cooked Dry Heat ☛ serving size: 3 oz = 85 g; Calories = 130

🦞 Salmon Salad ☛ serving size: 1 cup = 208 g; Calories = 441

🦞 Salmon Sockeye Raw ☛ serving size: 1 oz, boneless = 28.4 g; Calories = 37

🦞 Salmon Steamed Or Poached ☛ serving size: 1 small fillet = 170 g; Calories = 272

🦞 Sardine Pacific Canned In Tomato Sauce Drained Solids With Bone ☛ serving size: 1 cup = 89 g; Calories = 165

🦞 Sardines Dried ☛ serving size: 1 oz = 28 g; Calories = 114

🦞 Scallops ☛ serving size: 3 oz = 85 g; Calories = 94

🦞 Scallops Cooked Ns As To Cooking Method ☛ serving size: 1 oz, cooked = 28 g; Calories = 32

🦞 Scup Cooked Dry Heat ☛ serving size: 1 fillet = 50 g; Calories = 68

🦞 Scup Raw ☛ serving size: 3 oz = 85 g; Calories = 89

🦞 Sea Bass Cooked Ns As To Cooking Method ☛ serving size: 1 small fillet = 113 g; Calories = 172

🦞 Sea Bass Mixed Species Raw ☛ serving size: 1 fillet = 129 g; Calories = 125

🦞 Sea Bass Pickled ☛ serving size: 1 oz, boneless = 28 g; Calories = 43

🦞 Sea Bass Steamed Or Poached ☛ serving size: 1 small fillet = 113 g; Calories = 138

🦞 Seafood Newburg ☛ serving size: 1 cup = 244 g; Calories = 598

🦞 Seafood Salad ☛ serving size: 1 cup = 208 g; Calories = 397

Seatrout Mixed Species Cooked Dry Heat ☛ serving size: 3 oz = 85 g; Calories = 113

Seatrout Mixed Species Raw ☛ serving size: 3 oz = 85 g; Calories = 88

Shad American Cooked Dry Heat ☛ serving size: 1 fillet = 144 g; Calories = 363

Shad American Raw ☛ serving size: 3 oz = 85 g; Calories = 168

Shark Cooked Ns As To Cooking Method ☛ serving size: 1 small fillet = 170 g; Calories = 326

Shark Mixed Species Cooked Batter-Dipped And Fried ☛ serving size: 3 oz = 85 g; Calories = 194

Shark Mixed Species Raw ☛ serving size: 3 oz = 85 g; Calories = 111

Shark Steamed Or Poached ☛ serving size: 1 small fillet = 170 g; Calories = 277

Sheepshead Cooked Dry Heat ☛ serving size: 3 oz = 85 g; Calories = 107

Sheepshead Raw ☛ serving size: 3 oz = 85 g; Calories = 92

Shrimp Cooked Ns As To Cooking Method ☛ serving size: 1 tiny shrimp ("popcorn") = 1 g; Calories = 2

Shrimp Creole No Rice ☛ serving size: 1 cup = 246 g; Calories = 305

Shrimp Creole With Rice ☛ serving size: 1 cup = 243 g; Calories = 301

Shrimp Curry ☛ serving size: 1 cup = 236 g; Calories = 177

Shrimp Dried ☛ serving size: 1 oz = 28 g; Calories = 71

Shrimp Gumbo ☛ serving size: 1 cup = 244 g; Calories = 149

Skipjack Tuna (Raw) ☛ serving size: 3 oz = 85 g; Calories = 88

🐟 Smelt Rainbow Raw ☞ serving size: 3 oz = 85 g; Calories = 83

🐟 Smoked Haddock ☞ serving size: 1 oz, boneless = 28.4 g; Calories = 33

🐟 Smoked Salmon ☞ serving size: 1 oz, boneless = 28.4 g; Calories = 33

🐟 Smoked Sturgeon ☞ serving size: 1 oz = 28.4 g; Calories = 49

🐟 Smoked Whitefish ☞ serving size: 1 cup, cooked = 136 g; Calories = 147

🐟 Snails Cooked Ns As To Cooking Method ☞ serving size: 1 oz, without shell, cooked = 28 g; Calories = 39

🐟 Snapper Mixed Species Raw ☞ serving size: 3 oz = 85 g; Calories = 85

🐟 Spot Cooked Dry Heat ☞ serving size: 1 fillet = 50 g; Calories = 79

🐟 Spot Raw ☞ serving size: 1 fillet = 64 g; Calories = 79

🐟 Squid (Raw) ☞ serving size: 1 oz, boneless = 28.4 g; Calories = 26

🐟 Squid Baked Or Broiled Fat Added In Cooking ☞ serving size: 1 squid = 272 g; Calories = 386

🐟 Squid Baked Or Broiled Fat Not Added In Cooking ☞ serving size: 1 squid = 272 g; Calories = 307

🐟 Squid Canned ☞ serving size: 1 cup = 187 g; Calories = 198

🐟 Squid Coated Baked Or Broiled Fat Added In Cooking ☞ serving size: 1 oz, cooked = 28 g; Calories = 55

🐟 Squid Coated Baked Or Broiled Fat Not Added In Cooking ☞ serving size: 1 oz, cooked = 28 g; Calories = 44

🐟 Squid Coated Fried ☞ serving size: 1 oz, cooked = 28 g; Calories = 65

🐟 Squid Dried ☞ serving size: 1 oz, boneless = 28 g; Calories = 97

🦑 Squid Pickled 🖝 serving size: 1 oz, boneless = 28 g; Calories = 26

🦑 Squid Steamed Or Boiled 🖝 serving size: 1 oz, boneless, cooked = 28 g; Calories = 51

🦑 Stewed Codfish No Potatoes Puerto Rican Style 🖝 serving size: 1 cup = 227 g; Calories = 238

🦑 Stewed Codfish Puerto Rican Style 🖝 serving size: 1 cup = 200 g; Calories = 226

🦑 Stewed Salmon Puerto Rican Style 🖝 serving size: 1 cup = 212 g; Calories = 307

🦑 Sticks Frozen Prepared 🖝 serving size: 1 piece (4 inch x 2 inch x 1/2 inch) = 57 g; Calories = 158

🦑 Striped Bass (Raw) 🖝 serving size: 3 oz = 85 g; Calories = 83

🦑 Sturgeon Cooked Ns As To Cooking Method 🖝 serving size: 1 oz, boneless, raw (yield after cooking) = 23 g; Calories = 37

🦑 Sturgeon Mixed Species Raw 🖝 serving size: 3 oz = 85 g; Calories = 89

🦑 Sturgeon Steamed 🖝 serving size: 1 oz, boneless, raw (yield after cooking) = 23 g; Calories = 30

🦑 Sucker White Cooked Dry Heat 🖝 serving size: 1 fillet = 124 g; Calories = 148

🦑 Sucker White Raw 🖝 serving size: 3 oz = 85 g; Calories = 78

🦑 Sunfish Pumpkin Seed Cooked Dry Heat 🖝 serving size: 1 fillet = 37 g; Calories = 42

🦑 Sunfish Pumpkin Seed Raw 🖝 serving size: 1 fillet = 48 g; Calories = 43

🦑 Surimi 🖝 serving size: 1 oz = 28.4 g; Calories = 28

🐟 Swordfish Cooked Ns As To Cooking Method ☞ serving size: 1 small fillet = 170 g; Calories = 355

🐟 Swordfish Raw ☞ serving size: 3 oz = 85 g; Calories = 122

🐟 Swordfish Steamed Or Poached ☞ serving size: 1 small fillet = 170 g; Calories = 308

🐟 Tilapia Cooked Ns As To Cooking Method ☞ serving size: 1 small fillet = 113 g; Calories = 170

🐟 Tilapia Steamed Or Poached ☞ serving size: 1 small fillet = 113 g; Calories = 137

🐟 Tilefish Raw ☞ serving size: 3 oz = 85 g; Calories = 82

🐟 Timbale Or Mousse ☞ serving size: 1 cup = 175 g; Calories = 259

🐟 Trout Cooked Ns As To Cooking Method ☞ serving size: 1 small fillet = 113 g; Calories = 232

🐟 Trout Mixed Species Cooked Dry Heat ☞ serving size: 1 fillet = 62 g; Calories = 118

🐟 Trout Mixed Species Raw ☞ serving size: 1 fillet = 79 g; Calories = 117

🐟 Trout Rainbow Wild Raw ☞ serving size: 3 oz = 85 g; Calories = 101

🐟 Trout Smoked ☞ serving size: 1 oz, boneless = 28 g; Calories = 70

🐟 Trout Steamed Or Poached ☞ serving size: 1 small fillet = 113 g; Calories = 200

🐟 Tuna Cake Or Patty ☞ serving size: 1 cake or patty = 120 g; Calories = 247

🐟 Tuna Fresh Cooked Ns As To Cooking Method ☞ serving size: 1 small fillet = 170 g; Calories = 282

🐟 Tuna Fresh Dried ☞ serving size: 1 cup, nfs = 42 g; Calories = 143

Tuna Fresh Smoked ☛ serving size: 1 oz, boneless = 28 g; Calories = 56

Tuna Fresh Steamed Or Poached ☛ serving size: 1 small fillet = 170 g; Calories = 233

Tuna Light Canned In Oil Drained Solids ☛ serving size: 1 cup, solid or chunks = 146 g; Calories = 289

Tuna Light Canned In Oil Without Salt Drained Solids ☛ serving size: 3 oz = 85 g; Calories = 168

Tuna Light Canned In Water Drained Solids ☛ serving size: 1 oz = 28.4 g; Calories = 24

Tuna Light Canned In Water Without Salt Drained Solids ☛ serving size: 3 oz = 85 g; Calories = 99

Tuna Loaf ☛ serving size: 1 slice = 105 g; Calories = 244

Tuna Pot Pie ☛ serving size: 1 pie = 769 g; Calories = 1692

Tuna Salad ☛ serving size: 3 oz = 85 g; Calories = 159

Tuna Salad Made With Any Type Of Fat Free Dressing ☛ serving size: 1 cup = 238 g; Calories = 174

Tuna Salad Made With Creamy Dressing ☛ serving size: 1 cup = 238 g; Calories = 352

Tuna Salad Made With Italian Dressing ☛ serving size: 1 cup = 238 g; Calories = 252

Tuna Salad Made With Light Creamy Dressing ☛ serving size: 1 cup = 238 g; Calories = 186

Tuna Salad Made With Light Italian Dressing ☛ serving size: 1 cup = 238 g; Calories = 181

Tuna Salad Made With Light Mayonnaise ☛ serving size: 1 cup = 238 g; Calories = 252

🦐 Tuna Salad Made With Light Mayonnaise-Type Salad Dressing ☛ serving size: 1 cup = 238 g; Calories = 252

🦐 Tuna Salad Made With Mayonnaise ☛ serving size: 1 cup = 238 g; Calories = 462

🦐 Tuna Salad Made With Mayonnaise-Type Salad Dressing ☛ serving size: 1 cup = 238 g; Calories = 257

🦐 Tuna Salad With Cheese ☛ serving size: 1 cup = 238 g; Calories = 509

🦐 Tuna Salad With Egg ☛ serving size: 1 cup = 238 g; Calories = 455

🦐 Tuna White Canned In Oil Without Salt Drained Solids ☛ serving size: 3 oz = 85 g; Calories = 158

🦐 Tuna White Canned In Water Without Salt Drained Solids ☛ serving size: 3 oz = 85 g; Calories = 109

🦐 Tuna With Cream Or White Sauce ☛ serving size: 1 cup = 237 g; Calories = 247

🦐 Turbot European Raw ☛ serving size: 3 oz = 85 g; Calories = 81

🦐 Turtle Cooked Ns As To Cooking Method ☛ serving size: 1 oz, boneless, cooked = 28 g; Calories = 39

🦐 Turtle Green Raw ☛ serving size: 3 oz = 85 g; Calories = 76

🦐 USDA Commodity Salmon Nuggets Breaded Frozen Heated ☛ serving size: 1 oz = 28.4 g; Calories = 60

🦐 USDA Commodity Salmon Nuggets Cooked As Purchased Unheated ☛ serving size: 1 oz = 28.4 g; Calories = 54

🦐 Whelk (Cooked) ☛ serving size: 3 oz = 85 g; Calories = 234

🦐 Whitefish (Raw) ☛ serving size: 3 oz = 85 g; Calories = 114

🦐 Whiting Cooked Ns As To Cooking Method ☛ serving size: 1 small fillet = 113 g; Calories = 250

Whiting Steamed Or Poached ☛ serving size: 1 oz, boneless, raw (yield after cooking) = 23 g; Calories = 26

Wild Atlantic Salmon (Cooked) ☛ serving size: 3 oz = 85 g; Calories = 155

Wild Atlantic Salmon (Raw) ☛ serving size: 3 oz = 85 g; Calories = 121

Wolffish Atlantic Cooked Dry Heat ☛ serving size: 1/2 fillet = 119 g; Calories = 146

Wolffish Atlantic Raw ☛ serving size: 3 oz = 85 g; Calories = 82

Yellowfin Tuna (Raw) ☛ serving size: 1 oz, boneless = 28.4 g; Calories = 31

Yellowtail (Raw) ☛ serving size: 3 oz = 85 g; Calories = 124

16

FRUITS & FRUITS PRODUCTS

Abiyuch ☛ serving size: 1/2 cup = 114 g; Calories = 79

Acerola Cherries (West Indian Cherry) ☛ serving size: 1 cup = 98 g; Calories = 31

Acerola Juice Raw ☛ serving size: 1 cup = 242 g; Calories = 56

Ambrosia ☛ serving size: 1 cup = 193 g; Calories = 135

Apple Baked Ns As To Added Sweetener ☛ serving size: 1 apple with liquid = 171 g; Calories = 163

Apple Baked Unsweetened ☛ serving size: 1 apple with liquid = 161 g; Calories = 90

Apple Baked With Sugar ☛ serving size: 1 apple with liquid = 171 g; Calories = 163

Apple Candied ☛ serving size: 1 small apple = 198 g; Calories = 255

Apple Chips ☛ serving size: 1 cup = 28 g; Calories = 129

Apple Dried Cooked Ns As To Sweetened Or Unsweetened;

Sweetened Ns As To Type Of Sweetener ☛ serving size: 1 cup = 255 g; Calories = 235

Apple Dried Cooked With Sugar ☛ serving size: 1 cup = 280 g; Calories = 258

Apple Fried ☛ serving size: 1 cup = 179 g; Calories = 247

Apple Juice ☛ serving size: 1 cup = 248 g; Calories = 114

Apple Juice Canned Or Bottled Unsweetened With Added Ascorbic Acid ☛ serving size: 1 cup = 248 g; Calories = 114

Apple Juice Canned Or Bottled Unsweetened With Added Ascorbic Acid Calcium And Potassium ☛ serving size: 6 fl oz = 177 g; Calories = 85

Apple Juice Frozen Concentrate Unsweetened Diluted With 3 Volume Water With Added Ascorbic Acid ☛ serving size: 1 cup = 239 g; Calories = 112

Apple Juice Frozen Concentrate Unsweetened Diluted With 3 Volume Water Without Added Ascorbic Acid ☛ serving size: 1 cup = 239 g; Calories = 112

Apple Juice Frozen Concentrate Unsweetened Undiluted With Added Ascorbic Acid ☛ serving size: 1 can (6 fl oz) = 211 g; Calories = 350

Apple Juice Frozen Concentrate Unsweetened Undiluted Without Added Ascorbic Acid ☛ serving size: 1 can (6 fl oz) = 211 g; Calories = 350

Apple Pickled ☛ serving size: 1 apple = 29 g; Calories = 37

Apple Rings Fried ☛ serving size: 1 ring = 19 g; Calories = 23

Apple Salad With Dressing ☛ serving size: 1 cup = 137 g; Calories = 236

Apples ☛ serving size: 1 cup, quartered or chopped = 125 g; Calories = 65

Apples (Without Skin) ☛ serving size: 1 cup slices = 110 g; Calories = 53

Apples Canned Sweetened Sliced Drained Heated ☛ serving size: 1 cup slices = 204 g; Calories = 137

Apples Dehydrated (Low Moisture) Sulfured Stewed ☛ serving size: 1 cup = 193 g; Calories = 143

Apples Dehydrated (Low Moisture) Sulfured Uncooked ☛ serving size: 1 cup = 60 g; Calories = 208

Apples Dried Sulfured Stewed With Added Sugar ☛ serving size: 1 cup = 280 g; Calories = 232

Apples Dried Sulfured Stewed Without Added Sugar ☛ serving size: 1 cup = 255 g; Calories = 145

Apples Frozen Unsweetened Heated ☛ serving size: 1 cup slices = 206 g; Calories = 97

Apples Frozen Unsweetened Unheated ☛ serving size: 1 cup slices = 173 g; Calories = 83

Apples Raw Without Skin Cooked Boiled ☛ serving size: 1 cup slices = 171 g; Calories = 91

Apples Raw Without Skin Cooked Microwave ☛ serving size: 1 cup slices = 170 g; Calories = 95

Applesauce Canned Sweetened With Salt ☛ serving size: 1 cup = 255 g; Calories = 194

Applesauce Canned Sweetened Without Salt (Includes USDA Commodity) ☛ serving size: 1 cup = 246 g; Calories = 167

Applesauce Canned Unsweetened With Added Ascorbic Acid ☛ serving size: 1 cup = 244 g; Calories = 103

Applesauce Canned Unsweetened Without Added Ascorbic Acid (Includes USDA Commodity) ☛ serving size: 1 cup = 244 g; Calories = 103

Apricot Dried Cooked Ns As To Sweetened Or Unsweetened; Sweetened Ns As To Type Of Sweetener ☛ serving size: 1 cup = 250 g; Calories = 293

Apricot Dried Cooked With Sugar ☛ serving size: 1 cup, nfs = 270 g; Calories = 316

Apricot Nectar Canned Without Added Ascorbic Acid ☛ serving size: 1 cup = 251 g; Calories = 141

Apricots ☛ serving size: 1 cup, halves = 155 g; Calories = 74

Apricots Canned Extra Heavy Syrup Pack Without Skin Solids And Liquids ☛ serving size: 1 cup, whole, without pits = 246 g; Calories = 236

Apricots Canned Extra Light Syrup Pack With Skin Solids And Liquids ☛ serving size: 1 cup, halves = 247 g; Calories = 121

Apricots Canned Heavy Syrup Drained ☛ serving size: 1 cup, halves = 219 g; Calories = 182

Apricots Canned Heavy Syrup Pack With Skin Solids And Liquids ☛ serving size: 1 cup, halves = 258 g; Calories = 214

Apricots Canned Heavy Syrup Pack Without Skin Solids And Liquids ☛ serving size: 1 cup, whole, without pits = 258 g; Calories = 214

Apricots Canned Juice Pack With Skin Solids And Liquids ☛ serving size: 1 cup, halves = 244 g; Calories = 117

Apricots Canned Light Syrup Pack With Skin Solids And Liquids ☛ serving size: 1 cup, halves = 253 g; Calories = 159

Apricots Canned Water Pack With Skin Solids And Liquids ☛ serving size: 1 cup, halves = 243 g; Calories = 66

Apricots Canned Water Pack Without Skin Solids And Liquids ☞ serving size: 1 cup, whole, without pits = 227 g; Calories = 50

Apricots Dehydrated (Low-Moisture) Sulfured Stewed ☞ serving size: 1 cup = 249 g; Calories = 314

Apricots Dried Sulfured Stewed With Added Sugar ☞ serving size: 1 cup, halves = 270 g; Calories = 305

Apricots Dried Sulfured Stewed Without Added Sugar ☞ serving size: 1 cup, halves = 250 g; Calories = 213

Apricots Frozen Sweetened ☞ serving size: 1 cup = 242 g; Calories = 237

Asian Pears ☞ serving size: 1 fruit 2-1/4 inch high x 2-1/2 inch dia = 122 g; Calories = 51

Avocados ☞ serving size: 1 cup, cubes = 150 g; Calories = 240

Banana Baked ☞ serving size: 1 banana (7-1/4" long) = 128 g; Calories = 163

Banana Batter-Dipped Fried ☞ serving size: 1 small = 108 g; Calories = 333

Banana Red Fried ☞ serving size: 1 fruit (7-1/4" long) = 94 g; Calories = 138

Banana Ripe Fried ☞ serving size: 1 small = 73 g; Calories = 107

Banana Whip ☞ serving size: 1 cup = 130 g; Calories = 177

Bananas ☞ serving size: 1 cup, mashed = 225 g; Calories = 200

Bartlett Pears ☞ serving size: 1 cup, sliced = 140 g; Calories = 88

Beans String Green Pickled ☞ serving size: 1 cup = 135 g; Calories = 38

Blackberries ☞ serving size: 1 cup = 144 g; Calories = 62

Blackberries Canned Heavy Syrup Solids And Liquids ☛ serving size: 1 cup = 256 g; Calories = 236

Blackberries Frozen Sweetened Ns As To Type Of Sweetener ☛ serving size: 1 cup = 145 g; Calories = 144

Blackberries Frozen Unsweetened ☛ serving size: 1 cup, unthawed = 151 g; Calories = 97

Blackberry Juice Canned ☛ serving size: 1 cup = 250 g; Calories = 95

Blueberries ☛ serving size: 1 cup = 148 g; Calories = 84

Blueberries (Frozen) ☛ serving size: 1 cup, unthawed = 155 g; Calories = 79

Blueberries Canned Heavy Syrup Solids And Liquids ☛ serving size: 1 cup = 256 g; Calories = 225

Blueberries Canned Light Syrup Drained ☛ serving size: 1 cup = 244 g; Calories = 215

Blueberries Cooked Or Canned Unsweetened Water Pack ☛ serving size: 1 cup = 244 g; Calories = 93

Blueberries Frozen Sweetened ☛ serving size: 1 cup, thawed = 230 g; Calories = 196

Blueberries Wild Canned Heavy Syrup Drained ☛ serving size: 1 cup = 319 g; Calories = 341

Bosc Pear ☛ serving size: 1 cup, sliced = 140 g; Calories = 94

Boysenberries (Frozen) ☛ serving size: 1 cup, unthawed = 132 g; Calories = 66

Boysenberries Canned Heavy Syrup ☛ serving size: 1 cup = 256 g; Calories = 225

Breadfruit ☛ serving size: 1 cup = 220 g; Calories = 227

Cabbage Red Pickled ☞ serving size: 1 cup = 150 g; Calories = 66

California Avocados ☞ serving size: 1 cup, pureed = 230 g; Calories = 384

California Grapefruit ☞ serving size: 1 cup sections, with juice = 230 g; Calories = 85

California Valencia Oranges ☞ serving size: 1 cup sections, without membranes = 180 g; Calories = 88

Canned Orange Juice ☞ serving size: 1 cup = 249 g; Calories = 117

Cantaloupe Melons ☞ serving size: 1 cup, balls = 177 g; Calories = 60

Carissa ☞ serving size: 1 cup slices = 150 g; Calories = 93

Casaba Melon ☞ serving size: 1 cup, cubes = 170 g; Calories = 48

Cauliflower Pickled ☞ serving size: 1 cup = 125 g; Calories = 54

Celery Pickled ☞ serving size: 1 cup = 150 g; Calories = 24

Cherimoya ☞ serving size: 1 cup, pieces = 160 g; Calories = 120

Cherries (Sweet) ☞ serving size: 1 cup, with pits, yields = 138 g; Calories = 87

Cherries Sour Canned Water Pack Drained ☞ serving size: 1 cup = 168 g; Calories = 71

Cherries Sour Red Canned Extra Heavy Syrup Pack Solids And Liquids ☞ serving size: 1 cup = 261 g; Calories = 298

Cherries Sour Red Canned Heavy Syrup Pack Solids And Liquids ☞ serving size: 1 cup = 256 g; Calories = 233

Cherries Sour Red Canned Light Syrup Pack Solids And Liquids ☞ serving size: 1 cup = 252 g; Calories = 189

Cherries Sour Red Canned Water Pack Solids And Liquids

(Includes USDA Commodity Red Tart Cherries Canned) ☛ serving size: 1 cup = 244 g; Calories = 88

🍒 Cherries Sweet Canned Extra Heavy Syrup Pack Solids And Liquids ☛ serving size: 1 cup, pitted = 261 g; Calories = 266

🍒 Cherries Sweet Canned Juice Pack Solids And Liquids ☛ serving size: 1 cup, pitted = 250 g; Calories = 135

🍒 Cherries Sweet Canned Light Syrup Pack Solids And Liquids ☛ serving size: 1 cup, pitted = 252 g; Calories = 169

🍒 Cherries Sweet Canned Pitted Heavy Syrup Drained ☛ serving size: 1 cup = 179 g; Calories = 149

🍒 Cherries Sweet Canned Pitted Heavy Syrup Pack Solids And Liquids ☛ serving size: 1 cup = 253 g; Calories = 210

🍒 Cherries Sweet Canned Water Pack Solids And Liquids ☛ serving size: 1 cup, pitted = 248 g; Calories = 114

🍒 Cherries Tart Dried Sweetened ☛ serving size: 1/4 cup = 40 g; Calories = 133

🍒 Chinese Preserved Sweet Vegetable ☛ serving size: 1 slice = 12 g; Calories = 45

🍒 Clementines ☛ serving size: 1 fruit = 74 g; Calories = 35

🍒 Corn Relish ☛ serving size: 1 cup = 245 g; Calories = 206

🍒 Crabapples ☛ serving size: 1 cup slices = 110 g; Calories = 84

🍒 Cranberries ☛ serving size: 1 cup, chopped = 110 g; Calories = 51

🍒 Cranberry Juice Blend 100% Juice Bottled With Added Vitamin C And Calcium ☛ serving size: 6 (3/4) fl oz = 200 g; Calories = 90

🍒 Cranberry Juice Unsweetened ☛ serving size: 1 cup = 253 g; Calories = 116

Cranberry Salad Congealed ☛ serving size: 1 cup = 253 g; Calories = 294

Cranberry Sauce Canned Sweetened ☛ serving size: 1 cup = 277 g; Calories = 440

Cranberry Sauce Jellied Canned Ocean Spray ☛ serving size: 1/4 cup = 70 g; Calories = 112

Cranberry Sauce Whole Canned Ocean Spray ☛ serving size: 1/4 cup = 70 g; Calories = 111

Cranberry-Orange Relish Canned ☛ serving size: 1 cup = 275 g; Calories = 490

Cranberry-Orange Relish Uncooked ☛ serving size: 1 cup = 275 g; Calories = 360

Cranberry-Raspberry Sauce ☛ serving size: 1 container (12 oz) = 340 g; Calories = 551

Dates (Deglet Noor) ☛ serving size: 1 cup, chopped = 147 g; Calories = 415

Dried Apples ☛ serving size: 1 cup = 86 g; Calories = 209

Dried Apricots ☛ serving size: 1 cup, halves = 130 g; Calories = 313

Dried Bananas ☛ serving size: 1 cup = 100 g; Calories = 346

Dried Blueberries (Sweetened) ☛ serving size: 1/4 cup = 40 g; Calories = 127

Dried Cranberries (Sweetened) ☛ serving size: 1/4 cup = 40 g; Calories = 123

Dried Figs ☛ serving size: 1 cup = 149 g; Calories = 371

Dried Litchis ☛ serving size: 1 fruit = 2.5 g; Calories = 7

Dried Longans ☛ serving size: 1 fruit = 1.7 g; Calories = 5

Dried Peaches ☛ serving size: 1 cup, halves = 160 g; Calories = 382

Dried Peaches (Low-Moisture) ☛ serving size: 1 cup = 116 g; Calories = 377

Dried Pears ☛ serving size: 1 cup, halves = 180 g; Calories = 472

Durian ☛ serving size: 1 cup, chopped or diced = 243 g; Calories = 357

Elderberries ☛ serving size: 1 cup = 145 g; Calories = 106

European Black Currants ☛ serving size: 1 cup = 112 g; Calories = 71

Feijoa ☛ serving size: 1 cup, pureed = 243 g; Calories = 148

Fig Dried Cooked Ns As To Sweetened Or Unsweetened; Sweetened Ns As To Type Of Sweetener ☛ serving size: 1 cup = 259 g; Calories = 355

Fig Dried Cooked With Sugar ☛ serving size: 1 cup = 270 g; Calories = 370

Figs ☛ serving size: 1 large (2-1/2 inch dia) = 64 g; Calories = 47

Figs Canned Extra Heavy Syrup Pack Solids And Liquids ☛ serving size: 1 cup = 261 g; Calories = 279

Figs Canned Heavy Syrup Pack Solids And Liquids ☛ serving size: 1 cup = 259 g; Calories = 228

Figs Canned Light Syrup Pack Solids And Liquids ☛ serving size: 1 cup = 252 g; Calories = 174

Figs Canned Water Pack Solids And Liquids ☛ serving size: 1 cup = 248 g; Calories = 131

Figs Dried Stewed ☛ serving size: 1 cup = 259 g; Calories = 277

Florida Avocados ☛ serving size: 1 cup, pureed = 230 g; Calories = 276

Florida Grapefruit ☛ serving size: 1 cup sections, with juice = 230 g; Calories = 69

Florida Oranges ☛ serving size: 1 cup sections, without membranes = 185 g; Calories = 85

Fortified Fruit Juice Smoothie ☛ serving size: 8 fl oz = 240 g; Calories = 170

Fried Dwarf Banana Puerto Rican Style ☛ serving size: 1 banana (4" x 1-1/2" x 1-1/2") = 36 g; Calories = 56

Fried Dwarf Banana With Cheese Puerto Rican Style ☛ serving size: 1 banana (4" x 1-1/2" x 1-1/2") = 40 g; Calories = 84

Fried Yellow Plantains ☛ serving size: 1 cup = 169 g; Calories = 399

Frozen Raspberries ☛ serving size: 1 cup, unthawed = 140 g; Calories = 78

Frozen Strawberries ☛ serving size: 1 cup, thawed = 221 g; Calories = 77

Fruit Cocktail (Peach And Pineapple And Pear And Grape And Cherry) Canned Extra Heavy Syrup Solids And Liquids ☛ serving size: 1/2 cup = 130 g; Calories = 114

Fruit Cocktail (Peach And Pineapple And Pear And Grape And Cherry) Canned Extra Light Syrup Solids And Liquids ☛ serving size: 1/2 cup = 123 g; Calories = 55

Fruit Cocktail (Peach And Pineapple And Pear And Grape And Cherry) Canned Heavy Syrup Solids And Liquids ☛ serving size: 1 cup = 248 g; Calories = 181

Fruit Cocktail (Peach And Pineapple And Pear And Grape And Cherry) Canned Juice Pack Solids And Liquids ☛ serving size: 1 cup = 237 g; Calories = 109

Fruit Cocktail (Peach And Pineapple And Pear And Grape And Cherry) Canned Light Syrup Solids And Liquids ☛ serving size: 1 cup = 242 g; Calories = 138

Fruit Cocktail (Peach And Pineapple And Pear And Grape And

Cherry) Canned Water Pack Solids And Liquids ☛ serving size: 1 cup = 237 g; Calories = 76

Fruit Cocktail Canned Heavy Syrup Drained ☛ serving size: 1 cup = 214 g; Calories = 150

Fruit Cocktail Or Mix Frozen ☛ serving size: 1 cup = 215 g; Calories = 105

Fruit Dessert With Cream And/or Pudding And Nuts ☛ serving size: 1 cup = 178 g; Calories = 361

Fruit Juice Smoothie Bolthouse Farms Berry Boost ☛ serving size: 1 cup = 252 g; Calories = 116

Fruit Juice Smoothie Bolthouse Farms Green Goodness ☛ serving size: 1 cup = 230 g; Calories = 129

Fruit Juice Smoothie Bolthouse Farms Strawberry Banana ☛ serving size: 1 cup = 233 g; Calories = 121

Fruit Juice Smoothie Naked Juice Green Machine ☛ serving size: 1 cup = 275 g; Calories = 146

Fruit Juice Smoothie Naked Juice Mighty Mango ☛ serving size: 8 fl oz = 240 g; Calories = 151

Fruit Juice Smoothie Naked Juice Strawberry Banana ☛ serving size: 1 cup = 228 g; Calories = 114

Fruit Juice Smoothie Odwalla Original Superfood ☛ serving size: 1 cup = 227 g; Calories = 114

Fruit Juice Smoothie Odwalla Strawberry Banana ☛ serving size: 1 cup = 233 g; Calories = 112

Fruit Ns As To Type ☛ serving size: 1 fruit = 138 g; Calories = 95

Fruit Salad (Peach And Pear And Apricot And Pineapple And Cherry) Canned Extra Heavy Syrup Solids And Liquids ☛ serving size: 1 cup = 259 g; Calories = 228

Fruit Salad (Peach And Pear And Apricot And Pineapple And Cherry) Canned Juice Pack Solids And Liquids ☞ serving size: 1 cup = 249 g; Calories = 125

Fruit Salad (Peach And Pear And Apricot And Pineapple And Cherry) Canned Light Syrup Solids And Liquids ☞ serving size: 1 cup = 252 g; Calories = 146

Fruit Salad (Peach And Pear And Apricot And Pineapple And Cherry) Canned Water Pack Solids And Liquids ☞ serving size: 1 cup = 245 g; Calories = 74

Fruit Salad (Pineapple And Papaya And Banana And Guava) Tropical Canned Heavy Syrup Solids And Liquids ☞ serving size: 1 cup = 257 g; Calories = 221

Fruit Salad Excluding Citrus Fruits With Marshmallows ☞ serving size: 1 cup = 171 g; Calories = 409

Fruit Salad Excluding Citrus Fruits With Nondairy Whipped Topping ☞ serving size: 1 cup = 175 g; Calories = 243

Fruit Salad Excluding Citrus Fruits With Pudding ☞ serving size: 1 cup = 182 g; Calories = 228

Fruit Salad Excluding Citrus Fruits With Salad Dressing Or Mayonnaise ☞ serving size: 1 cup = 188 g; Calories = 442

Fruit Salad Excluding Citrus Fruits With Whipped Cream ☞ serving size: 1 cup = 182 g; Calories = 273

Fruit Salad Fresh Or Raw Excluding Citrus Fruits No Dressing ☞ serving size: 1 cup = 175 g; Calories = 93

Fruit Salad Fresh Or Raw Including Citrus Fruits No Dressing ☞ serving size: 1 cup = 175 g; Calories = 91

Fruit Salad Including Citrus Fruit With Whipped Cream ☞ serving size: 1 cup = 182 g; Calories = 268

Fruit Salad Including Citrus Fruits With Marshmallows ☛ serving size: 1 cup = 171 g; Calories = 402

Fruit Salad Including Citrus Fruits With Nondairy Whipped Topping ☛ serving size: 1 cup = 175 g; Calories = 238

Fruit Salad Including Citrus Fruits With Pudding ☛ serving size: 1 cup = 182 g; Calories = 224

Fruit Salad Including Citrus Fruits With Salad Dressing Or Mayonnaise ☛ serving size: 1 cup = 188 g; Calories = 432

Fruit Salad Puerto Rican Style ☛ serving size: 1 cup = 247 g; Calories = 143

Fuji Apples ☛ serving size: 1 cup, sliced = 109 g; Calories = 69

Fuyu Persimmon ☛ serving size: 1 fruit (2-1/2 inch dia) = 168 g; Calories = 118

Gala Apples ☛ serving size: 1 cup, sliced = 109 g; Calories = 62

Goji Berries Dried ☛ serving size: 5 tbsp = 28 g; Calories = 98

Golden Delicious Apples ☛ serving size: 1 cup, sliced = 109 g; Calories = 62

Golden Seedless Raisins ☛ serving size: 1 cup, packed = 165 g; Calories = 497

Gooseberries ☛ serving size: 1 cup = 150 g; Calories = 66

Gooseberries Canned Light Syrup Pack Solids And Liquids ☛ serving size: 1 cup = 252 g; Calories = 184

Granny Smith Apples ☛ serving size: 1 cup, sliced = 109 g; Calories = 63

Grape Juice ☛ serving size: 1 cup = 253 g; Calories = 152

Grape Juice (With Added Vitamin C) ☛ serving size: 1 cup = 253 g; Calories = 152

Grape Juice Canned Or Bottled Unsweetened With Added Ascorbic Acid And Calcium ☞ serving size: 1 cup = 253 g; Calories = 157

Grapefruit ☞ serving size: 1 cup sections, with juice = 230 g; Calories = 74

Grapefruit And Orange Sections Cooked Canned Or Frozen In Light Syrup ☞ serving size: 1 cup = 254 g; Calories = 152

Grapefruit And Orange Sections Cooked Canned Or Frozen Ns As To Added Sweetener ☞ serving size: 1 cup = 254 g; Calories = 152

Grapefruit And Orange Sections Cooked Canned Or Frozen Unsweetened Water Pack ☞ serving size: 1 cup = 244 g; Calories = 66

Grapefruit And Orange Sections Raw ☞ serving size: 1 section = 16 g; Calories = 6

Grapefruit Juice ☞ serving size: 8 fl oz = 240 g; Calories = 94

Grapefruit Juice 100% With Calcium Added ☞ serving size: 1 fl oz (no ice) = 31 g; Calories = 12

Grapefruit Juice White Bottled Unsweetened Ocean Spray ☞ serving size: 1 cup = 247 g; Calories = 91

Grapefruit Juice White Canned Or Bottled Unsweetened ☞ serving size: 1 cup = 247 g; Calories = 91

Grapefruit Juice White Canned Sweetened ☞ serving size: 1 cup = 250 g; Calories = 115

Grapefruit Juice White Frozen Concentrate Unsweetened Diluted With 3 Volume Water ☞ serving size: 1 cup = 247 g; Calories = 101

Grapefruit Juice White Frozen Concentrate Unsweetened Undiluted ☞ serving size: 1 can (6 fl oz) = 207 g; Calories = 302

Grapefruit Sections Canned Juice Pack Solids And Liquids ☞ serving size: 1 cup = 249 g; Calories = 92

Grapefruit Sections Canned Light Syrup Pack Solids And Liquids ☛ serving size: 1 cup = 254 g; Calories = 152

Grapefruit Sections Canned Water Pack Solids And Liquids ☛ serving size: 1 cup = 244 g; Calories = 88

Grapes ☛ serving size: 1 cup = 92 g; Calories = 62

Grapes Canned Thompson Seedless Heavy Syrup Pack Solids And Liquids ☛ serving size: 1 cup = 256 g; Calories = 195

Grapes Canned Thompson Seedless Water Pack Solids And Liquids ☛ serving size: 1 cup = 245 g; Calories = 98

Green Anjou Pear ☛ serving size: 1 cup, sliced = 140 g; Calories = 92

Green Olives ☛ serving size: 1 olive = 2.7 g; Calories = 4

Groundcherries ☛ serving size: 1 cup = 140 g; Calories = 74

Guanabana Nectar Canned ☛ serving size: 1 cup = 251 g; Calories = 148

Guava Nectar Canned With Added Ascorbic Acid ☛ serving size: 1 cup = 251 g; Calories = 158

Guava Nectar With Sucralose Canned ☛ serving size: fl oz = 335 g; Calories = 161

Guava Sauce Cooked ☛ serving size: 1 cup = 238 g; Calories = 86

Guava Shell Canned In Heavy Syrup ☛ serving size: 1 cup = 310 g; Calories = 338

Guavas ☛ serving size: 1 cup = 165 g; Calories = 112

Honeydew Melon ☛ serving size: 1 cup, diced (approx 20 pieces per cup) = 170 g; Calories = 61

Horned Melon (Kiwano) ☛ serving size: 1 cup = 233 g; Calories = 103

Jackfruit ☞ serving size: 1 cup, sliced = 165 g; Calories = 157

Jackfruit Canned Syrup Pack ☞ serving size: 1 cup, drained = 178 g; Calories = 164

Java Plum ☞ serving size: 1 cup = 135 g; Calories = 81

Juice Apple And Grape Blend With Added Ascorbic Acid ☞ serving size: 8 fl oz = 250 g; Calories = 125

Juice Apple Grape And Pear Blend With Added Ascorbic Acid And Calcium ☞ serving size: 8 fl oz = 250 g; Calories = 130

Jumbo Olives ☞ serving size: 1 super colossal = 15 g; Calories = 12

Kiwifruit ☞ serving size: 1 cup, sliced = 180 g; Calories = 110

Kiwifruit Zespri Sungold Raw ☞ serving size: 1 fruit = 81 g; Calories = 51

Kumquat Cooked Or Canned In Syrup ☞ serving size: 1 kumquat = 14 g; Calories = 14

Kumquats ☞ serving size: 1 fruit without refuse = 19 g; Calories = 14

Lemon Juice From Concentrate Bottled Concord ☞ serving size: 1 tbsp = 15 g; Calories = 4

Lemon Juice From Concentrate Bottled Real Lemon ☞ serving size: 1 tbsp = 15 g; Calories = 3

Lemon Juice From Concentrate Canned Or Bottled ☞ serving size: 1 tbsp = 15 g; Calories = 3

Lemon Juice Raw ☞ serving size: 1 cup = 244 g; Calories = 54

Lemon Peel Raw ☞ serving size: 1 tbsp = 6 g; Calories = 3

Lemons ☞ serving size: 1 cup, sections = 212 g; Calories = 62

Lime Juice ☞ serving size: 1 cup = 242 g; Calories = 61

Lime Juice Canned Or Bottled Unsweetened ☛ serving size: 1 cup = 246 g; Calories = 52

Limes ☛ serving size: 1 fruit (2 inch dia) = 67 g; Calories = 20

Litchis ☛ serving size: 1 cup = 190 g; Calories = 125

Loganberries (Frozen) ☛ serving size: 1 cup, unthawed = 147 g; Calories = 81

Longans ☛ serving size: 1 fruit without refuse = 3.2 g; Calories = 2

Loquats ☛ serving size: 1 cup, cubed = 149 g; Calories = 70

Low-Moisture Dried Apricots ☛ serving size: 1 cup = 119 g; Calories = 381

Lychee Cooked Or Canned In Sugar Or Syrup ☛ serving size: 1 lychee with liquid = 21 g; Calories = 20

Mamey Sapote ☛ serving size: 1 cup 1 inch pieces = 175 g; Calories = 217

Mammy Apple ☛ serving size: 1 fruit without refuse = 846 g; Calories = 432

Mango Cooked ☛ serving size: 1 oz = 28 g; Calories = 17

Mango Nectar Canned ☛ serving size: 1 cup = 251 g; Calories = 128

Mango Pickled ☛ serving size: 1 slice = 28 g; Calories = 37

Mangos ☛ serving size: 1 cup pieces = 165 g; Calories = 99

Mangosteen Canned Syrup Pack ☛ serving size: 1 cup, drained = 196 g; Calories = 143

Maraschino Cherries (Canned) ☛ serving size: 1 cherry (nlea serving) = 5 g; Calories = 8

Medjool Dates ☛ serving size: 1 date, pitted = 24 g; Calories = 67

Melon Balls ☛ serving size: 1 cup, unthawed = 173 g; Calories = 57

Mulberries ☛ serving size: 1 cup = 140 g; Calories = 60

Muscadine Grapes ☛ serving size: 1 grape = 6 g; Calories = 3

Mushrooms Pickled ☛ serving size: 1 cup = 156 g; Calories = 33

Nance Canned Syrup Drained ☛ serving size: 3 fruit without pits = 11.1 g; Calories = 11

Nance Frozen Unsweetened ☛ serving size: 1 cup without pits, thawed = 112 g; Calories = 82

Naranjilla (Lulo) Pulp Frozen Unsweetened ☛ serving size: 1 cup thawed = 120 g; Calories = 30

Navel Oranges ☛ serving size: 1 cup sections, without membranes = 165 g; Calories = 81

Nectarine Cooked ☛ serving size: 1 cup = 262 g; Calories = 223

Nectarines ☛ serving size: 1 cup slices = 143 g; Calories = 63

Oheloberries ☛ serving size: 1 cup = 140 g; Calories = 39

Okra Pickled ☛ serving size: 1 pod = 11 g; Calories = 3

Olives ☛ serving size: 1 tbsp = 8.4 g; Calories = 10

Olives Black ☛ serving size: 1 slice = 1 g; Calories = 1

Olives Green Stuffed ☛ serving size: 1 cup = 147 g; Calories = 188

Olives Nfs ☛ serving size: 1 slice = 1 g; Calories = 1

Orange Juice ☛ serving size: 1 cup = 248 g; Calories = 112

Orange Juice 100% Nfs ☛ serving size: 1 fl oz (no ice) = 31 g; Calories = 15

Orange Juice Chilled Includes From Concentrate With Added Calcium And Vitamins A D E ☛ serving size: 1 cup = 249 g; Calories = 122

Orange Juice From Concentrate ☛ serving size: 1 cup = 249 g; Calories = 122

Orange Juice Frozen Concentrate Unsweetened Diluted With 3 Volume Water ☛ serving size: 1 cup = 249 g; Calories = 92

Orange Juice Frozen Concentrate Unsweetened Diluted With 3 Volume Water With Added Calcium ☛ serving size: 1 cup = 249 g; Calories = 92

Orange Juice Frozen Concentrate Unsweetened Undiluted ☛ serving size: 1 cup = 262 g; Calories = 388

Orange Juice Frozen Concentrate Unsweetened Undiluted With Added Calcium ☛ serving size: 1 cup = 262 g; Calories = 385

Orange Juice With Added Calcium ☛ serving size: 1 cup = 249 g; Calories = 117

Orange Juice With Added Calcium And Vitamin D ☛ serving size: 1 cup = 249 g; Calories = 117

Orange Peel Raw ☛ serving size: 1 tbsp = 6 g; Calories = 6

Orange Pineapple Juice Blend ☛ serving size: 8 fl oz = 246 g; Calories = 126

Orange Sections Canned Juice Pack ☛ serving size: 1 cup = 204 g; Calories = 96

Orange-Grapefruit Juice Canned Or Bottled Unsweetened ☛ serving size: 1 cup = 247 g; Calories = 106

Oranges ☛ serving size: 1 cup, sections = 180 g; Calories = 85

Oranges Raw With Peel ☛ serving size: 1 cup = 170 g; Calories = 107

Papaya ☛ serving size: 1 cup 1 inch pieces = 145 g; Calories = 62

Papaya Canned Heavy Syrup Drained ☛ serving size: 1 piece = 39 g; Calories = 80

Papaya Cooked Or Canned In Sugar Or Syrup ☞ serving size: 1 cup = 244 g; Calories = 193

Papaya Dried ☞ serving size: 1 strip = 23 g; Calories = 68

Papaya Green Cooked ☞ serving size: 1 cup = 244 g; Calories = 105

Papaya Nectar Canned ☞ serving size: 1 cup = 250 g; Calories = 143

Passion Fruit (Granadilla) ☞ serving size: 1 cup = 236 g; Calories = 229

Peach Dried Cooked Ns As To Sweetened Or Unsweetened; Sweetened Ns As To Type Of Sweetener ☞ serving size: 1 cup = 258 g; Calories = 284

Peach Dried Cooked With Sugar ☞ serving size: 1 cup = 270 g; Calories = 297

Peach Nectar Canned With Added Ascorbic Acid ☞ serving size: 1 cup = 249 g; Calories = 125

Peach Nectar Canned Without Added Ascorbic Acid ☞ serving size: 1 cup = 249 g; Calories = 122

Peach Pickled ☞ serving size: 1 fruit = 88 g; Calories = 104

Peaches Canned Extra Heavy Syrup Pack Solids And Liquids ☞ serving size: 1 cup, halves or slices = 262 g; Calories = 252

Peaches Canned Extra Light Syrup Solids And Liquids ☞ serving size: 1 cup, halves or slices = 247 g; Calories = 104

Peaches Canned Heavy Syrup Drained ☞ serving size: 1 cup = 222 g; Calories = 160

Peaches Canned Heavy Syrup Pack Solids And Liquids ☞ serving size: 1 cup = 262 g; Calories = 194

Peaches Canned Juice Pack Solids And Liquids ☞ serving size: 1 cup = 250 g; Calories = 110

Peaches Canned Light Syrup Pack Solids And Liquids ☞ serving size: 1 cup, halves or slices = 251 g; Calories = 136

Peaches Canned Water Pack Solids And Liquids ☞ serving size: 1 cup, halves or slices = 244 g; Calories = 59

Peaches Dehydrated (Low-Moisture) Sulfured Stewed ☞ serving size: 1 cup = 242 g; Calories = 322

Peaches Dried Sulfured Stewed With Added Sugar ☞ serving size: 1 cup = 270 g; Calories = 278

Peaches Dried Sulfured Stewed Without Added Sugar ☞ serving size: 1 cup = 258 g; Calories = 199

Peaches Frozen Sliced Sweetened ☞ serving size: 1 cup, thawed = 250 g; Calories = 235

Peaches Spiced Canned Heavy Syrup Pack Solids And Liquids ☞ serving size: 1 cup, whole = 242 g; Calories = 182

Pear Dried Cooked Ns As To Sweetened Or Unsweetened; Sweetened Ns As To Type Of Sweetener ☞ serving size: 1 cup = 255 g; Calories = 395

Pear Dried Cooked With Sugar ☞ serving size: 1 cup = 280 g; Calories = 434

Pear Nectar Canned With Added Ascorbic Acid ☞ serving size: 1 cup = 250 g; Calories = 150

Pear Nectar Canned Without Added Ascorbic Acid ☞ serving size: 1 cup = 250 g; Calories = 150

Pears ☞ serving size: 1 cup, slices = 140 g; Calories = 80

Pears Canned Extra Light Syrup Pack Solids And Liquids ☞ serving size: 1 cup, halves = 247 g; Calories = 116

Pears Canned Heavy Syrup Drained ☞ serving size: 1 cup = 201 g; Calories = 149

Pears Canned Heavy Syrup Pack Solids And Liquids ☞ serving size: 1 cup = 266 g; Calories = 197

Pears Canned In Syrup ☞ serving size: 1 cup, halves = 266 g; Calories = 258

Pears Canned Juice Pack Solids And Liquids ☞ serving size: 1 cup, halves = 248 g; Calories = 124

Pears Canned Light Syrup Pack Solids And Liquids ☞ serving size: 1 cup, halves = 251 g; Calories = 143

Pears Canned Water Pack Solids And Liquids ☞ serving size: 1 cup, halves = 244 g; Calories = 71

Pears Dried Sulfured Stewed With Added Sugar ☞ serving size: 1 cup, halves = 280 g; Calories = 392

Pears Dried Sulfured Stewed Without Added Sugar ☞ serving size: 1 cup, halves = 255 g; Calories = 324

Peppers Pickled ☞ serving size: 1 cup = 135 g; Calories = 54

Persimmons Japanese Dried ☞ serving size: 1 fruit without refuse = 34 g; Calories = 93

Persimmons Native Raw ☞ serving size: 1 fruit without refuse = 25 g; Calories = 32

Pickled Green Bananas Puerto Rican Style ☞ serving size: 1 cup = 150 g; Calories = 480

Pineapple ☞ serving size: 1 cup, chunks = 165 g; Calories = 83

Pineapple (Traditional) ☞ serving size: 1 cup, chunks = 165 g; Calories = 74

Pineapple Canned Extra Heavy Syrup Pack Solids And Liquids ☞ serving size: 1 cup, crushed, sliced, or chunks = 260 g; Calories = 216

Pineapple Canned Heavy Syrup Pack Solids And Liquids ☞ serving size: 1 cup, crushed, sliced, or chunks = 254 g; Calories = 198

Pineapple Canned Juice Pack Drained ☛ serving size: 1 cup, chunks = 181 g; Calories = 109

Pineapple Canned Juice Pack Solids And Liquids ☛ serving size: 1 cup, crushed, sliced, or chunks = 249 g; Calories = 149

Pineapple Canned Light Syrup Pack Solids And Liquids ☛ serving size: 1 cup, crushed, sliced, or chunks = 252 g; Calories = 131

Pineapple Canned Water Pack Solids And Liquids ☛ serving size: 1 cup, crushed, sliced, or chunks = 246 g; Calories = 79

Pineapple Dried ☛ serving size: 1 piece = 28 g; Calories = 75

Pineapple Frozen Chunks Sweetened ☛ serving size: 1 cup, chunks = 245 g; Calories = 211

Pineapple Juice Canned Not From Concentrate Unsweetened With Added Vitamins A C And E ☛ serving size: 1 cup = 250 g; Calories = 125

Pineapple Juice Canned Or Bottled Unsweetened With Added Ascorbic Acid ☛ serving size: 1 cup = 250 g; Calories = 133

Pineapple Juice Canned Or Bottled Unsweetened Without Added Ascorbic Acid ☛ serving size: 1 cup = 250 g; Calories = 133

Pineapple Juice Frozen Concentrate Unsweetened Diluted With 3 Volume Water ☛ serving size: 1 cup = 250 g; Calories = 128

Pineapple Juice Frozen Concentrate Unsweetened Undiluted ☛ serving size: 1 can (6 fl oz) = 216 g; Calories = 387

Pineapple Raw Extra Sweet Variety ☛ serving size: 1 cup, chunks = 165 g; Calories = 84

Pineapple Salad With Dressing ☛ serving size: 1 serving (lettuce, 1 cup diced pineapple, dressing) = 184 g; Calories = 177

Pink Grapefruit ☛ serving size: 1 cup sections, with juice = 230 g; Calories = 97

Pink Grapefruit Juice ☛ serving size: 1 cup = 247 g; Calories = 96

Pitanga ☛ serving size: 1 cup = 173 g; Calories = 57

Plantains ☛ serving size: 1 cup, sliced = 148 g; Calories = 181

Plantains Cooked ☛ serving size: 1 cup, mashed = 200 g; Calories = 310

Plantains Green Fried ☛ serving size: 1 cup = 118 g; Calories = 365

Plum Pickled ☛ serving size: 1 plum = 28 g; Calories = 34

Plums ☛ serving size: 1 cup, sliced = 165 g; Calories = 76

Plums Canned Heavy Syrup Drained ☛ serving size: 1 cup, with pits, yields = 183 g; Calories = 163

Plums Canned Purple Extra Heavy Syrup Pack Solids And Liquids ☛ serving size: 1 cup, pitted = 261 g; Calories = 264

Plums Canned Purple Heavy Syrup Pack Solids And Liquids ☛ serving size: 1 cup, pitted = 258 g; Calories = 230

Plums Canned Purple Juice Pack Solids And Liquids ☛ serving size: 1 cup, pitted = 252 g; Calories = 146

Plums Canned Purple Light Syrup Pack Solids And Liquids ☛ serving size: 1 cup, pitted = 252 g; Calories = 159

Plums Canned Purple Water Pack Solids And Liquids ☛ serving size: 1 cup, pitted = 249 g; Calories = 102

Plums Dried (Prunes) Stewed With Added Sugar ☛ serving size: 1 cup, pitted = 248 g; Calories = 308

Plums Dried (Prunes) Stewed Without Added Sugar ☛ serving size: 1 cup, pitted = 248 g; Calories = 265

Pomegranate Juice Bottled ☛ serving size: 1 cup = 249 g; Calories = 135

Pomegranates ☞ serving size: 1/2 cup arils (seed/juice sacs) = 87 g; Calories = 72

Prickly Pears ☞ serving size: 1 cup = 149 g; Calories = 61

Prune Dried Cooked Ns As To Sweetened Or Unsweetened; Sweetened Ns As To Type Of Sweetener ☞ serving size: 1 prune = 10 g; Calories = 14

Prune Dried Cooked With Sugar ☞ serving size: 1 prune = 10 g; Calories = 14

Prune Puree ☞ serving size: 2 tbsp = 36 g; Calories = 93

Prune Whip ☞ serving size: 1 cup = 130 g; Calories = 191

Prunes (Dried Plums) ☞ serving size: 1 cup, pitted = 174 g; Calories = 418

Prunes (Low-Moisture) ☞ serving size: 1 cup = 132 g; Calories = 448

Prunes Canned Heavy Syrup Pack Solids And Liquids ☞ serving size: 1 cup = 234 g; Calories = 246

Prunes Dehydrated (Low-Moisture) Stewed ☞ serving size: 1 cup = 280 g; Calories = 316

Pummelo ☞ serving size: 1 cup, sections = 190 g; Calories = 72

Purple Passion Fruit Juice ☞ serving size: 1 cup = 247 g; Calories = 126

Quinces ☞ serving size: 1 fruit without refuse = 92 g; Calories = 52

Raisins ☞ serving size: 1 cup, packed = 165 g; Calories = 493

Raisins Cooked ☞ serving size: 1 cup = 295 g; Calories = 646

Raisins Seeded ☞ serving size: 1 cup, packed = 165 g; Calories = 488

Rambutan Canned Syrup Pack ☞ serving size: 1 cup, drained = 150 g; Calories = 123

Raspberries ☛ serving size: 1 cup = 123 g; Calories = 64

Raspberries Canned Red Heavy Syrup Pack Solids And Liquids ☛ serving size: 1 cup = 256 g; Calories = 233

Raspberries Cooked Or Canned Unsweetened Water Pack ☛ serving size: 1 cup = 243 g; Calories = 85

Raspberries Frozen Red Sweetened ☛ serving size: 1 cup, thawed = 250 g; Calories = 258

Raspberries Frozen Unsweetened ☛ serving size: 1 cup = 250 g; Calories = 130

Red And White Currants ☛ serving size: 1 cup = 112 g; Calories = 63

Red Anjou Pears ☛ serving size: 1 small = 126 g; Calories = 78

Red Delicious Apples ☛ serving size: 1 cup, sliced = 109 g; Calories = 64

Red Or Green Grapes (European) ☛ serving size: 1 cup = 151 g; Calories = 104

Rhubarb ☛ serving size: 1 cup, diced = 122 g; Calories = 26

Rhubarb Cooked Or Canned Drained Solids ☛ serving size: 1 cup = 240 g; Calories = 278

Rhubarb Cooked Or Canned In Light Syrup ☛ serving size: 1 cup = 240 g; Calories = 144

Rhubarb Cooked Or Canned Unsweetened ☛ serving size: 1 cup = 240 g; Calories = 50

Rhubarb Frozen Cooked With Sugar ☛ serving size: 1 cup = 240 g; Calories = 278

Rhubarb Frozen Uncooked ☛ serving size: 1 cup, diced = 137 g; Calories = 29

Roselle ☛ serving size: 1 cup, without refuse = 57 g; Calories = 28

Rowal ☛ serving size: 1/2 cup = 114 g; Calories = 127

Ruby Red Grapefruit Juice Blend (Grapefruit Grape Apple) Ocean Spray Bottled With Added Vitamin C ☛ serving size: 8 fl oz = 248 g; Calories = 109

Sapodilla ☛ serving size: 1 cup, pulp = 241 g; Calories = 200

Sauerkraut Cooked Fat Added In Cooking ☛ serving size: 1 cup = 147 g; Calories = 46

Sauerkraut Cooked Ns As To Fat Added In Cooking ☛ serving size: 1 cup = 142 g; Calories = 55

Seaweed Pickled ☛ serving size: 1 cup = 150 g; Calories = 234

Shredded Coconut Meat (Sweetened) ☛ serving size: 1 cup = 256 g; Calories = 182

Sour Red Cherries ☛ serving size: 1 cup, without pits = 155 g; Calories = 78

Sour Red Cherries (Frozen) ☛ serving size: 1 cup, unthawed = 155 g; Calories = 71

Soursop ☛ serving size: 1 cup, pulp = 225 g; Calories = 149

Starfruit (Carambola) ☛ serving size: 1 cup, cubes = 132 g; Calories = 41

Starfruit Cooked With Sugar ☛ serving size: 1 cup = 205 g; Calories = 142

Strawberries ☛ serving size: 1 cup, halves = 152 g; Calories = 49

Strawberries Canned Heavy Syrup Pack Solids And Liquids ☛ serving size: 1 cup = 254 g; Calories = 234

Strawberries Cooked Or Canned Unsweetened Water Pack ☛ serving size: 1 cup = 242 g; Calories = 51

◔ Strawberries Frozen Sweetened Sliced ☛ serving size: 1 cup, thawed = 255 g; Calories = 245

◔ Strawberries Raw With Sugar ☛ serving size: 1 cup, nfs = 160 g; Calories = 80

◔ Strawberry Guavas ☛ serving size: 1 cup = 244 g; Calories = 168

◔ Sugar Apples ☛ serving size: 1 cup, pulp = 250 g; Calories = 235

◔ Tamarind Nectar Canned ☛ serving size: 1 cup = 251 g; Calories = 143

◔ Tamarinds ☛ serving size: 1 cup, pulp = 120 g; Calories = 287

◔ Tangerine Juice ☛ serving size: 1 cup = 247 g; Calories = 106

◔ Tangerines ☛ serving size: 1 cup, sections = 195 g; Calories = 103

◔ Tangerines (Mandarin Oranges) Canned Juice Pack ☛ serving size: 1 cup = 249 g; Calories = 92

◔ Tangerines (Mandarin Oranges) Canned Juice Pack Drained ☛ serving size: 1 cup = 189 g; Calories = 72

◔ Tangerines (Mandarin Oranges) Canned Light Syrup Pack ☛ serving size: 1 cup = 252 g; Calories = 154

◔ Tomato Green Pickled ☛ serving size: 1 tomato (2-3/8" dia) = 74 g; Calories = 27

◔ Tsukemono Japanese Pickles ☛ serving size: 1 cup = 135 g; Calories = 39

◔ Turnip Pickled ☛ serving size: 1 cup = 155 g; Calories = 67

◔ Vegetable Relish ☛ serving size: 1 cup = 140 g; Calories = 50

◔ Vegetables Pickled ☛ serving size: 1 cup = 163 g; Calories = 44

◔ Vegetables Pickled Hawaiian Style ☛ serving size: 1 cup = 150 g; Calories = 53

Watermelon ☛ serving size: 1 cup, balls = 154 g; Calories = 46

White California Grapefruit ☛ serving size: 1 cup sections, with juice = 230 g; Calories = 85

White Florida Grapefruit ☛ serving size: 1 cup sections, with juice = 230 g; Calories = 74

White Grapefruit ☛ serving size: 1 cup sections, with juice = 230 g; Calories = 76

White Grapefruit Juice ☛ serving size: 1 cup = 247 g; Calories = 96

Wild Blueberries (Frozen) ☛ serving size: 1 cup, frozen = 140 g; Calories = 80

Yellow Passion Fruit Juice ☛ serving size: 1 cup = 247 g; Calories = 148

Yellow Peaches ☛ serving size: 1 cup slices = 154 g; Calories = 60

Zante Currants ☛ serving size: 1 cup = 144 g; Calories = 418

Zucchini Pickled ☛ serving size: 1 cup = 170 g; Calories = 65

17

GRAINS AND PASTA

Amaranth Grain Uncooked ☛ serving size: 1 cup = 193 g; Calories = 716

Arrowroot Flour ☛ serving size: 1 cup = 128 g; Calories = 457

Barley Fat Added In Cooking ☛ serving size: 1 cup, cooked = 170 g; Calories = 235

Barley Fat Not Added In Cooking ☛ serving size: 1 cup, cooked = 170 g; Calories = 207

Barley Flour Or Meal ☛ serving size: 1 cup = 148 g; Calories = 511

Barley Hulled ☛ serving size: 1 cup = 184 g; Calories = 651

Barley Malt Flour ☛ serving size: 1 cup = 162 g; Calories = 585

Barley Ns As To Fat Added In Cooking ☛ serving size: 1 cup, cooked = 170 g; Calories = 207

Barley Pearled Raw ☛ serving size: 1 cup = 200 g; Calories = 704

Brown Rice ☛ serving size: 1 cup = 202 g; Calories = 249

Buckwheat (Uncooked) ☛ serving size: 1 cup = 170 g; Calories = 583

🌑 Buckwheat Flour Whole-Groat 🐄 serving size: 1 cup = 120 g; Calories = 402

🌑 Buckwheat Groats Fat Added In Cooking 🐄 serving size: 1 cup, cooked = 170 g; Calories = 190

🌑 Buckwheat Groats Fat Not Added In Cooking 🐄 serving size: 1 cup, cooked = 170 g; Calories = 156

🌑 Buckwheat Groats Ns As To Fat Added In Cooking 🐄 serving size: 1 cup, cooked = 170 g; Calories = 156

🌑 Buckwheat Groats Roasted Dry 🐄 serving size: 1 cup = 164 g; Calories = 567

🌑 Bulgur Dry 🐄 serving size: 1 cup = 140 g; Calories = 479

🌑 Bulgur Fat Added In Cooking 🐄 serving size: 1 cup, cooked = 140 g; Calories = 157

🌑 Bulgur Fat Not Added In Cooking 🐄 serving size: 1 cup, cooked = 140 g; Calories = 116

🌑 Bulgur Ns As To Fat Added In Cooking 🐄 serving size: 1 cup, cooked = 140 g; Calories = 116

🌑 Canned Hominy 🐄 serving size: 1 cup = 165 g; Calories = 119

🌑 Congee 🐄 serving size: 1 cup = 249 g; Calories = 82

🌑 Cooked Amaranth 🐄 serving size: 1 cup = 246 g; Calories = 251

🌑 Cooked Brown Rice 🐄 serving size: 1 cup = 195 g; Calories = 218

🌑 Cooked Bulgur 🐄 serving size: 1 cup = 182 g; Calories = 151

🌑 Cooked Couscous 🐄 serving size: 1 cup, cooked = 157 g; Calories = 176

🌑 Cooked Japanese Somen 🐄 serving size: 1 cup = 176 g; Calories = 231

🌑 Cooked Millet 🐄 serving size: 1 cup = 174 g; Calories = 207

☀ Cooked Oat Bran ☛ serving size: 1 cup = 219 g; Calories = 88

☀ Cooked Oatmeal ☛ serving size: 1 cup = 234 g; Calories = 166

☀ Cooked Pasta (Unenriched) ☛ serving size: 1 cup spaghetti not packed = 124 g; Calories = 196

☀ Cooked Pearled Barley ☛ serving size: 1 cup = 157 g; Calories = 193

☀ Cooked Spelt ☛ serving size: 1 cup = 194 g; Calories = 246

☀ Cooked Teff ☛ serving size: 1 cup = 252 g; Calories = 255

☀ Cooked Wild Rice ☛ serving size: 1 cup = 164 g; Calories = 166

☀ Corn Bran Crude ☛ serving size: 1 cup = 76 g; Calories = 170

☀ Corn Flour Masa Enriched White ☛ serving size: 1 cup = 114 g; Calories = 414

☀ Corn Flour Masa Unenriched White ☛ serving size: 1 cup = 114 g; Calories = 414

☀ Corn Flour Whole-Grain Blue (Harina De Maiz Morado) ☛ serving size: 1 tbsp = 6.9 g; Calories = 25

☀ Corn Flour Whole-Grain White ☛ serving size: 1 cup = 117 g; Calories = 422

☀ Corn Flour Whole-Grain Yellow ☛ serving size: 1 cup = 117 g; Calories = 422

☀ Corn Flour Yellow Degermed Unenriched ☛ serving size: 1 cup = 126 g; Calories = 473

☀ Corn Flour Yellow Masa Enriched ☛ serving size: 1 cup = 114 g; Calories = 414

☀ Corn Grain White ☛ serving size: 1 cup = 166 g; Calories = 606

☀ Corn Grain Yellow ☛ serving size: 1 cup = 166 g; Calories = 606

🐜 Cornmeal Degermed Enriched White ☞ serving size: 1 cup = 157 g; Calories = 581

🐜 Cornmeal Degermed Enriched Yellow ☞ serving size: 1 cup = 157 g; Calories = 581

🐜 Cornmeal Degermed Unenriched White ☞ serving size: 1 cup = 157 g; Calories = 581

🐜 Cornmeal Degermed Unenriched Yellow ☞ serving size: 1 cup = 157 g; Calories = 581

🐜 Cornmeal White Self-Rising Bolted Plain Enriched ☞ serving size: 1 cup = 122 g; Calories = 408

🐜 Cornmeal White Self-Rising Bolted With Wheat Flour Added Enriched ☞ serving size: 1 cup = 170 g; Calories = 592

🐜 Cornmeal White Self-Rising Degermed Enriched ☞ serving size: 1 cup = 138 g; Calories = 490

🐜 Cornmeal Yellow Self-Rising Bolted Plain Enriched ☞ serving size: 1 cup = 122 g; Calories = 408

🐜 Cornmeal Yellow Self-Rising Bolted With Wheat Flour Added Enriched ☞ serving size: 1 cup = 170 g; Calories = 592

🐜 Cornmeal Yellow Self-Rising Degermed Enriched ☞ serving size: 1 cup = 138 g; Calories = 490

🐜 Cornstarch ☞ serving size: 1 cup = 128 g; Calories = 488

🐜 Couscous Dry ☞ serving size: 1 cup = 173 g; Calories = 651

🐜 Couscous Plain Cooked ☞ serving size: 1 cup, cooked = 160 g; Calories = 178

🐜 Egg Noodles (Cooked) ☞ serving size: 1 cup = 160 g; Calories = 221

🐜 Gluten Free Corn Noodles (Cooked) ☞ serving size: 1 cup = 140 g; Calories = 176

🍚 Hominy Canned Yellow ☛ serving size: 1 cup = 160 g; Calories = 115

🍚 Japanese Soba Noodles (Buckwheat) ☛ serving size: 1 cup = 114 g; Calories = 113

🍚 Kamut Cooked ☛ serving size: 1 cup = 172 g; Calories = 227

🍚 Long Rice Noodles Made From Mung Beans Cooked ☛ serving size: 1 cup, cooked = 190 g; Calories = 160

🍚 Macaroni Vegetable Enriched Cooked ☛ serving size: 1 cup spiral shaped = 134 g; Calories = 172

🍚 Macaroni Vegetable Enriched Dry ☛ serving size: 1 cup spiral shaped = 84 g; Calories = 308

🍚 Medium Grain White Rice ☛ serving size: 1 cup = 186 g; Calories = 242

🍚 Millet Fat Added In Cooking ☛ serving size: 1 cup, cooked = 170 g; Calories = 238

🍚 Millet Fat Not Added In Cooking ☛ serving size: 1 cup, cooked = 170 g; Calories = 201

🍚 Millet Flour ☛ serving size: 1 cup = 119 g; Calories = 455

🍚 Millet Ns As To Fat Added In Cooking ☛ serving size: 1 cup, cooked = 170 g; Calories = 201

🍚 Millet Raw ☛ serving size: 1 cup = 200 g; Calories = 756

🍚 Noodles Chinese Chow Mein ☛ serving size: 1/2 cup dry = 28 g; Calories = 132

🍚 Noodles Cooked ☛ serving size: 1 cup, cooked = 160 g; Calories = 219

🍚 Noodles Egg Cooked Enriched With Added Salt ☛ serving size: 1 cup = 160 g; Calories = 221

Noodles Egg Cooked Unenriched With Added Salt ☛ serving size: 1 cup = 160 g; Calories = 221

Noodles Egg Dry Enriched ☛ serving size: 1 cup = 38 g; Calories = 146

Noodles Egg Dry Unenriched ☛ serving size: 1 cup = 38 g; Calories = 146

Noodles Egg Spinach Enriched Dry ☛ serving size: 1 cup = 38 g; Calories = 145

Noodles Egg Unenriched Cooked Without Added Salt ☛ serving size: 1 cup = 160 g; Calories = 221

Noodles Flat Crunchy Chinese Restaurant ☛ serving size: 1 cup = 45 g; Calories = 235

Noodles Japanese Soba Dry ☛ serving size: 2 oz = 57 g; Calories = 192

Noodles Japanese Somen Dry ☛ serving size: 2 oz = 57 g; Calories = 203

Noodles Vegetable Cooked ☛ serving size: 1 cup, cooked = 160 g; Calories = 210

Noodles Whole Grain Cooked ☛ serving size: 1 cup, cooked = 160 g; Calories = 237

Oat Bran ☛ serving size: 1 cup = 94 g; Calories = 231

Oat Flour Partially Debranned ☛ serving size: 1 cup = 104 g; Calories = 420

Pasta Cooked ☛ serving size: 1 cup, cooked = 140 g; Calories = 220

Pasta Cooked Enriched With Added Salt ☛ serving size: 1 cup spaghetti not packed = 124 g; Calories = 195

Pasta Cooked Enriched Without Added Salt ☛ serving size: 1 cup spaghetti not packed = 124 g; Calories = 196

🐾 Pasta Cooked Unenriched With Added Salt 🖙 serving size: 1 cup spaghetti not packed = 124 g; Calories = 195

🐾 Pasta Dry Enriched 🖙 serving size: 1 cup spaghetti = 91 g; Calories = 338

🐾 Pasta Dry Unenriched 🖙 serving size: 1 cup spaghetti = 91 g; Calories = 338

🐾 Pasta Fresh-Refrigerated Plain As Purchased 🖙 serving size: 4 (1/2) oz = 128 g; Calories = 369

🐾 Pasta Fresh-Refrigerated Plain Cooked 🖙 serving size: 2 oz = 128 g; Calories = 168

🐾 Pasta Fresh-Refrigerated Spinach As Purchased 🖙 serving size: 4 (1/2) oz = 128 g; Calories = 370

🐾 Pasta Fresh-Refrigerated Spinach Cooked 🖙 serving size: 2 oz = 57 g; Calories = 74

🐾 Pasta Gluten-Free Brown Rice Flour Cooked Tinkyada 🖙 serving size: 1 cup spaghetti not packed = 169 g; Calories = 233

🐾 Pasta Gluten-Free Corn And Rice Flour Cooked 🖙 serving size: 1 cup spaghetti = 141 g; Calories = 252

🐾 Pasta Gluten-Free Corn Dry 🖙 serving size: 1 cup = 105 g; Calories = 375

🐾 Pasta Gluten-Free Corn Flour And Quinoa Flour Cooked Ancient Harvest 🖙 serving size: 1 cup spaghetti packed = 166 g; Calories = 252

🐾 Pasta Gluten-Free Rice Flour And Rice Bran Extract Cooked De Boles 🖙 serving size: 1 cup spaghetti = 121 g; Calories = 242

🐾 Pasta Homemade Made With Egg Cooked 🖙 serving size: 2 oz = 57 g; Calories = 74

🐾 Pasta Homemade Made Without Egg Cooked 🖙 serving size: 2 oz = 57 g; Calories = 71

Pasta Vegetable Cooked ☛ serving size: 1 cup, cooked = 140 g; Calories = 179

Pasta Whole Grain 51% Whole Wheat Remaining Enriched Semolina Cooked ☛ serving size: 1 cup spaghetti not packed = 116 g; Calories = 181

Pasta Whole Grain 51% Whole Wheat Remaining Enriched Semolina Dry ☛ serving size: 1 cup spaghetti = 91 g; Calories = 329

Pasta Whole Grain 51% Whole Wheat Remaining Unenriched Semolina Cooked ☛ serving size: 1 cup spaghetti not packed = 116 g; Calories = 184

Pasta Whole Grain 51% Whole Wheat Remaining Unenriched Semolina Dry ☛ serving size: 1 cup spaghetti = 91 g; Calories = 329

Pasta Whole Grain Cooked ☛ serving size: 1 cup, cooked = 140 g; Calories = 207

Pasta Whole-Wheat Dry ☛ serving size: 1 cup spaghetti = 91 g; Calories = 320

Quinoa Cooked ☛ serving size: 1 cup = 185 g; Calories = 222

Quinoa Fat Added In Cooking ☛ serving size: 1 cup, cooked = 170 g; Calories = 238

Quinoa Fat Not Added In Cooking ☛ serving size: 1 cup, cooked = 170 g; Calories = 204

Quinoa Ns As To Fat Added In Cooking ☛ serving size: 1 cup, cooked = 170 g; Calories = 238

Quinoa Uncooked ☛ serving size: 1 cup = 170 g; Calories = 626

Rice Bran ☛ serving size: 1 cup = 118 g; Calories = 373

Rice Brown And Wild Cooked Fat Added In Cooking ☛ serving size: 1 cup, cooked = 155 g; Calories = 212

Rice Brown And Wild Cooked Fat Not Added In Cooking ☛ serving size: 1 cup, cooked = 151 g; Calories = 181

Rice Brown And Wild Cooked Ns As To Fat Added In Cooking ☛ serving size: 1 cup, cooked = 150 g; Calories = 170

Rice Brown Cooked Fat Added In Cooking Made With Butter ☛ serving size: 1 cup, cooked = 196 g; Calories = 267

Rice Brown Cooked Fat Added In Cooking Made With Margarine ☛ serving size: 1 cup, cooked = 196 g; Calories = 259

Rice Brown Cooked Fat Added In Cooking Made With Oil ☛ serving size: 1 cup, cooked = 196 g; Calories = 274

Rice Brown Cooked Fat Added In Cooking Ns As To Type Of Fat ☛ serving size: 1 cup, cooked = 196 g; Calories = 269

Rice Brown Cooked Ns As To Fat Added In Cooking ☛ serving size: 1 cup, cooked = 196 g; Calories = 239

Rice Brown Long-Grain Raw ☛ serving size: 1 cup = 185 g; Calories = 679

Rice Brown Medium-Grain Raw ☛ serving size: 1 cup = 190 g; Calories = 688

Rice Brown Parboiled Cooked Uncle Bens ☛ serving size: 1 cup = 155 g; Calories = 228

Rice Brown Parboiled Dry Uncle Bens ☛ serving size: 1/4 cup = 48 g; Calories = 178

Rice Cooked Nfs ☛ serving size: 1 cup, cooked = 158 g; Calories = 204

Rice Cooked With Milk ☛ serving size: 1 cup, cooked = 200 g; Calories = 286

Rice Flour Brown ☛ serving size: 1 cup = 158 g; Calories = 574

Rice Flour White Unenriched ☛ serving size: 1 cup = 158 g; Calories = 578

Rice Noodles (Cooked) ☛ serving size: 1 cup = 176 g; Calories = 190

Rice Noodles Dry ☛ serving size: 2 oz = 57 g; Calories = 208

Rice Sweet Cooked With Honey ☛ serving size: 1 cup, cooked = 175 g; Calories = 245

Rice White Cooked Fat Added In Cooking Made With Butter ☛ serving size: 1 cup, cooked = 163 g; Calories = 238

Rice White Cooked Fat Added In Cooking Made With Margarine ☛ serving size: 1 cup, cooked = 163 g; Calories = 230

Rice White Cooked Fat Added In Cooking Made With Oil ☛ serving size: 1 cup, cooked = 163 g; Calories = 245

Rice White Cooked Fat Added In Cooking Ns As To Type Of Fat ☛ serving size: 1 cup, cooked = 163 g; Calories = 240

Rice White Cooked Fat Not Added In Cooking ☛ serving size: 1 cup, cooked = 158 g; Calories = 204

Rice White Cooked Glutinous ☛ serving size: 1 cup, cooked = 174 g; Calories = 167

Rice White Cooked Ns As To Fat Added In Cooking ☛ serving size: 1 cup, cooked = 163 g; Calories = 210

Rice White Cooked With Fat Puerto Rican Style ☛ serving size: 1 cup, cooked = 155 g; Calories = 307

Rice White Glutinous Unenriched Cooked ☛ serving size: 1 cup = 174 g; Calories = 169

Rice White Glutinous Unenriched Uncooked ☛ serving size: 1 cup = 185 g; Calories = 685

Rice White Long-Grain Parboiled Enriched Cooked ☛ serving size: 1 cup = 158 g; Calories = 194

🌡 Rice White Long-Grain Parboiled Enriched Dry ☞ serving size: 1 cup = 185 g; Calories = 692

🌡 Rice White Long-Grain Parboiled Unenriched Cooked ☞ serving size: 1 cup = 158 g; Calories = 194

🌡 Rice White Long-Grain Parboiled Unenriched Dry ☞ serving size: 1 cup = 185 g; Calories = 692

🌡 Rice White Long-Grain Precooked Or Instant Enriched Dry ☞ serving size: 1 cup = 95 g; Calories = 361

🌡 Rice White Long-Grain Precooked Or Instant Enriched Prepared ☞ serving size: 1 cup = 165 g; Calories = 205

🌡 Rice White Long-Grain Regular Cooked Enriched With Salt ☞ serving size: 1 cup = 158 g; Calories = 205

🌡 Rice White Long-Grain Regular Cooked Unenriched With Salt ☞ serving size: 1 cup = 158 g; Calories = 205

🌡 Rice White Long-Grain Regular Raw Enriched ☞ serving size: 1 cup = 185 g; Calories = 675

🌡 Rice White Long-Grain Regular Raw Unenriched ☞ serving size: 1 cup = 185 g; Calories = 675

🌡 Rice White Long-Grain Regular Unenriched Cooked Without Salt ☞ serving size: 1 cup = 158 g; Calories = 205

🌡 Rice White Medium-Grain Cooked Unenriched ☞ serving size: 1 cup = 186 g; Calories = 242

🌡 Rice White Medium-Grain Raw Enriched ☞ serving size: 1 cup = 195 g; Calories = 702

🌡 Rice White Medium-Grain Raw Unenriched ☞ serving size: 1 cup = 195 g; Calories = 702

🌡 Rice White Short-Grain Cooked Unenriched ☞ serving size: 1 cup = 205 g; Calories = 267

Rice White Short-Grain Enriched Cooked ☛ serving size: 1 cup = 186 g; Calories = 242

Rice White Short-Grain Enriched Uncooked ☛ serving size: 1 cup = 200 g; Calories = 716

Rice White Short-Grain Raw Unenriched ☛ serving size: 1 cup = 200 g; Calories = 716

Rice White Steamed Chinese Restaurant ☛ serving size: 1 cup, loosely packed = 132 g; Calories = 199

Rice Wild 100% Cooked Fat Added In Cooking ☛ serving size: 1 cup, cooked = 164 g; Calories = 198

Rice Wild 100% Cooked Fat Not Added In Cooking ☛ serving size: 1 cup, cooked = 164 g; Calories = 164

Rice Wild 100% Cooked Ns As To Fat Added In Cooking ☛ serving size: 1 cup, cooked = 164 g; Calories = 198

Roasted Buckwheat Groats ☛ serving size: 1 cup = 168 g; Calories = 155

Rye Flour Dark ☛ serving size: 1 cup = 128 g; Calories = 416

Rye Flour Light ☛ serving size: 1 cup = 102 g; Calories = 364

Rye Flour Medium ☛ serving size: 1 cup = 102 g; Calories = 356

Rye Grain ☛ serving size: 1 cup = 169 g; Calories = 571

Semolina Enriched ☛ serving size: 1 cup = 167 g; Calories = 601

Semolina Unenriched ☛ serving size: 1 cup = 167 g; Calories = 601

Sorghum Flour Refined Unenriched ☛ serving size: 1 cup = 161 g; Calories = 575

Sorghum Grain ☛ serving size: 1 cup = 192 g; Calories = 632

Spaghetti Protein-Fortified Cooked Enriched (N X 6.25) ☛ serving size: 1 cup = 140 g; Calories = 230

☀ Spaghetti Protein-Fortified Dry Enriched (N X 6.25) ☞ serving size: 2 oz = 57 g; Calories = 213

☀ Spaghetti Spinach Cooked ☞ serving size: 1 cup = 140 g; Calories = 182

☀ Spaghetti Spinach Dry ☞ serving size: 2 oz = 57 g; Calories = 212

☀ Spelt Uncooked ☞ serving size: 1 cup = 174 g; Calories = 588

☀ Spinach Egg Noodles (Cooked) ☞ serving size: 1 cup = 160 g; Calories = 211

☀ Tapioca Pearl Dry ☞ serving size: 1 cup = 152 g; Calories = 544

☀ Teff Uncooked ☞ serving size: 1 cup = 193 g; Calories = 708

☀ Triticale ☞ serving size: 1 cup = 192 g; Calories = 645

☀ Triticale Flour Whole-Grain ☞ serving size: 1 cup = 130 g; Calories = 439

☀ Uncooked Oats ☞ serving size: 1 cup = 156 g; Calories = 607

☀ Uncooked Whole-Grain Cornmeal ☞ serving size: 1 cup = 122 g; Calories = 442

☀ Uncooked Yellow Cornmeal ☞ serving size: 1 cup = 122 g; Calories = 442

☀ Vermicelli Made From Soybeans ☞ serving size: 1 cup = 140 g; Calories = 176

☀ Wheat Bran Crude ☞ serving size: 1 cup = 58 g; Calories = 125

☀ Wheat Durum ☞ serving size: 1 cup = 192 g; Calories = 651

☀ Wheat Flour White All-Purpose Enriched Bleached ☞ serving size: 1 cup = 125 g; Calories = 455

☀ Wheat Flour White All-Purpose Enriched Calcium-Fortified ☞ serving size: 1 cup = 125 g; Calories = 455

Wheat Flour White All-Purpose Enriched Unbleached ☛ serving size: 1 cup = 125 g; Calories = 455

Wheat Flour White All-Purpose Self-Rising Enriched ☛ serving size: 1 cup = 125 g; Calories = 443

Wheat Flour White All-Purpose Unenriched ☛ serving size: 1 cup = 125 g; Calories = 455

Wheat Flour White Bread Enriched ☛ serving size: 1 cup = 137 g; Calories = 495

Wheat Flour White Cake Enriched ☛ serving size: 1 cup unsifted, dipped = 137 g; Calories = 496

Wheat Flour White Tortilla Mix Enriched ☛ serving size: 1 cup = 111 g; Calories = 450

Wheat Flour Whole-Grain ☛ serving size: 1 cup = 120 g; Calories = 408

Wheat Flours Bread Unenriched ☛ serving size: 1 cup unsifted, dipped = 137 g; Calories = 495

Wheat Germ Crude ☛ serving size: 1 cup = 115 g; Calories = 414

Wheat Hard Red Spring ☛ serving size: 1 cup = 192 g; Calories = 632

Wheat Hard Red Winter ☛ serving size: 1 cup = 192 g; Calories = 628

Wheat Hard White ☛ serving size: 1 cup = 192 g; Calories = 657

Wheat Kamut Khorasan Uncooked ☛ serving size: 1 cup = 186 g; Calories = 627

Wheat Soft Red Winter ☛ serving size: 1 cup = 168 g; Calories = 556

Wheat Soft White ☛ serving size: 1 cup = 168 g; Calories = 571

Wheat Sprouted ☛ serving size: 1 cup = 108 g; Calories = 214

White Rice ☞ serving size: 1 cup = 158 g; Calories = 205

Whole Grain Sorghum Flour ☞ serving size: 1 cup = 121 g; Calories = 434

Whole Wheat Pasta ☞ serving size: 1 cup spaghetti not packed = 117 g; Calories = 174

Wild Rice Raw ☞ serving size: 1 cup = 160 g; Calories = 571

Yellow Cornmeal (Grits) ☞ serving size: 1 cup = 233 g; Calories = 152

Yellow Rice Cooked Fat Added In Cooking ☞ serving size: 1 cup, cooked = 163 g; Calories = 170

Yellow Rice Cooked Fat Not Added In Cooking ☞ serving size: 1 cup, cooked = 158 g; Calories = 139

Yellow Rice Cooked Ns As To Fat Added In Cooking ☞ serving size: 1 cup, cooked = 158 g; Calories = 139

18

MEATS AND POULTRY

Bacon (Pan-Fried) ☛ serving size: 1 slice = 11.5 g; Calories = 54

Bacon (Raw) ☛ serving size: 1 slice raw = 28 g; Calories = 110

Bacon And Beef Sticks ☛ serving size: 1 oz = 28 g; Calories = 145

Bacon Turkey Low Sodium ☛ serving size: 1 serving = 15 g; Calories = 38

Bear Cooked ☛ serving size: 1 oz, boneless, cooked = 28 g; Calories = 72

Beaver Cooked ☛ serving size: 1 oz, boneless, cooked = 28 g; Calories = 59

Beef And Chicken Polish Sausage ☛ serving size: 1 serving 5 pieces = 55 g; Calories = 143

Beef Australian Imported Grass-Fed Ground 85% Lean / 15% Fat Raw ☛ serving size: 4 oz (4 oz) = 114 g; Calories = 273

Beef Baloney (Bologna) ☛ serving size: 1 slice = 30 g; Calories = 90

Beef Bologna Reduced Sodium ☛ serving size: 1 cup pieces = 138 g; Calories = 428

Beef Brisket Cooked Lean And Fat Eaten ☛ serving size: 1 thin slice (approx 4-1/2" x 2-1/2" x 1/8") = 21 g; Calories = 61

Beef Burgundy ☛ serving size: 1 cup = 244 g; Calories = 356

Beef Carcass Separable Lean And Fat Choice Raw ☛ serving size: 1 oz = 28.4 g; Calories = 83

Beef Carcass Separable Lean And Fat Select Raw ☛ serving size: 1 oz = 28.4 g; Calories = 79

Beef Chuck For Stew Separable Lean And Fat All Grades Raw ☛ serving size: 3 oz = 85 g; Calories = 109

Beef Chuck For Stew Separable Lean And Fat Choice Cooked Braised ☛ serving size: 3 oz = 85 g; Calories = 165

Beef Chuck Pot Roast ☛ serving size: 3 oz = 85 g; Calories = 180

Beef Composite Separable Lean Only Trimmed To 1/8 Inch Fat Choice Cooked ☛ serving size: 3 oz = 85 g; Calories = 173

Beef Cured Breakfast Strips Cooked ☛ serving size: 3 slices = 34 g; Calories = 153

Beef Cured Breakfast Strips Raw Or Unheated ☛ serving size: 3 slices = 68 g; Calories = 276

Beef Cured Corned Beef Brisket Cooked ☛ serving size: 3 oz = 85 g; Calories = 213

Beef Cured Corned Beef Brisket Raw ☛ serving size: 1 oz = 28.4 g; Calories = 56

Beef Cured Corned Beef Canned ☛ serving size: 1 oz = 28.4 g; Calories = 71

Beef Cured Dried ☛ serving size: 10 slices = 28 g; Calories = 43

🐄 Beef Cured Luncheon Meat Jellied 🖛 serving size: 1 slice (1 oz) (4 inch x 4 inch x 3/32 inch thick) = 28 g; Calories = 31

🐄 Beef Cured Pastrami 🖛 serving size: 1 package, 2.5 oz = 71 g; Calories = 104

🐄 Beef Cured Sausage Cooked Smoked 🖛 serving size: 1 sausage = 43 g; Calories = 134

🐄 Beef Dried Chipped Cooked In Fat 🖛 serving size: 1 oz, cooked = 28 g; Calories = 64

🐄 Beef Flank Steak Separable Lean And Fat Trimmed To 0 Inch Fat All Grades Cooked Broiled 🖛 serving size: 3 oz = 85 g; Calories = 163

🐄 Beef Flank Steak Separable Lean And Fat Trimmed To 0 Inch Fat All Grades Raw 🖛 serving size: 3 oz = 85 g; Calories = 132

🐄 Beef Flank Steak Separable Lean And Fat Trimmed To 0 Inch Fat Choice Cooked Braised 🖛 serving size: 3 oz = 85 g; Calories = 224

🐄 Beef Flank Steak Separable Lean And Fat Trimmed To 0 Inch Fat Choice Cooked Broiled 🖛 serving size: 3 oz = 85 g; Calories = 172

🐄 Beef Flank Steak Separable Lean And Fat Trimmed To 0 Inch Fat Choice Raw 🖛 serving size: 1 oz = 28.4 g; Calories = 47

🐄 Beef Ground 70% Lean Meat / 30% Fat Loaf Cooked Baked 🖛 serving size: 3 oz = 85 g; Calories = 205

🐄 Beef Ground 70% Lean Meat / 30% Fat Patty Cooked Broiled 🖛 serving size: 3 oz = 85 g; Calories = 236

🐄 Beef Ground 70% Lean Meat / 30% Fat Patty Cooked Pan-Broiled 🖛 serving size: 3 oz = 85 g; Calories = 202

🐄 Beef Ground 70% Lean Meat / 30% Fat Raw 🖛 serving size: 4 oz = 113 g; Calories = 375

🐄 Beef Ground 75% Lean Meat / 25% Fat Crumbles Cooked Pan-Browned 🖛 serving size: 3 oz = 85 g; Calories = 236

🐄 Beef Ground 75% Lean Meat / 25% Fat Loaf Cooked Baked ☞ serving size: 3 oz = 85 g; Calories = 216

🐄 Beef Ground 75% Lean Meat / 25% Fat Patty Cooked Broiled ☞ serving size: 3 oz = 85 g; Calories = 237

🐄 Beef Ground 75% Lean Meat / 25% Fat Patty Cooked Pan-Broiled ☞ serving size: 3 oz = 85 g; Calories = 211

🐄 Beef Ground 75% Lean Meat / 25% Fat Raw ☞ serving size: 4 oz = 113 g; Calories = 331

🐄 Beef Ground 80% Lean Meat / 20% Fat Crumbles Cooked Pan-Browned ☞ serving size: 3 oz = 85 g; Calories = 231

🐄 Beef Ground 80% Lean Meat / 20% Fat Loaf Cooked Baked ☞ serving size: 3 oz = 85 g; Calories = 216

🐄 Beef Ground 80% Lean Meat / 20% Fat Patty Cooked Pan-Broiled ☞ serving size: 3 oz = 85 g; Calories = 209

🐄 Beef Ground 80% Lean Meat / 20% Fat Raw ☞ serving size: 4 oz = 113 g; Calories = 287

🐄 Beef Ground 85% Lean Meat / 15% Fat Crumbles Cooked Pan-Browned ☞ serving size: 3 oz = 85 g; Calories = 218

🐄 Beef Ground 85% Lean Meat / 15% Fat Loaf Cooked Baked ☞ serving size: 3 oz = 85 g; Calories = 204

🐄 Beef Ground 85% Lean Meat / 15% Fat Patty Cooked Broiled ☞ serving size: 3 oz = 85 g; Calories = 213

🐄 Beef Ground 85% Lean Meat / 15% Fat Patty Cooked Pan-Broiled ☞ serving size: 3 oz = 85 g; Calories = 197

🐄 Beef Ground 85% Lean Meat / 15% Fat Raw ☞ serving size: 3 oz = 85 g; Calories = 183

🐄 Beef Ground 90% Lean Meat / 10% Fat Crumbles Cooked Pan-Browned ☞ serving size: 3 oz = 85 g; Calories = 196

Beef Ground 90% Lean Meat / 10% Fat Loaf Cooked Baked ☞ serving size: 3 oz = 85 g; Calories = 182

Beef Ground 90% Lean Meat / 10% Fat Patty Cooked Broiled ☞ serving size: 3 oz = 85 g; Calories = 185

Beef Ground 90% Lean Meat / 10% Fat Patty Cooked Pan-Broiled ☞ serving size: 3 oz = 85 g; Calories = 173

Beef Ground 90% Lean Meat / 10% Fat Raw ☞ serving size: 4 oz = 113 g; Calories = 199

Beef Ground 93% Lean Meat / 7% Fat Crumbles Cooked Pan-Browned ☞ serving size: 3 oz = 85 g; Calories = 178

Beef Ground 93% Lean Meat / 7% Fat Loaf Cooked Baked ☞ serving size: 3 oz = 85 g; Calories = 163

Beef Ground 93% Lean Meat / 7% Fat Raw ☞ serving size: 4 oz = 113 g; Calories = 172

Beef Ground 93% Lean Meat /7% Fat Patty Cooked Pan-Broiled ☞ serving size: 3 oz = 85 g; Calories = 155

Beef Ground 95% Lean Meat / 5% Fat Crumbles Cooked Pan-Browned ☞ serving size: 3 oz = 85 g; Calories = 164

Beef Ground 95% Lean Meat / 5% Fat Loaf Cooked Baked ☞ serving size: 3 oz = 85 g; Calories = 148

Beef Ground 95% Lean Meat / 5% Fat Patty Cooked Broiled ☞ serving size: 3 oz = 85 g; Calories = 148

Beef Ground 95% Lean Meat / 5% Fat Patty Cooked Pan-Broiled ☞ serving size: 3 oz = 85 g; Calories = 139

Beef Ground 95% Lean Meat / 5% Fat Raw ☞ serving size: 4 oz = 113 g; Calories = 155

Beef Ground 97% Lean Meat / 3% Fat Crumbles Cooked Pan-Browned ☞ serving size: 3 oz = 85 g; Calories = 149

Beef Ground 97% Lean Meat / 3% Fat Loaf Cooked Baked ☛ serving size: 3 oz = 85 g; Calories = 131

Beef Ground 97% Lean Meat / 3% Fat Raw ☛ serving size: 4 oz = 113 g; Calories = 137

Beef Ground Patties Frozen Cooked Broiled ☛ serving size: 3 oz = 85 g; Calories = 251

Beef Liver Braised ☛ serving size: 1 oz, raw (yield after cooking) = 19 g; Calories = 36

Beef Liver Fried ☛ serving size: 1 oz, raw (yield after cooking) = 21 g; Calories = 37

Beef Loin Tenderloin Roast Boneless Separable Lean And Fat Trimmed To 0 Inch Fat Choice Cooked Roasted ☛ serving size: 3 oz = 85 g; Calories = 160

Beef Loin Top Loin Steak Boneless Lip Off Separable Lean Only Trimmed To 0 Inch Fat Select Raw ☛ serving size: 3 oz = 85 g; Calories = 115

Beef Loin Top Sirloin Cap Steak Boneless Separable Lean Only Trimmed To 1/8 Inch Fat Choice Cooked Grilled ☛ serving size: 3 oz = 85 g; Calories = 161

Beef Neck Bones Cooked ☛ serving size: 1 oz, with bone, cooked (yield after bone removed) = 11 g; Calories = 33

Beef New Zealand Imported Bolar Blade Separable Lean And Fat Raw ☛ serving size: 4 oz = 114 g; Calories = 181

Beef Rib Back Ribs Bone-In Separable Lean Only Trimmed To 0 Inch Fat Select Raw ☛ serving size: 3 oz = 85 g; Calories = 188

Beef Rib Eye Roast Boneless Lip-On Separable Lean And Fat Trimmed To 1/8 Inch Fat All Grades Cooked Roasted ☛ serving size: 3 oz = 85 g; Calories = 248

🐄 Beef Roast Roasted Lean And Fat Eaten 🐄 serving size: 1 thin slice (approx 4-1/2" x 2-1/2" x 1/8") = 21 g; Calories = 33

🐄 Beef Roast Roasted Lean Only Eaten 🐄 serving size: 1 thin slice (approx 4-1/2" x 2-1/2" x 1/8") = 21 g; Calories = 32

🐄 Beef Salad 🐄 serving size: 1 cup = 182 g; Calories = 473

🐄 Beef Sandwich Steak Flaked Formed Thinly Sliced 🐄 serving size: 1 sandwich steak = 41 g; Calories = 135

🐄 Beef Sandwich Steaks Flaked Chopped Formed And Thinly Sliced Raw 🐄 serving size: 3 oz = 85 g; Calories = 263

🐄 Beef Sausage 🐄 serving size: 1 patty = 35 g; Calories = 142

🐄 Beef Sausage Fresh Cooked 🐄 serving size: 1 serving = 43 g; Calories = 143

🐄 Beef Sausage Pre-Cooked 🐄 serving size: 1 serving = 48 g; Calories = 157

🐄 Beef Sausage With Cheese 🐄 serving size: 1 link = 76 g; Calories = 306

🐄 Beef Shoulder Pot Roast Or Steak Boneless Separable Lean Only Trimmed To 0 Inch Fat Choice Raw 🐄 serving size: 3 oz = 85 g; Calories = 106

🐄 Beef Steak Battered Fried Lean And Fat Eaten 🐄 serving size: 1 oz, boneless, cooked = 28 g; Calories = 71

🐄 Beef Steak Battered Fried Lean Only Eaten 🐄 serving size: 1 oz, boneless, cooked, lean only = 28 g; Calories = 66

🐄 Beef Steak Battered Fried Ns As To Fat Eaten 🐄 serving size: 1 oz, boneless, cooked = 28 g; Calories = 65

🐄 Beef Steak Braised Lean And Fat Eaten 🐄 serving size: 1 oz, with bone, cooked (yield after bone removed) = 22 g; Calories = 55

🐄 Beef Steak Braised Lean Only Eaten 🐄 serving size: 1 oz, with bone, cooked, lean only (yield after bone removed) = 21 g; Calories = 34

Beef Steak Fried Lean And Fat Eaten serving size: 1 oz, with bone, cooked (yield after bone removed) = 23 g; Calories = 54

Beef Steak Fried Lean Only Eaten serving size: 1 oz, with bone, cooked, lean only (yield after bone removed) = 23 g; Calories = 42

Beef Steak With Onions Puerto Rican Style serving size: 1 cup = 179 g; Calories = 571

Beef Stew Meat Cooked Lean And Fat Eaten serving size: 1 oz, boneless, cooked = 28 g; Calories = 66

Beef Stew Meat Cooked Lean Only Eaten serving size: 1 oz, boneless, cooked, lean only = 28 g; Calories = 70

Beef Stew Meat Cooked Ns As To Fat Eaten serving size: 1 oz, boneless, cooked = 28 g; Calories = 70

Beef Stew Meat With Gravy No Potatoes Puerto Rican Style serving size: 1 cup = 235 g; Calories = 545

Beef Top Sirloin Steak Separable Lean And Fat Trimmed To 0 Inch Fat Choice Cooked Broiled serving size: 3 oz = 85 g; Calories = 186

Beef Variety Meats And By-Products Brain Cooked Pan-Fried serving size: 3 oz = 85 g; Calories = 167

Beef Variety Meats And By-Products Brain Cooked Simmered serving size: 3 oz = 85 g; Calories = 128

Beef Variety Meats And By-Products Brain Raw serving size: 1 oz = 28.4 g; Calories = 41

Beef Variety Meats And By-Products Heart Cooked Simmered serving size: 3 oz = 85 g; Calories = 140

Beef Variety Meats And By-Products Heart Raw ☛ serving size: 1 oz = 28.4 g; Calories = 32

Beef Variety Meats And By-Products Kidneys Cooked Simmered ☛ serving size: 3 oz = 85 g; Calories = 134

Beef Variety Meats And By-Products Kidneys Raw ☛ serving size: 1 oz = 28.4 g; Calories = 28

Beef Variety Meats And By-Products Liver Cooked Braised ☛ serving size: 1 slice = 68 g; Calories = 130

Beef Variety Meats And By-Products Liver Raw ☛ serving size: 3 oz = 85 g; Calories = 115

Beef Variety Meats And By-Products Lungs Cooked Braised ☛ serving size: 3 oz = 85 g; Calories = 102

Beef Variety Meats And By-Products Lungs Raw ☛ serving size: 1 oz = 28.4 g; Calories = 26

Beef Variety Meats And By-Products Mechanically Separated Beef Raw ☛ serving size: 1 oz = 28.4 g; Calories = 78

Beef Variety Meats And By-Products Pancreas Cooked Braised ☛ serving size: 3 oz = 85 g; Calories = 230

Beef Variety Meats And By-Products Pancreas Raw ☛ serving size: 1 oz = 28.4 g; Calories = 67

Beef Variety Meats And By-Products Spleen Cooked Braised ☛ serving size: 3 oz = 85 g; Calories = 123

Beef Variety Meats And By-Products Spleen Raw ☛ serving size: 1 oz = 28.4 g; Calories = 30

Beef Variety Meats And By-Products Suet Raw ☛ serving size: 1 oz = 28.4 g; Calories = 243

Beef Variety Meats And By-Products Thymus Cooked Braised ☛ serving size: 3 oz = 85 g; Calories = 271

🐾 Beef Variety Meats And By-Products Thymus Raw 🐄 serving size: 1 oz = 28.4 g; Calories = 67

🐾 Beef Variety Meats And By-Products Tongue Cooked Simmered 🐄 serving size: 3 oz = 85 g; Calories = 241

🐾 Beef Variety Meats And By-Products Tongue Raw 🐄 serving size: 1 oz = 28.4 g; Calories = 64

🐾 Beef Variety Meats And By-Products Tripe Cooked Simmered 🐄 serving size: 1 serving = 85 g; Calories = 80

🐾 Beef Variety Meats And By-Products Tripe Raw 🐄 serving size: 1 oz = 28.4 g; Calories = 24

🐾 Beerwurst Pork And Beef 🐄 serving size: 1 serving 2 oz = 56 g; Calories = 155

🐾 Berliner Sausage 🐄 serving size: 1 slice = 23 g; Calories = 53

🐾 Bison Cooked 🐄 serving size: 1 cup, cooked = 134 g; Calories = 190

🐾 Bison Ground Grass-Fed Raw 🐄 serving size: 1 patty (cooked from 4 oz raw) = 85 g; Calories = 124

🐾 Blood Sausage 🐄 serving size: 4 slices = 100 g; Calories = 379

🐾 Bockwurst Pork Veal Raw 🐄 serving size: 1 sausage = 91 g; Calories = 274

🐾 Bologna Beef And Pork Low Fat 🐄 serving size: 1 cup pieces = 138 g; Calories = 317

🐾 Bologna Beef Low Fat 🐄 serving size: 1 slice = 28 g; Calories = 57

🐾 Bologna Chicken Pork 🐄 serving size: 1 serving = 28 g; Calories = 94

🐾 Bologna Chicken Pork Beef 🐄 serving size: 1 serving = 28 g; Calories = 76

Bologna Chicken Turkey Pork ☞ serving size: 1 serving = 28 g; Calories = 83

Bologna Meat And Poultry ☞ serving size: 1 slice = 33 g; Calories = 93

Bologna Pork And Turkey Lite ☞ serving size: 1 serving 2 oz = 56 g; Calories = 118

Bologna Pork Turkey And Beef ☞ serving size: 1 oz = 28.4 g; Calories = 95

Boneless Skinless Chicken Leg (Raw) ☞ serving size: 3 oz = 85 g; Calories = 102

Boston Steak (Pork) ☞ serving size: 3 oz = 85 g; Calories = 220

Brains Cooked ☞ serving size: 1 oz, raw (yield after cooking) = 24 g; Calories = 36

Bratwurst Beef And Pork Smoked ☞ serving size: 1 serving 2.33 oz = 66 g; Calories = 196

Bratwurst Chicken Cooked ☞ serving size: 1 serving 2.96 oz = 84 g; Calories = 148

Bratwurst Pork Beef And Turkey Lite Smoked ☞ serving size: 1 serving 2.33 oz = 66 g; Calories = 123

Bratwurst With Cheese ☞ serving size: 1 bun-size or griller link = 75 g; Calories = 253

Braunschweiger Pork Liver Sausage ☞ serving size: 1 oz = 28.4 g; Calories = 93

Brotwurst Pork Beef Link ☞ serving size: 1 link = 70 g; Calories = 226

Brunswick Stew ☞ serving size: 1 cup = 243 g; Calories = 292

Buffalo Sirloin Steak ☞ serving size: 1 serving (3 oz) = 85 g; Calories = 145

Canada Goose Breast Meat Skinless Raw ☛ serving size: 3 oz = 85 g; Calories = 113

Canadian Bacon (Pan-Fried) ☛ serving size: 1 slice = 13.8 g; Calories = 20

Canadian Bacon (Raw) ☛ serving size: 3 oz = 85 g; Calories = 94

Canned Ham ☛ serving size: 1 oz = 28.4 g; Calories = 68

Caribou Cooked ☛ serving size: 1 oz, boneless, cooked = 28 g; Calories = 47

Cassava Pasteles Puerto Rican Style ☛ serving size: 1 pastel (6" x 2" x 1/2") = 145 g; Calories = 368

Cheesefurter Cheese Smokie Pork Beef ☛ serving size: 2 (1/3) links = 100 g; Calories = 328

Chicken "wings" Boneless With Hot Sauce From Other Sources ☛ serving size: 1 boneless wing = 35 g; Calories = 81

Chicken "wings" Plain From Fast Food / Restaurant ☛ serving size: 1 drummette = 22 g; Calories = 71

Chicken "wings" Plain From Other Sources ☛ serving size: 1 drummette = 22 g; Calories = 69

Chicken (Light Meat) ☛ serving size: 1 cup, chopped or diced = 140 g; Calories = 214

Chicken Back ☛ serving size: 1 small back (yield after cooking, bone removed) = 110 g; Calories = 328

Chicken Breast Baked Broiled Or Roasted Skin Eaten From Raw ☛ serving size: 1 cup, cooked, diced = 135 g; Calories = 259

Chicken Breast Baked Broiled Or Roasted Skin Not Eaten From Raw ☛ serving size: 1 cup, cooked, diced = 135 g; Calories = 217

Chicken Breast Sauteed Skin Eaten ☛ serving size: 1 cup, cooked, diced = 135 g; Calories = 278

🦃 Chicken Breast Tenders Breaded Cooked Microwaved ☞ serving size: 1 piece = 15 g; Calories = 38

🦃 Chicken Breast Tenders Breaded Uncooked ☞ serving size: 1 piece = 15 g; Calories = 40

🦃 Chicken Broiler Rotisserie BBQ Drumstick Meat Only ☞ serving size: 1 drumstick = 71 g; Calories = 122

🦃 Chicken Broiler Rotisserie BBQ Skin ☞ serving size: 1 serving = 85 g; Calories = 321

🦃 Chicken Canned Meat Only With Broth ☞ serving size: 1 can (5 oz) = 142 g; Calories = 234

🦃 Chicken Canned No Broth ☞ serving size: 1 oz = 28 g; Calories = 52

🦃 Chicken Capons Giblets Cooked Simmered ☞ serving size: 1 cup, chopped or diced = 145 g; Calories = 238

🦃 Chicken Capons Giblets Raw ☞ serving size: 1 giblets = 115 g; Calories = 150

🦃 Chicken Chicken Roll Roasted ☞ serving size: 1 slice = 28 g; Calories = 53

🦃 Chicken Cornbread ☞ serving size: 1 piece (2-1/2" x 2-1/2" x 1-1/2") = 67 g; Calories = 112

🦃 Chicken Cornish Game Hens Meat And Skin Cooked Roasted ☞ serving size: 3 oz = 85 g; Calories = 220

🦃 Chicken Cornish Game Hens Meat And Skin Raw ☞ serving size: 3 oz = 85 g; Calories = 170

🦃 Chicken Cornish Game Hens Meat Only Cooked Roasted ☞ serving size: 3 oz = 85 g; Calories = 114

🦃 Chicken Cornish Game Hens Meat Only Raw ☞ serving size: 3 oz = 85 g; Calories = 99

🖐 Chicken Dark Meat Drumstick Meat Only With Added Solution Raw 🖝 serving size: 1 drumstick with skin = 143 g; Calories = 152

🖐 Chicken Fillet Grilled 🖝 serving size: 1 fillet = 100 g; Calories = 145

🖐 Chicken Ground Raw 🖝 serving size: 4 oz crumbled = 112 g; Calories = 160

🖐 Chicken Heart All Classes Cooked Simmered 🖝 serving size: 1 cup, chopped or diced = 145 g; Calories = 268

🖐 Chicken Heart All Classes Raw 🖝 serving size: 1 heart = 6.1 g; Calories = 9

🖐 Chicken Hotdog 🖝 serving size: 3 oz = 85 g; Calories = 190

🖐 Chicken Leg Drumstick And Thigh Baked Coated Skin / Coating Not Eaten 🖝 serving size: 1 cup, cooked, diced = 135 g; Calories = 246

🖐 Chicken Liver Braised 🖝 serving size: 1 oz, raw (yield after cooking) = 18 g; Calories = 30

🖐 Chicken Liver Fried 🖝 serving size: 1 oz, raw (yield after cooking) = 19 g; Calories = 36

🖐 Chicken Neck Or Ribs 🖝 serving size: 1 neck (yield after cooking, bone removed) = 35 g; Calories = 86

🖐 Chicken Thigh Baked Or Broiled Skin Not Eaten From Fast Food / Restaurant 🖝 serving size: 1 cup, cooked, diced = 135 g; Calories = 258

🖐 Chicken Thigh Fried Coated Prepared Skinless Coating Eaten From Raw 🖝 serving size: 1 cup, cooked, diced = 135 g; Calories = 311

🖐 Chicken Wing Fried Coated From Pre-Cooked 🖝 serving size: 1 wing, any size = 55 g; Calories = 161

🖐 Chicken Wing Fried Coated From Raw 🖝 serving size: 1 wing, any size = 55 g; Calories = 158

🖐 Chorizo 🖝 serving size: 1 oz = 28.4 g; Calories = 84

Chuck Steak (Mock Tender) ☛ serving size: 1 steak = 141 g; Calories = 268

Cooked Deer Tenderloin ☛ serving size: 1 serving (3 oz) = 85 g; Calories = 127

Cooked Grass Fed Ground Bison (Buffalo) ☛ serving size: 3 oz = 85 g; Calories = 152

Cooked Ground Pork ☛ serving size: 3 oz = 85 g; Calories = 253

Corned Beef Loaf Jellied ☛ serving size: 1 slice (1 oz) (4 inch x 4 inch x 3/32 inch thick) = 28 g; Calories = 43

Cornish Game Hen Roasted Skin Not Eaten ☛ serving size: 1 hen (1-1/4 lb, raw) (yield after cooking, bone and skin removed) = 250 g; Calories = 333

Cured Ham ☛ serving size: 1 cup = 140 g; Calories = 316

Cured Smoked Beef ☛ serving size: 1 slice (1 oz) = 28 g; Calories = 37

Deer Chop Cooked ☛ serving size: 1 oz, with bone, cooked (yield after bone removed) = 23 g; Calories = 44

Dove Cooked (Includes Squab) ☛ serving size: 1 cup, chopped or diced = 140 g; Calories = 298

Dove Cooked Ns As To Cooking Method ☛ serving size: 1 dove (yield after cooking, bone removed) = 110 g; Calories = 233

Dove Fried ☛ serving size: 1 dove (yield after cooking, bone removed) = 110 g; Calories = 245

Dry Pork And Beef Salami ☛ serving size: 1 slice = 9.8 g; Calories = 37

Dry Pork Salami ☛ serving size: 1 package (4 oz) = 113 g; Calories = 460

🦆 Duck Coated Fried 🖝 serving size: 1 leg (drumstick and thigh) (yield after cooking, bone removed) = 115 g; Calories = 259

🦆 Duck Cooked Skin Eaten 🖝 serving size: 1/2 duck (yield after cooking, bone removed) = 380 g; Calories = 1277

🦆 Game Meat Antelope Raw 🖝 serving size: 1 oz = 28.4 g; Calories = 32

🦆 Game Meat Bear Cooked Simmered 🖝 serving size: 3 oz = 85 g; Calories = 220

🦆 Game Meat Bear Raw 🖝 serving size: 1 oz = 28.4 g; Calories = 46

🦆 Goat Raw 🖝 serving size: 1 oz = 28.4 g; Calories = 31

🦆 Goat Ribs Cooked 🖝 serving size: 1 rib (yield after cooking, bone removed) = 46 g; Calories = 65

🦆 Goose Domesticated Meat And Skin Cooked Roasted 🖝 serving size: 1 cup, chopped or diced = 140 g; Calories = 427

🦆 Goose Domesticated Meat And Skin Raw 🖝 serving size: 3 oz = 85 g; Calories = 315

🦆 Goose Domesticated Meat Only Raw 🖝 serving size: 3 oz = 85 g; Calories = 137

🦆 Grilled Beef Tenderloin Steak 🖝 serving size: 3 oz = 85 g; Calories = 168

🦆 Grilled Porterhouse Steak 🖝 serving size: 3 oz = 85 g; Calories = 181

🦆 Grilled Porterhouse Steak (Choice) 🖝 serving size: 3 oz = 85 g; Calories = 188

🦆 Grilled T-Bone Steak 🖝 serving size: 3 oz = 85 g; Calories = 180

🦆 Grilled T-Bone Steak (Choice) 🖝 serving size: 3 oz = 85 g; Calories = 185

🦆 Grilled Top Round Steak 🖝 serving size: 3 oz = 85 g; Calories = 138

Ground Beef Cooked ☛ serving size: 1 oz, cooked = 28 g; Calories = 73

Ground Beef Patty Cooked ☛ serving size: 1 miniature patty = 20 g; Calories = 54

Ground Beef Raw ☛ serving size: 1 oz = 28 g; Calories = 69

Ground Hog Cooked ☛ serving size: 1 oz, with bone, cooked (yield after bone removed) = 23 g; Calories = 54

Ground Meat Nfs ☛ serving size: 1 small patty (3.33 oz, raw, 5 patties per lb) (yield after cooking) = 68 g; Calories = 177

Ground Turkey 85% Lean 15% Fat Pan-Broiled Crumbles ☛ serving size: 3 oz = 85 g; Calories = 219

Ground Turkey 85% Lean 15% Fat Raw ☛ serving size: 1 patty (cooked from 4 oz raw) = 85 g; Calories = 153

Ground Turkey 93% Lean 7% Fat Pan-Broiled Crumbles ☛ serving size: 3 oz = 85 g; Calories = 181

Ground Turkey 93% Lean 7% Fat Raw ☛ serving size: 1 oz = 28.4 g; Calories = 43

Ground Turkey Cooked ☛ serving size: 1 patty (4 oz, raw) (yield after cooking) = 82 g; Calories = 167

Ground Turkey Raw ☛ serving size: 1 lb = 453.6 g; Calories = 671

Lamb Australian Imported Fresh Separable Fat Cooked ☛ serving size: 3 oz = 85 g; Calories = 543

Lamb Australian Imported Fresh Separable Fat Raw ☛ serving size: 1 oz = 28.4 g; Calories = 184

Lamb Domestic Shoulder Arm Separable Lean Only Trimmed To 1/4 Inch Fat Choice Raw ☛ serving size: 1 oz = 28.4 g; Calories = 38

Lamb Domestic Shoulder Blade Separable Lean And Fat

Trimmed To 1/4 Inch Fat Choice Cooked Braised ☞ serving size: 3 oz = 85 g; Calories = 293

🐑 Lamb Ground Or Patty Cooked ☞ serving size: 1 patty (4 oz, raw) (yield after cooking) = 77 g; Calories = 216

🐑 Lamb Ground Raw ☞ serving size: 1 oz = 28.4 g; Calories = 80

🐑 Lamb Hocks Cooked ☞ serving size: 1 oz, with bone, cooked (yield after bone removed) = 19 g; Calories = 46

🐑 Lamb Liver (Cooked) ☞ serving size: 3 oz = 85 g; Calories = 202

🐑 Lamb Loin Chop Cooked Lean And Fat Eaten ☞ serving size: 1 small (4 oz, with bone, raw) (yield after cooking, bone removed) = 71 g; Calories = 222

🐑 Lamb Ribs Cooked Lean And Fat Eaten ☞ serving size: 1 rib (yield after cooking, bone removed) = 46 g; Calories = 165

🐑 Lamb Ribs Cooked Lean Only Eaten ☞ serving size: 1 rib (yield after cooking, bone and fat removed) = 25 g; Calories = 58

🐑 Liver Sausage Liverwurst Pork ☞ serving size: 1 slice (2-1/2 inch dia x 1/4 inch thick) = 18 g; Calories = 59

🐑 Luncheon Meat Pork And Chicken Minced Canned Includes Spam Lite ☞ serving size: 2 oz (1 serving) = 56 g; Calories = 110

🐑 Luncheon Meat Pork Canned ☞ serving size: 1 oz = 28.4 g; Calories = 95

🐑 Meat Loaf Made With Beef ☞ serving size: 1 small or thin slice = 86 g; Calories = 171

🐑 Meat Loaf Made With Beef And Pork ☞ serving size: 1 small or thin slice = 86 g; Calories = 169

🐑 Moose Cooked ☞ serving size: 1 oz, boneless, cooked = 28 g; Calories = 37

🐑 Mortadella Beef Pork ☞ serving size: 1 oz = 28.4 g; Calories = 88

Ostrich Cooked ☛ serving size: 1 oz, cooked = 28 g; Calories = 49

Ostrich Fan Raw ☛ serving size: 1 serving (cooked from 4oz raw) = 85 g; Calories = 100

Ostrich Ground Cooked Pan-Broiled ☛ serving size: 1 patty = 93 g; Calories = 163

Ostrich Ground Raw ☛ serving size: 1 patty = 109 g; Calories = 180

Pastrami Turkey ☛ serving size: 2 slices = 57 g; Calories = 79

Pate Chicken Liver Canned ☛ serving size: 1 tbsp = 13 g; Calories = 26

Pate De Foie Gras Canned (Goose Liver Pate) Smoked ☛ serving size: 1 tbsp = 13 g; Calories = 60

Pate Goose Liver Smoked Canned ☛ serving size: 1 tbsp = 13 g; Calories = 60

Pepperoni ☛ serving size: 3 oz = 85 g; Calories = 428

Pheasant Breast Meat Only Raw ☛ serving size: 3 oz = 85 g; Calories = 113

Pheasant Cooked ☛ serving size: 1/2 pheasant breast (yield after cooking, bone removed) = 130 g; Calories = 309

Pheasant Raw Meat And Skin ☛ serving size: 3 oz = 85 g; Calories = 154

Pork Beerwurst ☛ serving size: 1 slice (4 inch dia x 1/8 inch thick) = 23 g; Calories = 55

Pork Bratwurst ☛ serving size: 1 link cooked = 85 g; Calories = 283

Pork Chop Battered Fried Lean And Fat Eaten ☛ serving size: 1 small or thin cut (3 oz, with bone, raw) (yield after cooking, bone removed) = 52 g; Calories = 146

Pork Chop Ns As To Cooking Method Lean Only Eaten ☛ serving

size: 1 small or thin cut (3 oz, with bone, raw) (yield after cooking, bone and fat removed) = 43 g; Calories = 71

🐖 Pork Cured Ham -- Water Added Rump Bone-In Separable Lean And Fat Unheated ☛ serving size: 1 oz = 28.4 g; Calories = 49

🐖 Pork Cured Ham Whole Separable Lean Only Unheated ☛ serving size: 1 cup = 140 g; Calories = 206

🐖 Pork Fresh Loin Blade (Roasts) Bone-In Separable Lean Only Cooked Roasted ☛ serving size: 3 oz = 85 g; Calories = 185

🐖 Pork Sausage Link/patty Reduced Fat Unprepared ☛ serving size: 3 oz = 85 g; Calories = 185

🐖 Pork Sausage Link/patty Unprepared ☛ serving size: 1 link = 25 g; Calories = 72

🐖 Pork Sausage Reduced Sodium Cooked ☛ serving size: 3 oz = 85 g; Calories = 230

🐖 Pork Steak Or Cutlet Breaded Or Floured Fried Lean And Fat Eaten ☛ serving size: 1 oz, with bone, raw (yield after cooking, bone removed) = 18 g; Calories = 58

🐖 Pork Tenderloin Baked ☛ serving size: 1 oz, boneless, raw (yield after cooking) = 21 g; Calories = 32

🐖 Pork Tenderloin Battered Fried ☛ serving size: 1 oz, boneless, raw (yield after cooking) = 25 g; Calories = 48

🐖 Quail Cooked ☛ serving size: 1 quail (yield after cooking, bone removed) = 75 g; Calories = 170

🐖 Quail Cooked Total Edible ☛ serving size: 1 oz = 28.4 g; Calories = 65

🐖 Quail Meat And Skin Raw ☛ serving size: 1 quail = 109 g; Calories = 209

🐖 Quail Meat Only Raw ☛ serving size: 1 quail = 92 g; Calories = 123

Rabbit Domestic Ns As To Cooking Method ☛ serving size: 1 oz, with bone, cooked (yield after bone removed) = 22 g; Calories = 45

Rabbit Ns As To Domestic Or Wild Breaded Fried ☛ serving size: 1 oz, boneless, cooked = 28 g; Calories = 69

Rabbit Ns As To Domestic Or Wild Cooked ☛ serving size: 1 oz, with bone, cooked (yield after bone removed) = 22 g; Calories = 45

Roast Beef Deli Style Prepackaged Sliced ☛ serving size: 1 slice oval = 9.3 g; Calories = 11

Roast Beef Spread ☛ serving size: 1 serving .25 cup = 57 g; Calories = 127

Roast Duck ☛ serving size: 1 cup, chopped or diced = 140 g; Calories = 281

Roast Goose ☛ serving size: 1 unit (yield from 1 lb ready-to-cook goose) = 143 g; Calories = 340

Roast Turkey (Without Skin) ☛ serving size: 3 oz = 85 g; Calories = 135

Roast Turkey Dark Meat ☛ serving size: 1 serving = 85 g; Calories = 147

Salami ☛ serving size: 1 oz = 28 g; Calories = 119

Salami Cooked Beef ☛ serving size: 1 slice = 26 g; Calories = 68

Salami Cooked Beef And Pork ☛ serving size: 1 slice round = 12.3 g; Calories = 41

Salami Italian Pork And Beef Dry Sliced 50% Less Sodium ☛ serving size: 1 serving 5 slices = 28 g; Calories = 98

Salami Pork Beef Less Sodium ☛ serving size: 3 (1/2) oz = 100 g; Calories = 396

Swedish Meatballs With Cream Or White Sauce ☛ serving size: 1 cup = 246 g; Calories = 418

Sweet Italian Sausage ☛ serving size: 1 link 3 oz = 84 g; Calories = 125

Swiss Steak ☛ serving size: 1 cup = 249 g; Calories = 326

Swisswurst Pork And Beef With Swiss Cheese Smoked ☛ serving size: 1 serving 2.7 oz = 77 g; Calories = 236

Tripe Cooked ☛ serving size: 1 oz, raw (yield after cooking) = 16 g; Calories = 14

Turkey All Classes Back Meat And Skin Cooked Roasted ☛ serving size: 1 cup, chopped or diced = 140 g; Calories = 342

Turkey Back From Whole Bird Meat Only Raw ☛ serving size: 4 oz = 114 g; Calories = 129

Turkey Back From Whole Bird Meat Only Roasted ☛ serving size: 3 oz = 85 g; Calories = 147

Turkey Back From Whole Bird Meat Only With Added Solution Raw ☛ serving size: 4 oz = 114 g; Calories = 131

Turkey Back From Whole Bird Meat Only With Added Solution Roasted ☛ serving size: 3 oz = 85 g; Calories = 108

Turkey Bacon Microwaved ☛ serving size: 1 slice = 8.1 g; Calories = 30

Turkey Baloney (Bologna) ☛ serving size: 0.99 oz 1 serving = 28 g; Calories = 59

Turkey Breast From Whole Bird Meat Only Raw ☛ serving size: 4 oz = 114 g; Calories = 130

Turkey Breast From Whole Bird Meat Only With Added Solution Raw ☛ serving size: 4 oz = 114 g; Calories = 116

Turkey Breast From Whole Bird Meat Only With Added Solution Roasted ☛ serving size: 3 oz = 85 g; Calories = 108

🦃 Turkey Canned Meat Only With Broth ☛ serving size: 1 cup, drained = 135 g; Calories = 228

🦃 Turkey Dark Meat From Whole Meat And Skin Cooked Roasted ☛ serving size: 1 serving = 85 g; Calories = 175

🦃 Turkey Drumstick From Whole Bird Meat Only With Added Solution Roasted ☛ serving size: 3 oz = 85 g; Calories = 134

🦃 Turkey From Whole Dark Meat Meat Only Raw ☛ serving size: 1 serving = 85 g; Calories = 92

🦃 Turkey Ground ☛ serving size: 1 cup, cooked = 130 g; Calories = 261

🦃 Turkey Ham Prepackaged Or Deli Luncheon Meat ☛ serving size: 1 slice, nfs = 28 g; Calories = 35

🦃 Turkey Ham Sliced Extra Lean Prepackaged Or Deli-Sliced ☛ serving size: 1 cup pieces = 138 g; Calories = 185

🦃 Turkey Whole Meat Only Raw ☛ serving size: 3 oz = 85 g; Calories = 98

🦃 Veal Breast Point Half Boneless Separable Lean And Fat Cooked Braised ☛ serving size: 3 oz = 85 g; Calories = 211

🦃 Veal Breast Separable Fat Cooked ☛ serving size: 1 oz = 28.4 g; Calories = 148

🦃 Veal Chop Ns As To Cooking Method Ns As To Fat Eaten ☛ serving size: 1 small (4.75 oz, with bone, raw) (yield after cooking, bone removed) = 78 g; Calories = 168

🦃 Veal Composite Of Trimmed Retail Cuts Separable Fat Raw ☛ serving size: 1 oz = 28.4 g; Calories = 181

🦃 Veal Cordon Bleu ☛ serving size: 1 roll (with ham and sauce) = 229 g; Calories = 593

🦃 Veal Cutlet Or Steak Broiled Lean And Fat Eaten ☛ serving size: 1 oz, boneless, cooked = 28 g; Calories = 45

Veal Cutlet Or Steak Broiled Lean Only Eaten ☛ serving size: 1 oz, boneless, cooked, lean only = 28 g; Calories = 51

Veal Ground Cooked Broiled ☛ serving size: 3 oz = 85 g; Calories = 146

Veal Ground Cooked Pan-Fried ☛ serving size: 3 oz = 85 g; Calories = 183

Veal Ground Raw ☛ serving size: 3 oz = 85 g; Calories = 168

Veal Leg (Top Round) Separable Lean And Fat Cooked Braised ☛ serving size: 3 oz = 85 g; Calories = 179

Veal Loin Chop Separable Lean And Fat Cooked Grilled ☛ serving size: 3 oz = 85 g; Calories = 168

Veal Marsala ☛ serving size: 1 slice with sauce = 96 g; Calories = 165

Veal Rib Separable Lean Only Raw ☛ serving size: 1 oz = 28.4 g; Calories = 34

Veal Shank (Fore And Hind) Separable Lean And Fat Raw ☛ serving size: 1 oz = 28.4 g; Calories = 32

Veal Shoulder Blade Chop Separable Lean And Fat Raw ☛ serving size: 3 oz = 85 g; Calories = 126

Veal Sirloin Separable Lean And Fat Cooked Braised ☛ serving size: 3 oz = 85 g; Calories = 214

Veal Variety Meats And By-Products Brain Raw ☛ serving size: 1 oz = 28.4 g; Calories = 34

Veal Variety Meats And By-Products Heart Raw ☛ serving size: 1 oz = 28.4 g; Calories = 31

Veal Variety Meats And By-Products Kidneys Raw ☛ serving size: 1 oz = 28.4 g; Calories = 28

Veal Variety Meats And By-Products Liver Raw ☛ serving size: 1 oz = 28.4 g; Calories = 40

Veal Variety Meats And By-Products Lungs Raw ☛ serving size: 1 oz = 28.4 g; Calories = 26

Veal Variety Meats And By-Products Pancreas Raw ☛ serving size: 1 oz = 28.4 g; Calories = 52

Veal Variety Meats And By-Products Spleen Raw ☛ serving size: 1 oz = 28.4 g; Calories = 28

Veal Variety Meats And By-Products Thymus Raw ☛ serving size: 1 oz = 28.4 g; Calories = 29

Veal Variety Meats And By-Products Tongue Raw ☛ serving size: 1 oz = 28.4 g; Calories = 37

Venison/deer Cured ☛ serving size: 1 oz, boneless, cooked = 28 g; Calories = 52

Venison/deer Jerky ☛ serving size: 1 strip or stick (4" long) = 14 g; Calories = 55

Venison/deer Roasted ☛ serving size: 1 oz, boneless, cooked = 28 g; Calories = 53

Venison/deer Stewed ☛ serving size: 1 oz, boneless, cooked = 28 g; Calories = 53

Vienna Sausages Stewed With Potatoes Puerto Rican Style ☛ serving size: 1 cup = 175 g; Calories = 376

Wild Pig Smoked ☛ serving size: 1 oz, boneless, cooked = 28 g; Calories = 44

Yachtwurst With Pistachio Nuts Cooked ☛ serving size: 1 serving 2 oz = 56 g; Calories = 150

19

NUTS AND SEEDS

Acorns (Dried) ☞ serving size: 1 oz = 28.4 g; Calories = 145

Almond Butter ☞ serving size: 1 tbsp = 16 g; Calories = 98

Almond Paste ☞ serving size: 1 oz = 28.4 g; Calories = 130

Almonds ☞ serving size: 1 cup, whole = 143 g; Calories = 828

Almonds Flavored ☞ serving size: 1 nut = 1 g; Calories = 6

Almonds Honey Roasted ☞ serving size: 1 nut = 1 g; Calories = 6

Almonds Salted ☞ serving size: 1 nut = 1 g; Calories = 6

Almonds Unsalted ☞ serving size: 1 nut = 1 g; Calories = 6

Black Walnuts (Dried) ☞ serving size: 1 cup, chopped = 125 g; Calories = 774

Boiled Chestnuts ☞ serving size: 1 oz = 28.4 g; Calories = 37

Boiled Chinese Chestnuts ☞ serving size: 1 oz = 28.4 g; Calories = 44

● Boiled Japanese Chestnuts ☛ serving size: 1 oz = 28.4 g; Calories = 16

● Brazilnuts ☛ serving size: 1 cup, whole = 133 g; Calories = 877

● Breadfruit Nuts (Seeds) ☛ serving size: 1 oz = 28.4 g; Calories = 48

● Butternuts (Dried) ☛ serving size: 1 cup = 120 g; Calories = 734

● Cashew Butter ☛ serving size: 1 tbsp = 16 g; Calories = 94

● Cashews (Raw) ☛ serving size: 1 oz = 28.4 g; Calories = 157

● Cashews Lightly Salted ☛ serving size: 1 nut = 2 g; Calories = 12

● Cashews Unsalted ☛ serving size: 1 nut = 2 g; Calories = 12

● Chestnuts ☛ serving size: 1 oz = 28.4 g; Calories = 56

● Chia Seeds ☛ serving size: 1 oz = 28.4 g; Calories = 138

● Chinese Chestnuts ☛ serving size: 1 oz = 28.4 g; Calories = 64

● Coconut Milk ☛ serving size: 1 cup = 226 g; Calories = 445

● Coconut Water ☛ serving size: 1 cup = 240 g; Calories = 46

● Dried Beechnuts ☛ serving size: 1 oz = 28.4 g; Calories = 164

● Dried Chinese Chestnuts ☛ serving size: 1 oz = 28.4 g; Calories = 103

● Dried Coconut ☛ serving size: 1 oz = 28.4 g; Calories = 168

● Dried Coconut (Unsweetened) ☛ serving size: 1 oz = 28.4 g; Calories = 187

● Dried Ginkgo Nuts ☛ serving size: 1 oz = 28.4 g; Calories = 99

● Dried Hickorynuts ☛ serving size: 1 cup = 120 g; Calories = 788

● Dried Japanese Chestnuts ☛ serving size: 1 cup = 155 g; Calories = 558

Dried Lotus Seeds ☞ serving size: 1 cup = 32 g; Calories = 106

Dried Pilinuts ☞ serving size: 1 cup = 120 g; Calories = 863

Dried Pine Nuts ☞ serving size: 1 oz = 28.4 g; Calories = 179

Dried Pumpkin And Squash Seeds ☞ serving size: 1 cup = 129 g; Calories = 721

Dried Sunflower Seeds ☞ serving size: 1 cup, with hulls, edible yield = 46 g; Calories = 269

Dry Roasted Almonds ☞ serving size: 1 cup whole kernels = 138 g; Calories = 825

Dry Roasted Hazelnuts ☞ serving size: 1 oz = 28.4 g; Calories = 184

Dry Roasted Macadamia Nuts ☞ serving size: 1 cup, whole or halves = 132 g; Calories = 948

Dry Roasted Peanuts ☞ serving size: 1 cup = 146 g; Calories = 857

Dry Roasted Pecans ☞ serving size: 1 oz = 28.4 g; Calories = 202

Dry Roasted Pistachio Nuts ☞ serving size: 1 cup = 123 g; Calories = 704

Dry Roasted Sunflower Seeds ☞ serving size: 1 cup = 128 g; Calories = 745

Dry Roasted Sunflower Seeds (With Salt) ☞ serving size: 1 cup = 128 g; Calories = 699

Dry-Roasted Cashews ☞ serving size: 1 cup, halves and whole = 137 g; Calories = 786

Dry-Roasted Mixed Nuts (Salted) ☞ serving size: 1 cup = 131 g; Calories = 795

Flax Seeds ☞ serving size: 1 tbsp, whole = 10.3 g; Calories = 55

Ginko Nuts ☞ serving size: 1 oz = 28.4 g; Calories = 52

Hazelnuts 🖝 serving size: 1 cup, chopped = 115 g; Calories = 722

Hemp Seeds 🖝 serving size: 3 tbsp = 30 g; Calories = 166

Lotus Seeds 🖝 serving size: 1 oz = 28.4 g; Calories = 25

Macadamia Nuts 🖝 serving size: 1 cup, whole or halves = 134 g; Calories = 962

Mixed Nuts Honey Roasted 🖝 serving size: 1 cup = 142 g; Calories = 822

Mixed Nuts Nfs 🖝 serving size: 1 cup = 142 g; Calories = 859

Mixed Nuts Unroasted 🖝 serving size: 1 cup = 142 g; Calories = 861

Mixed Nuts With Peanuts Unsalted 🖝 serving size: 1 cup = 142 g; Calories = 866

Mixed Nuts Without Peanuts Salted 🖝 serving size: 1 cup = 142 g; Calories = 866

Mixed Nuts Without Peanuts Unsalted 🖝 serving size: 1 cup = 142 g; Calories = 873

Mixed Seeds 🖝 serving size: 1 cup = 145 g; Calories = 841

Nuts Acorn Flour Full Fat 🖝 serving size: 1 oz = 28.4 g; Calories = 142

Nuts Acorns Raw 🖝 serving size: 1 oz = 28.4 g; Calories = 110

Nuts Almond Butter Plain With Salt Added 🖝 serving size: 1 tbsp = 16 g; Calories = 98

Nuts Almonds Blanched 🖝 serving size: 1 cup whole kernels = 145 g; Calories = 856

Nuts Almonds Dry Roasted With Salt Added 🖝 serving size: 1 cup whole kernels = 138 g; Calories = 825

Nuts Almonds Honey Roasted Unblanched 🖝 serving size: 1 cup whole kernels = 144 g; Calories = 855

🔘 Nuts Almonds Oil Roasted Lightly Salted ☞ serving size: 1 cup whole kernels = 157 g; Calories = 953

🔘 Nuts Almonds Oil Roasted With Salt Added ☞ serving size: 1 cup whole kernels = 157 g; Calories = 953

🔘 Nuts Almonds Oil Roasted With Salt Added Smoke Flavor ☞ serving size: 1 oz (28 almonds) = 28 g; Calories = 170

🔘 Nuts Almonds Oil Roasted Without Salt Added ☞ serving size: 1 cup whole kernels = 157 g; Calories = 953

🔘 Nuts Cashew Butter Plain With Salt Added ☞ serving size: 1 tbsp = 16 g; Calories = 97

🔘 Nuts Cashew Nuts Dry Roasted With Salt Added ☞ serving size: 1 cup, halves and whole = 137 g; Calories = 786

🔘 Nuts Cashew Nuts Oil Roasted With Salt Added ☞ serving size: 1 cup, whole = 129 g; Calories = 750

🔘 Nuts Chestnuts European Dried Peeled ☞ serving size: 1 oz = 28.4 g; Calories = 105

🔘 Nuts Chestnuts European Dried Unpeeled ☞ serving size: 1 oz = 28.4 g; Calories = 106

🔘 Nuts Chestnuts European Raw Unpeeled ☞ serving size: 1 cup = 145 g; Calories = 309

🔘 Nuts Chestnuts Japanese Raw ☞ serving size: 1 oz = 28.4 g; Calories = 44

🔘 Nuts Chestnuts Japanese Roasted ☞ serving size: 1 oz = 28.4 g; Calories = 57

🔘 Nuts Coconut Cream Canned Sweetened ☞ serving size: 1 tbsp = 19 g; Calories = 68

🔘 Nuts Coconut Cream Raw (Liquid Expressed From Grated Meat) ☞ serving size: 1 tbsp = 15 g; Calories = 50

Nuts Coconut Meat Dried (Desiccated) Creamed ☛ serving size: 1 oz = 28.4 g; Calories = 194

Nuts Coconut Meat Dried (Desiccated) Sweetened Flaked Canned ☛ serving size: 1 cup = 77 g; Calories = 341

Nuts Coconut Meat Dried (Desiccated) Sweetened Flaked Packaged ☛ serving size: 1 cup = 85 g; Calories = 388

Nuts Coconut Meat Raw ☛ serving size: 1 cup, shredded = 80 g; Calories = 283

Nuts Coconut Milk Frozen (Liquid Expressed From Grated Meat And Water) ☛ serving size: 1 cup = 240 g; Calories = 485

Nuts Coconut Milk Raw (Liquid Expressed From Grated Meat And Water) ☛ serving size: 1 cup = 240 g; Calories = 552

Nuts Formulated Wheat-Based All Flavors Except Macadamia Without Salt ☛ serving size: 1 oz = 28.4 g; Calories = 184

Nuts Formulated Wheat-Based Unflavored With Salt Added ☛ serving size: 1 oz = 28.4 g; Calories = 177

Nuts Ginkgo Nuts Canned ☛ serving size: 1 cup (78 kernels) = 155 g; Calories = 172

Nuts Hazelnuts Or Filberts Blanched ☛ serving size: 1 oz = 28.4 g; Calories = 179

Nuts Macadamia Nuts Dry Roasted With Salt Added ☛ serving size: 1 cup, whole or halves = 132 g; Calories = 945

Nuts Mixed Nuts Dry Roasted With Peanuts Salt Added Chosen Roaster ☛ serving size: 1 cup = 132 g; Calories = 803

Nuts Mixed Nuts Dry Roasted With Peanuts Salt Added Planters Pistachio Blend ☛ serving size: 1 cup = 147 g; Calories = 841

Nuts Mixed Nuts Dry Roasted With Peanuts With Salt Added ☛ serving size: 1 cup = 137 g; Calories = 814

Nuts Mixed Nuts Oil Roasted With Peanuts Lightly Salted ☞ serving size: 1 oz = 28.4 g; Calories = 172

Nuts Mixed Nuts Oil Roasted With Peanuts With Salt Added ☞ serving size: 1 cup = 134 g; Calories = 813

Nuts Mixed Nuts Oil Roasted With Peanuts Without Salt Added ☞ serving size: 1 cup = 134 g; Calories = 813

Nuts Mixed Nuts Oil Roasted Without Peanuts Lightly Salted ☞ serving size: 1 oz = 28.4 g; Calories = 172

Nuts Mixed Nuts Oil Roasted Without Peanuts With Salt Added ☞ serving size: 1 cup = 144 g; Calories = 886

Nuts Mixed Nuts Oil Roasted Without Peanuts Without Salt Added ☞ serving size: 1 cup = 144 g; Calories = 886

Nuts Nfs ☞ serving size: 1 cup = 142 g; Calories = 859

Nuts Pecans Dry Roasted With Salt Added ☞ serving size: 1 oz = 28.4 g; Calories = 202

Nuts Pecans Oil Roasted With Salt Added ☞ serving size: 1 cup = 110 g; Calories = 787

Nuts Pecans Oil Roasted Without Salt Added ☞ serving size: 1 cup = 110 g; Calories = 787

Nuts Pistachio Nuts Dry Roasted With Salt Added ☞ serving size: 1 cup = 123 g; Calories = 700

Nuts Walnuts Dry Roasted With Salt Added ☞ serving size: 1 oz = 28 g; Calories = 180

Nuts Walnuts Glazed ☞ serving size: 1 oz = 28 g; Calories = 140

Oil Roasted Cashews ☞ serving size: 1 cup, whole = 129 g; Calories = 748

Peanut Butter And Chocolate Spread ☞ serving size: 1 tablespoon = 16 g; Calories = 80

⬤ Peanut Butter And Jelly ☛ serving size: 1 tablespoon = 16 g; Calories = 69

⬤ Peanut Butter Lower Sodium And Lower Sugar ☛ serving size: 1 tablespoon = 16 g; Calories = 100

⬤ Peanuts Dry Roasted Lightly Salted ☛ serving size: 1 peanut, without shell = 1 g; Calories = 6

⬤ Pecans ☛ serving size: 1 cup, chopped = 109 g; Calories = 753

⬤ Pecans Honey Roasted ☛ serving size: 1 nut = 2 g; Calories = 13

⬤ Pecans Salted ☛ serving size: 1 nut = 2 g; Calories = 14

⬤ Pecans Unsalted ☛ serving size: 1 nut = 2 g; Calories = 14

⬤ Pine Nuts (Dried) ☛ serving size: 1 cup = 135 g; Calories = 909

⬤ Pistachio Nuts ☛ serving size: 1 cup = 123 g; Calories = 689

⬤ Pistachio Nuts Lightly Salted ☛ serving size: 1 nut = 1 g; Calories = 6

⬤ Pistachio Nuts Salted ☛ serving size: 1 nut = 1 g; Calories = 6

⬤ Pistachio Nuts Unsalted ☛ serving size: 1 nut = 1 g; Calories = 6

⬤ Pumpkin Seeds Salted ☛ serving size: 1 cup, without shell = 144 g; Calories = 817

⬤ Raw Sesame Butter (Tahini) ☛ serving size: 1 tbsp = 15 g; Calories = 86

⬤ Roasted Chestnuts ☛ serving size: 1 cup = 143 g; Calories = 350

⬤ Roasted Chinese Chestnuts ☛ serving size: 1 oz = 28.4 g; Calories = 68

⬤ Roasted Squash And Pumpkin Seeds (Salted) ☛ serving size: 1 cup = 118 g; Calories = 677

🔘 Roasted Squash And Pumpkin Seeds (Unsalted) ☞ serving size: 1 cup = 118 g; Calories = 677

🔘 Roasted Squash And Pumpkin Seeds (With Shells) ☞ serving size: 1 cup = 64 g; Calories = 285

🔘 Safflower Seeds ☞ serving size: 1 oz = 28.4 g; Calories = 147

🔘 Seeds Breadfruit Seeds Raw ☞ serving size: 1 oz = 28.4 g; Calories = 54

🔘 Seeds Breadfruit Seeds Roasted ☞ serving size: 1 oz = 28.4 g; Calories = 59

🔘 Seeds Breadnut Tree Seeds Dried ☞ serving size: 1 cup = 160 g; Calories = 587

🔘 Seeds Breadnut Tree Seeds Raw ☞ serving size: 1 oz (8-14 seeds) = 28.4 g; Calories = 62

🔘 Seeds Cottonseed Flour Low Fat (Glandless) ☞ serving size: 1 oz = 28.4 g; Calories = 94

🔘 Seeds Cottonseed Flour Partially Defatted (Glandless) ☞ serving size: 1 cup = 94 g; Calories = 338

🔘 Seeds Cottonseed Kernels Roasted (Glandless) ☞ serving size: 1 cup = 149 g; Calories = 754

🔘 Seeds Cottonseed Meal Partially Defatted (Glandless) ☞ serving size: 1 oz = 28.4 g; Calories = 104

🔘 Seeds Pumpkin And Squash Seeds Whole Roasted With Salt Added ☞ serving size: 1 cup = 64 g; Calories = 285

🔘 Seeds Safflower Seed Meal Partially Defatted ☞ serving size: 1 oz = 28.4 g; Calories = 97

🔘 Seeds Sesame Butter Paste ☞ serving size: 1 tbsp = 16 g; Calories = 94

⬤ Seeds Sesame Butter Tahini From Unroasted Kernels (Non-Chemically Removed Seed Coat) ☛ serving size: 1 tbsp = 14 g; Calories = 85

⬤ Seeds Sesame Butter Tahini Type Of Kernels Unspecified ☛ serving size: 1 tbsp = 15 g; Calories = 89

⬤ Seeds Sesame Flour High-Fat ☛ serving size: 1 oz = 28.4 g; Calories = 149

⬤ Seeds Sesame Flour Low-Fat ☛ serving size: 1 oz = 28.4 g; Calories = 95

⬤ Seeds Sesame Flour Partially Defatted ☛ serving size: 1 oz = 28.4 g; Calories = 109

⬤ Seeds Sesame Meal Partially Defatted ☛ serving size: 1 oz = 28.4 g; Calories = 161

⬤ Seeds Sesame Seed Kernels Dried (Decorticated) ☛ serving size: 1 cup = 150 g; Calories = 947

⬤ Seeds Sesame Seed Kernels Toasted With Salt Added (Decorticated) ☛ serving size: 1 cup = 128 g; Calories = 726

⬤ Seeds Sesame Seed Kernels Toasted Without Salt Added (Decorticated) ☛ serving size: 1 cup = 128 g; Calories = 726

⬤ Seeds Sesame Seeds Whole Dried ☛ serving size: 1 cup = 144 g; Calories = 825

⬤ Seeds Sisymbrium Sp. Seeds Whole Dried ☛ serving size: 1 cup = 74 g; Calories = 235

⬤ Seeds Sunflower Seed Butter With Salt Added ☛ serving size: 1 tbsp = 16 g; Calories = 99

⬤ Seeds Sunflower Seed Butter Without Salt ☛ serving size: 1 tbsp = 16 g; Calories = 99

⬤ Seeds Sunflower Seed Flour Partially Defatted ☛ serving size: 1 cup = 64 g; Calories = 209

Seeds Sunflower Seed Kernels Dry Roasted With Salt Added ☛ serving size: 1 cup = 128 g; Calories = 745

Seeds Sunflower Seed Kernels Oil Roasted With Salt Added ☛ serving size: 1 cup = 135 g; Calories = 799

Seeds Sunflower Seed Kernels Oil Roasted Without Salt ☛ serving size: 1 cup = 135 g; Calories = 799

Seeds Sunflower Seed Kernels Toasted With Salt Added ☛ serving size: 1 cup = 134 g; Calories = 830

Seeds Sunflower Seed Kernels Toasted Without Salt ☛ serving size: 1 cup = 134 g; Calories = 830

Seeds Watermelon Seed Kernels Dried ☛ serving size: 1 cup = 108 g; Calories = 602

Sesame Butter (Tahini) ☛ serving size: 1 tbsp = 15 g; Calories = 89

Sesame Seeds (Toasted) ☛ serving size: 1 oz = 28.4 g; Calories = 161

Shredded Coconut Meat ☛ serving size: 1 cup, shredded = 93 g; Calories = 466

Sunflower Seeds Flavored ☛ serving size: 1 cup, without shell = 144 g; Calories = 817

Sunflower Seeds Plain Salted ☛ serving size: 1 cup, without shell = 144 g; Calories = 828

Trail Mix Nfs ☛ serving size: 1 cup = 140 g; Calories = 633

Trail Mix With Chocolate ☛ serving size: 1 cup = 140 g; Calories = 701

Trail Mix With Nuts ☛ serving size: 1 cup = 140 g; Calories = 840

Trail Mix With Nuts And Fruit ☛ serving size: 1 cup = 140 g; Calories = 633

Trail Mix With Pretzels Cereal Or Granola ☞ serving size: 1 cup = 140 g; Calories = 662

Walnuts ☞ serving size: 1 cup, chopped = 117 g; Calories = 765

Walnuts Honey Roasted ☞ serving size: 1 nut = 2 g; Calories = 12

20

PREPARED MEALS

Almond Chicken ☞ serving size: 1 cup = 242 g; Calories = 477

Banquet Salisbury Steak With Gravy Family Size Frozen Unprepared ☞ serving size: 1 patty = 72 g; Calories = 112

Beans String Green Cooked Szechuan-Style ☞ serving size: 1 cup = 185 g; Calories = 176

Beef And Broccoli ☞ serving size: 1 cup = 217 g; Calories = 336

Beef And Noodles With Soy-Based Sauce ☞ serving size: 1 cup = 249 g; Calories = 426

Beef And Rice With Soy-Based Sauce ☞ serving size: 1 cup = 244 g; Calories = 429

Beef And Vegetables Excluding Carrots Broccoli And Dark-Green Leafy; No Potatoes Soy-Based Sauce ☞ serving size: 1 cup = 217 g; Calories = 310

Beef And Vegetables Including Carrots Broccoli And/or Dark-Green Leafy; No Potatoes Soy-Based Sauce ☞ serving size: 1 cup = 217 g; Calories = 306

Beef Chow Mein Or Chop Suey No Noodles ☛ serving size: 1 cup = 220 g; Calories = 180

Beef Chow Mein Or Chop Suey With Noodles ☛ serving size: 1 cup = 220 g; Calories = 286

Beef Corned Beef Hash With Potato Canned ☛ serving size: 1 cup = 236 g; Calories = 387

Beef Egg Foo Yung ☛ serving size: 1 patty = 86 g; Calories = 126

Beef Enchilada Chili Gravy Rice Refried Beans Frozen Meal ☛ serving size: 1 meal (15 oz) = 425 g; Calories = 527

Beef Enchilada Dinner NFS Frozen Meal ☛ serving size: 1 meal (15 oz) = 425 g; Calories = 527

Beef Macaroni With Tomato Sauce Frozen Entree Reduced Fat ☛ serving size: 1 serving = 269 g; Calories = 304

Beef Noodles And Vegetables Excluding Carrots Broccoli And Dark-Green Leafy; Soy-Based Sauce ☛ serving size: 1 cup = 217 g; Calories = 302

Beef Noodles And Vegetables Including Carrots Broccoli And/or Dark-Green Leafy; Soy-Based Sauce ☛ serving size: 1 cup = 217 g; Calories = 297

Beef Pot Pie Frozen Entree Prepared ☛ serving size: 1 pie, cooked (average weight) = 268 g; Calories = 590

Beef Potatoes And Vegetables Excluding Carrots Broccoli And Dark-Green Leafy; Soy-Based Sauce ☛ serving size: 1 cup = 252 g; Calories = 365

Beef Potatoes And Vegetables Including Carrots Broccoli And/or Dark-Green Leafy; Soy-Based Sauce ☛ serving size: 1 cup = 252 g; Calories = 368

Beef Rice And Vegetables Excluding Carrots Broccoli And Dark-

Green Leafy; Soy-Based Sauce ☛ serving size: 1 cup = 217 g; Calories = 310

🥄 Beef Rice And Vegetables Including Carrots Broccoli And/or Dark-Green Leafy; Soy-Based Sauce ☛ serving size: 1 cup = 217 g; Calories = 304

🥄 Beef Stew Canned Entree ☛ serving size: 1 cup (1 serving) = 196 g; Calories = 194

🥄 Beef Taco Filling: Beef Cheese Tomato Taco Sauce ☛ serving size: 1 cup = 204 g; Calories = 367

🥄 Beef Tofu And Vegetables Excluding Carrots Broccoli And Dark-Green Leafy; No Potatoes Soy-Based Sauce ☛ serving size: 1 cup = 217 g; Calories = 247

🥄 Beef Tofu And Vegetables Including Carrots Broccoli And/or Dark-Green Leafy; No Potatoes Soy-Based Sauce ☛ serving size: 1 cup = 217 g; Calories = 243

🥄 Beef With Soy-Based Sauce ☛ serving size: 1 cup = 244 g; Calories = 449

🥄 Beef With Sweet And Sour Sauce ☛ serving size: 1 cup = 252 g; Calories = 461

🥄 Bibimbap Korean ☛ serving size: 1 cup = 162 g; Calories = 128

🥄 Biryani With Chicken ☛ serving size: 1 cup = 196 g; Calories = 200

🥄 Biryani With Meat ☛ serving size: 1 cup = 196 g; Calories = 282

🥄 Biryani With Vegetables ☛ serving size: 1 cup = 172 g; Calories = 205

🥄 Bread Stuffing Made With Egg ☛ serving size: 1 cup = 170 g; Calories = 326

🥄 Burrito Bean And Cheese Frozen ☛ serving size: 1 burrito = 129 g; Calories = 285

Burrito Beef And Bean Frozen ☞ serving size: 1 burrito frozen = 139 g; Calories = 332

Burrito Beef And Bean Microwaved ☞ serving size: 1 burrito cooked = 116 g; Calories = 346

Burrito With Beans And Rice Meatless ☞ serving size: 1 small burrito = 182 g; Calories = 384

Burrito With Beans Meatless ☞ serving size: 1 small burrito = 170 g; Calories = 369

Burrito With Beans Rice And Sour Cream Meatless ☞ serving size: 1 small burrito = 208 g; Calories = 437

Burrito With Chicken ☞ serving size: 1 small burrito = 142 g; Calories = 344

Burrito With Chicken And Beans ☞ serving size: 1 small burrito = 153 g; Calories = 349

Burrito With Chicken And Sour Cream ☞ serving size: 1 small burrito = 162 g; Calories = 381

Burrito With Chicken Beans And Rice ☞ serving size: 1 small burrito = 165 g; Calories = 365

Burrito With Chicken Beans And Sour Cream ☞ serving size: 1 small burrito = 179 g; Calories = 401

Burrito With Chicken Beans Rice And Sour Cream ☞ serving size: 1 small burrito = 191 g; Calories = 416

Burrito With Meat ☞ serving size: 1 small burrito = 161 g; Calories = 390

Burrito With Meat And Beans ☞ serving size: 1 small burrito = 166 g; Calories = 380

Burrito With Meat And Sour Cream ☞ serving size: 1 small burrito = 187 g; Calories = 441

🥄 Burrito With Meat Beans And Rice 🐖 serving size: 1 small burrito = 177 g; Calories = 395

🥄 Burrito With Meat Beans And Sour Cream 🐖 serving size: 1 small burrito = 192 g; Calories = 432

🥄 Burrito With Meat Beans And Sour Cream From Fast Food 🐖 serving size: 1 small burrito = 192 g; Calories = 401

🥄 Burrito With Meat Beans Rice And Sour Cream 🐖 serving size: 1 small burrito = 203 g; Calories = 445

🥄 Cake Made With Glutinous Rice 🐖 serving size: 1 oz = 28 g; Calories = 77

🥄 Cake Made With Glutinous Rice And Dried Beans 🐖 serving size: 1 piece = 16 g; Calories = 30

🥄 Cake Or Pancake Made With Rice Flour And/or Dried Beans 🐖 serving size: 1 idli (2-1/4" dia) = 38 g; Calories = 49

🥄 Cannelloni Cheese- And Spinach-Filled No Sauce 🐖 serving size: 1 cannelloni = 74 g; Calories = 117

🥄 Cannelloni Cheese-Filled With Tomato Sauce Diet Frozen Meal 🐖 serving size: 1 meal (9.125 oz) = 259 g; Calories = 298

🥄 Cheese Enchilada Frozen Meal 🐖 serving size: 1 meal (10 oz) = 284 g; Calories = 537

🥄 Cheese Quiche Meatless 🐖 serving size: 1 piece (1/8 of 9" dia) = 192 g; Calories = 699

🥄 Cheese Turnover Puerto Rican Style 🐖 serving size: 1 turnover = 21 g; Calories = 88

🥄 Chicken Burritos Diet Frozen Meal 🐖 serving size: 1 meal (10 oz) = 284 g; Calories = 500

🥄 Chicken Chow Mein With Rice Diet Frozen Meal 🐖 serving size: 1 lean cuisine meal (11.25 oz) = 319 g; Calories = 290

Chicken Egg Foo Yung ☛ serving size: 1 patty = 86 g; Calories = 116

Chicken Enchilada Diet Frozen Meal ☛ serving size: 1 meal (8.5 oz) = 241 g; Calories = 352

Chicken Fajitas Diet Frozen Meal ☛ serving size: 1 meal (6.75 oz) = 191 g; Calories = 235

Chicken In Orange Sauce With Almond Rice Diet Frozen Meal ☛ serving size: 1 meal (8 oz) = 227 g; Calories = 302

Chicken In Soy-Based Sauce Rice And Vegetables Frozen Meal ☛ serving size: 1 meal (9 oz) = 255 g; Calories = 278

Chicken Nuggets Dark And White Meat Precooked Frozen Not Reheated ☛ serving size: 1 serving = 87 g; Calories = 233

Chicken Nuggets White Meat Precooked Frozen Not Reheated ☛ serving size: 1 serving = 82 g; Calories = 214

Chicken Or Turkey And Noodles With Soy-Based Sauce ☛ serving size: 1 cup = 224 g; Calories = 347

Chicken Or Turkey And Rice With Soy-Based Sauce ☛ serving size: 1 cup = 244 g; Calories = 390

Chicken Or Turkey And Vegetables Excluding Carrots Broccoli And Dark-Green Leafy; No Potatoes Soy-Based Sauce ☛ serving size: 1 cup = 217 g; Calories = 280

Chicken Or Turkey Chow Mein Or Chop Suey No Noodles ☛ serving size: 1 cup = 220 g; Calories = 183

Chicken Or Turkey Chow Mein Or Chop Suey With Noodles ☛ serving size: 1 cup = 220 g; Calories = 288

Chicken Or Turkey Rice And Vegetables Excluding Carrots Broccoli And Dark-Green Leafy; Soy-Based Sauce ☛ serving size: 1 cup = 217 g; Calories = 282

Chicken Or Turkey Rice And Vegetables Including Carrots Broccoli And/or Dark-Green Leafy; Soy-Based Sauce ☛ serving size: 1 cup = 217 g; Calories = 278

Chicken Or Turkey With Teriyaki ☛ serving size: 1 cup = 244 g; Calories = 398

Chicken Pot Pie Frozen Entree Prepared ☛ serving size: 1 pie = 302 g; Calories = 616

Chicken Tenders Breaded Frozen Prepared ☛ serving size: 1 piece = 21 g; Calories = 50

Chicken Thighs Frozen Breaded Reheated ☛ serving size: 1 thigh with bone and breading = 133 g; Calories = 444

Chilaquiles Tortilla Casserole With Salsa And Cheese No Egg ☛ serving size: 1 cup = 232 g; Calories = 694

Chilaquiles Tortilla Casserole With Salsa Cheese And Egg ☛ serving size: 1 cup = 232 g; Calories = 677

Chiles Rellenos Cheese-Filled ☛ serving size: 1 chili = 143 g; Calories = 313

Chiles Rellenos Filled With Meat And Cheese ☛ serving size: 1 chili = 143 g; Calories = 293

Chili Con Carne With Beans Canned Entree ☛ serving size: 1 cup = 242 g; Calories = 259

Chili No Beans Canned Entree ☛ serving size: 1 cup = 240 g; Calories = 283

Chili With Beans Microwavable Bowls ☛ serving size: 1 cup = 244 g; Calories = 244

Chimichanga Meatless ☛ serving size: 1 small chimichanga = 128 g; Calories = 288

Chimichanga Meatless With Sour Cream ☛ serving size: 1 small chimichanga = 136 g; Calories = 303

Chimichanga With Chicken ☛ serving size: 1 small chimichanga = 97 g; Calories = 264

Chimichanga With Chicken And Sour Cream ☛ serving size: 1 small chimichanga = 108 g; Calories = 287

Chimichanga With Meat ☛ serving size: 1 small chimichanga = 105 g; Calories = 273

Chimichanga With Meat And Sour Cream ☛ serving size: 1 small chimichanga = 92 g; Calories = 259

Chow Fun Noodles With Meat And Vegetables ☛ serving size: 1 cup = 152 g; Calories = 155

Chow Fun Noodles With Vegetables Meatless ☛ serving size: 1 cup = 152 g; Calories = 113

Chow Mein Or Chop Suey Meatless With Noodles ☛ serving size: 1 cup = 220 g; Calories = 257

Chow Mein Or Chop Suey Ns As To Type Of Meat No Noodles ☛ serving size: 1 cup = 220 g; Calories = 183

Chow Mein Or Chop Suey Ns As To Type Of Meat With Noodles ☛ serving size: 1 cup = 220 g; Calories = 288

Chow Mein Or Chop Suey Various Types Of Meat With Noodles ☛ serving size: 1 cup = 220 g; Calories = 297

Congee With Meat Poultry And/or Seafood ☛ serving size: 1 cup = 249 g; Calories = 132

Congee With Meat Poultry And/or Seafood And Vegetables ☛ serving size: 1 cup = 249 g; Calories = 130

Congee With Vegetables ☛ serving size: 1 cup = 249 g; Calories = 87

Corn Dogs Frozen Prepared ☛ serving size: 1 corndog = 78 g; Calories = 195

Cornmeal Dressing With Chicken Or Turkey And Vegetables ☞ serving size: 1 cup = 161 g; Calories = 380

Crepe Filled With Meat Poultry Or Seafood No Sauce ☞ serving size: 1 crepe with filling, any size = 125 g; Calories = 243

Crepe Filled With Meat Poultry Or Seafood With Sauce ☞ serving size: 1 crepe with filling, any size = 155 g; Calories = 285

Dirty Rice ☞ serving size: 1 cup = 198 g; Calories = 222

Dosa (Indian) With Filling ☞ serving size: 1 small = 113 g; Calories = 207

Dressing With Chicken Or Turkey And Vegetables ☞ serving size: 1 cup = 161 g; Calories = 349

Dressing With Meat And Vegetables ☞ serving size: 1 cup = 161 g; Calories = 420

Dressing With Oysters ☞ serving size: 1 cup = 161 g; Calories = 304

Dukboki Or Tteokbokki Korean ☞ serving size: 1 cup = 250 g; Calories = 330

Dumpling Fried Puerto Rican Style ☞ serving size: 1 small dumpling = 16 g; Calories = 59

Dumpling Meat-Filled ☞ serving size: 1 dumpling, any size = 97 g; Calories = 348

Dumpling Potato- Or Cheese-Filled Frozen ☞ serving size: 3 pieces pierogies = 114 g; Calories = 222

Dumpling Vegetable ☞ serving size: 1 dumpling, any size = 97 g; Calories = 159

Egg Foo Yung Nfs ☞ serving size: 1 patty = 86 g; Calories = 106

Egg Roll Meatless ☞ serving size: 1 miniature egg roll = 13 g; Calories = 35

Egg Roll With Beef And/or Pork ☛ serving size: 1 miniature roll = 13 g; Calories = 36

Egg Roll With Chicken Or Turkey ☛ serving size: 1 miniature egg roll = 13 g; Calories = 33

Egg Roll With Shrimp ☛ serving size: 1 miniature egg roll = 13 g; Calories = 35

Egg Rolls Chicken Refrigerated Heated ☛ serving size: 1 roll = 80 g; Calories = 158

Egg Rolls Pork Refrigerated Heated ☛ serving size: 1 roll = 85 g; Calories = 193

Egg Rolls Vegetable Frozen Prepared ☛ serving size: 1 egg roll = 68 g; Calories = 146

Empanada Mexican Turnover Filled With Cheese And Vegetables ☛ serving size: 1 small/appetizer = 81 g; Calories = 258

Empanada Mexican Turnover Filled With Chicken And Vegetables ☛ serving size: 1 small/appetizer = 81 g; Calories = 231

Enchilada Just Cheese Meatless No Beans Green-Chile Or Enchilada Sauce ☛ serving size: 1 enchilada, any size = 111 g; Calories = 210

Enchilada Just Cheese Meatless No Beans Red-Chile Or Enchilada Sauce ☛ serving size: 1 enchilada, any size = 119 g; Calories = 199

Enchilada With Beans Green-Chile Or Enchilada Sauce ☛ serving size: 1 enchilada, any size = 132 g; Calories = 195

Enchilada With Beans Meatless Red-Chile Or Enchilada Sauce ☛ serving size: 1 enchilada, any size = 141 g; Calories = 185

Enchilada With Chicken And Beans Green-Chile Or Enchilada Sauce ☛ serving size: 1 enchilada, any size = 132 g; Calories = 197

Enchilada With Chicken And Beans Red-Chile Or Enchilada Sauce ☛ serving size: 1 enchilada, any size = 132 g; Calories = 173

🥄 Enchilada With Chicken Green-Chile Or Enchilada Sauce 🐾 serving size: 1 enchilada, any size = 114 g; Calories = 171

🥄 Enchilada With Chicken Red-Chile Or Enchilada Sauce 🐾 serving size: 1 enchilada, any size = 123 g; Calories = 160

🥄 Enchilada With Meat And Beans Green-Chile Or Enchilada Sauce 🐾 serving size: 1 enchilada, any size = 123 g; Calories = 193

🥄 Enchilada With Meat And Beans Red-Chile Or Enchilada Sauce 🐾 serving size: 1 enchilada, any size = 132 g; Calories = 184

🥄 Enchilada With Meat Green-Chile Or Enchilada Sauce 🐾 serving size: 1 enchilada, any size = 114 g; Calories = 192

🥄 Enchilada With Meat Red-Chile Or Enchilada Sauce 🐾 serving size: 1 enchilada, any size = 122 g; Calories = 179

🥄 Fajita With Vegetables 🐾 serving size: 1 fajita = 141 g; Calories = 227

🥄 Fish And Vegetables Excluding Carrots Broccoli And Dark-Green Leafy; No Potatoes Soy-Based Sauce 🐾 serving size: 1 cup = 217 g; Calories = 221

🥄 Fish And Vegetables Including Carrots Broccoli And/or Dark-Green Leafy; No Potatoes Soy-Based Sauce 🐾 serving size: 1 cup = 217 g; Calories = 219

🥄 Flavored Pasta 🐾 serving size: 1 cup = 185 g; Calories = 161

🥄 Flavored Rice And Pasta Mixture 🐾 serving size: 1 cup, beef flavor = 184 g; Calories = 219

🥄 Flavored Rice And Pasta Mixture Reduced Sodium 🐾 serving size: 1 cup = 196 g; Calories = 220

🥄 Flavored Rice Brown And Wild 🐾 serving size: 1 cup = 217 g; Calories = 230

🥄 Flavored Rice Mixture 🐾 serving size: 1 cup = 218 g; Calories = 277

Flavored Rice Mixture With Cheese ☞ serving size: 1 cup = 230 g; Calories = 285

Fried Rice Puerto Rican Style ☞ serving size: 1 cup = 173 g; Calories = 206

Fried Stuffed Potatoes Puerto Rican Style ☞ serving size: 1 fritter (4" x 2-1/4" x 3/4") = 95 g; Calories = 178

Gnocchi Cheese ☞ serving size: 1 cup = 70 g; Calories = 125

Gnocchi Potato ☞ serving size: 1 cup = 188 g; Calories = 250

Gordita Sope Or Chalupa With Beans ☞ serving size: 1 small = 150 g; Calories = 314

Gordita Sope Or Chalupa With Beans And Sour Cream ☞ serving size: 1 small = 165 g; Calories = 343

Gordita Sope Or Chalupa With Chicken ☞ serving size: 1 small = 115 g; Calories = 285

Gordita Sope Or Chalupa With Chicken And Sour Cream ☞ serving size: 1 small = 124 g; Calories = 300

Gordita Sope Or Chalupa With Meat ☞ serving size: 1 small = 115 g; Calories = 288

Gordita Sope Or Chalupa With Meat And Sour Cream ☞ serving size: 1 small = 132 g; Calories = 326

Grape Leaves Stuffed With Rice ☞ serving size: 1 roll = 56 g; Calories = 91

Ground Beef With Tomato Sauce And Taco Seasonings On A Cornbread Crust ☞ serving size: 1 cup = 179 g; Calories = 347

Hopping John ☞ serving size: 1 cup = 224 g; Calories = 282

Hot Pockets Croissant Pockets Chicken Broccoli And Cheddar Stuffed Sandwich Frozen ☞ serving size: 1 serving (1 hot pocket) = 127 g; Calories = 299

Hot Pockets Ham N Cheese Stuffed Sandwich Frozen ☞ serving size: 1 serving (1 hot pocket) = 127 g; Calories = 343

Hot Pockets Meatballs & Mozzarella Stuffed Sandwich Frozen ☞ serving size: 1 hot pocket (1 nlea serving) = 127 g; Calories = 320

Hungry Man Salisbury Steak With Gravy Frozen Unprepared ☞ serving size: 1 patty = 64 g; Calories = 87

Jalapeno Pepper Stuffed With Cheese Breaded Or Battered Fried ☞ serving size: 1 jalapeno pepper = 25 g; Calories = 60

Jambalaya With Meat And Rice ☞ serving size: 1 cup = 244 g; Calories = 434

Jimmy Dean Sausage Egg And Cheese Breakfast Biscuit Frozen Unprepared ☞ serving size: 1 biscuit = 128 g; Calories = 420

Kishke Stuffed Derma ☞ serving size: 1 cubic inch, cooked = 18 g; Calories = 83

Knish Cheese ☞ serving size: 1 knish = 60 g; Calories = 205

Knish Meat ☞ serving size: 1 knish = 50 g; Calories = 175

Knish Potato ☞ serving size: 1 knish = 61 g; Calories = 213

Kung Pao Beef ☞ serving size: 1 cup = 162 g; Calories = 353

Kung Pao Pork ☞ serving size: 1 cup = 162 g; Calories = 358

Kung Pao Shrimp ☞ serving size: 1 cup = 162 g; Calories = 284

Lasagna Cheese Frozen Prepared ☞ serving size: 1 cup 1 serving = 225 g; Calories = 293

Lasagna Cheese Frozen Unprepared ☞ serving size: 1 cup 1 serving = 237 g; Calories = 344

Lasagna Meatless Spinach Noodles ☞ serving size: 1 piece (1/6 of 8" square, approx 2-1/2" x 4") = 227 g; Calories = 386

Lasagna Meatless Whole Wheat Noodles ☞ serving size: 1 piece (1/6 of 8" square, approx 2-1/2" x 4") = 227 g; Calories = 406

Lasagna Meatless With Vegetables ☞ serving size: 1 piece (1/6 of 8" square, approx 2-1/2" x 4") = 227 g; Calories = 402

Lasagna Vegetable Frozen Baked ☞ serving size: 1 serving = 227 g; Calories = 316

Lasagna With Cheese And Meat Sauce Diet Frozen Meal ☞ serving size: 1 weight watchers meal (11 oz) = 312 g; Calories = 368

Lasagna With Cheese And Sauce Diet Frozen Meal ☞ serving size: 1 meal (11 oz) = 312 g; Calories = 427

Lasagna With Chicken Or Turkey ☞ serving size: 1 piece (1/6 of 8" square, approx 2-1/2" x 4") = 206 g; Calories = 402

Lasagna With Chicken Or Turkey And Spinach ☞ serving size: 1 piece (1/6 of 8" square, approx 2-1/2" x 4") = 206 g; Calories = 394

Lasagna With Meat ☞ serving size: 1 piece (1/6 of 8" square, approx 2-1/2" x 4") = 206 g; Calories = 286

Lasagna With Meat & Sauce Frozen Entree ☞ serving size: 1 piece side = 134 g; Calories = 166

Lasagna With Meat & Sauce Low-Fat Frozen Entree ☞ serving size: 1 package = 309 g; Calories = 312

Lasagna With Meat And Spinach ☞ serving size: 1 piece (1/6 of 8" square, approx 2-1/2" x 4") = 206 g; Calories = 406

Lasagna With Meat Home Recipe ☞ serving size: 1 piece (1/6 of 8" square, approx 2-1/2" x 4") = 206 g; Calories = 404

Lasagna With Meat Sauce Frozen Prepared ☞ serving size: 1 piece side = 123 g; Calories = 166

Lasagna With Meat Spinach Noodles ☞ serving size: 1 piece (1/6 of 8" square, approx 2-1/2" x 4") = 206 g; Calories = 400

🥄 Lasagna With Meat Whole Wheat Noodles ☞ serving size: 1 piece (1/6 of 8" square, approx 2-1/2" x 4") = 206 g; Calories = 408

🥄 Lean Pockets Ham N Cheddar ☞ serving size: 1 hot pocket (1 nlea serving) = 127 g; Calories = 292

🥄 Lean Pockets Meatballs & Mozzarella ☞ serving size: 1 each = 128 g; Calories = 307

🥄 Lefse (Norwegian) ☞ serving size: 1 lefse, any size = 80 g; Calories = 173

🥄 Linguini With Vegetables And Seafood In White Wine Sauce Diet Frozen Meal ☞ serving size: 1 meal (9.5 oz) = 269 g; Calories = 307

🥄 Lo Mein With Beef ☞ serving size: 1 cup = 200 g; Calories = 258

🥄 Lo Mein With Chicken ☞ serving size: 1 cup = 200 g; Calories = 260

🥄 Lo Mein With Pork ☞ serving size: 1 cup = 200 g; Calories = 276

🥄 Lo Mein With Shrimp ☞ serving size: 1 cup = 200 g; Calories = 242

🥄 Macaroni And Cheese Box Mix With Cheese Sauce Prepared ☞ serving size: 1 cup prepared = 189 g; Calories = 310

🥄 Macaroni And Cheese Box Mix With Cheese Sauce Unprepared ☞ serving size: 1 serving (3.5 oz) = 25 g; Calories = 84

🥄 Macaroni And Cheese Canned Entree ☞ serving size: 1 serving = 244 g; Calories = 200

🥄 Macaroni And Cheese Canned Microwavable ☞ serving size: 7 (1/2) oz 1 serving = 213 g; Calories = 285

🥄 Macaroni And Cheese Diet Frozen Meal ☞ serving size: 1 meal (9 oz) = 255 g; Calories = 332

🥄 Macaroni And Cheese Dinner With Dry Sauce Mix Boxed Uncooked ☞ serving size: 1 serving (makes about 1 cup prepared) = 70 g; Calories = 265

Macaroni And Cheese Dry Mix Prepared With 2% Milk And 80% Stick Margarine From Dry Mix ☞ serving size: 1 cup = 198 g; Calories = 376

Macaroni And Cheese Frozen Entree ☞ serving size: 1 cup = 137 g; Calories = 204

Macaroni Or Noodles Creamed With Cheese ☞ serving size: 1 cup = 230 g; Calories = 361

Macaroni Or Noodles Creamed With Cheese And Tuna ☞ serving size: 1 cup = 230 g; Calories = 329

Macaroni Or Noodles With Cheese ☞ serving size: 1 cup = 230 g; Calories = 508

Macaroni Or Noodles With Cheese And Chicken Or Turkey ☞ serving size: 1 cup = 230 g; Calories = 405

Macaroni Or Noodles With Cheese And Egg ☞ serving size: 1 cup = 230 g; Calories = 430

Macaroni Or Noodles With Cheese And Frankfurters Or Hot Dogs ☞ serving size: 1 cup = 230 g; Calories = 488

Macaroni Or Noodles With Cheese And Meat ☞ serving size: 1 cup = 230 g; Calories = 481

Macaroni Or Noodles With Cheese And Meat Prepared From Hamburger Helper Mix ☞ serving size: 1 cup = 230 g; Calories = 331

Macaroni Or Noodles With Cheese And Tomato ☞ serving size: 1 cup = 230 g; Calories = 336

Macaroni Or Noodles With Cheese And Tuna ☞ serving size: 1 cup = 230 g; Calories = 373

Macaroni Or Noodles With Cheese Easy Mac Type ☞ serving size: 1 cup = 230 g; Calories = 253

Macaroni Or Noodles With Cheese Made From Packaged Mix ☛ serving size: 1 cup = 230 g; Calories = 407

Macaroni Or Noodles With Cheese Made From Reduced Fat Packaged Mix ☛ serving size: 1 cup = 230 g; Calories = 297

Macaroni Or Noodles With Cheese Made From Reduced Fat Packaged Mix Unprepared ☛ serving size: 1 serving (3.5 oz) = 99 g; Calories = 294

Macaroni Or Noodles With Cheese Microwaveable Unprepared ☛ serving size: 1 serving 1 pouch = 61 g; Calories = 237

Macaroni Or Pasta Salad Made With Any Type Of Fat Free Dressing ☛ serving size: 1 cup = 204 g; Calories = 273

Macaroni Or Pasta Salad Made With Creamy Dressing ☛ serving size: 1 cup = 204 g; Calories = 316

Macaroni Or Pasta Salad Made With Italian Dressing ☛ serving size: 1 cup = 204 g; Calories = 269

Macaroni Or Pasta Salad Made With Light Creamy Dressing ☛ serving size: 1 cup = 204 g; Calories = 249

Macaroni Or Pasta Salad Made With Light Italian Dressing ☛ serving size: 1 cup = 204 g; Calories = 235

Macaroni Or Pasta Salad Made With Light Mayonnaise ☛ serving size: 1 cup = 204 g; Calories = 324

Macaroni Or Pasta Salad Made With Light Mayonnaise-Type Salad Dressing ☛ serving size: 1 cup = 204 g; Calories = 324

Macaroni Or Pasta Salad Made With Mayonnaise ☛ serving size: 1 cup = 204 g; Calories = 451

Macaroni Or Pasta Salad Made With Mayonnaise-Type Salad Dressing ☛ serving size: 1 cup = 204 g; Calories = 326

Macaroni Or Pasta Salad With Cheese ☛ serving size: 1 cup = 204 g; Calories = 500

Macaroni Or Pasta Salad With Chicken ☛ serving size: 1 cup = 204 g; Calories = 435

Macaroni Or Pasta Salad With Crab Meat ☛ serving size: 1 cup = 204 g; Calories = 408

Macaroni Or Pasta Salad With Egg ☛ serving size: 1 cup = 204 g; Calories = 439

Macaroni Or Pasta Salad With Meat ☛ serving size: 1 cup = 204 g; Calories = 430

Macaroni Or Pasta Salad With Shrimp ☛ serving size: 1 cup = 204 g; Calories = 416

Macaroni Or Pasta Salad With Tuna ☛ serving size: 1 cup = 204 g; Calories = 410

Macaroni Or Pasta Salad With Tuna And Egg ☛ serving size: 1 cup = 204 g; Calories = 402

Macaroni With Tuna Puerto Rican Style ☛ serving size: 1 cup = 225 g; Calories = 331

Manicotti Cheese-Filled No Sauce ☛ serving size: 1 manicotti = 127 g; Calories = 269

Manicotti Cheese-Filled With Meat Sauce ☛ serving size: 1 manicotti = 143 g; Calories = 235

Manicotti Cheese-Filled With Tomato Sauce Diet Frozen Meal ☛ serving size: 1 meal (9.25 oz) = 262 g; Calories = 322

Manicotti Cheese-Filled With Tomato Sauce Meatless ☛ serving size: 1 manicotti = 143 g; Calories = 225

Manicotti Vegetable- And Cheese-Filled With Tomato Sauce Meatless ☛ serving size: 1 manicotti = 143 g; Calories = 196

Meat Pie Puerto Rican Style ☛ serving size: 1 pie (9" dia) = 1110 g;

Calories = 5273

🥄 Meat Turnover Puerto Rican Style ☛ serving size: 1 turnover = 28 g; Calories = 72

🥄 Mexican Casserole Made With Ground Beef Beans Tomato Sauce Cheese Taco Seasonings And Corn Chips ☛ serving size: 1 cup = 144 g; Calories = 337

🥄 Mexican Casserole Made With Ground Beef Tomato Sauce Cheese Taco Seasonings And Corn Chips ☛ serving size: 1 cup = 144 g; Calories = 386

🥄 Moo Goo Gai Pan ☛ serving size: 1 cup = 216 g; Calories = 160

🥄 Moo Shu Pork Without Chinese Pancake ☛ serving size: 1 cup = 151 g; Calories = 228

🥄 Nachos With Cheese And Sour Cream ☛ serving size: 1 nacho = 7 g; Calories = 16

🥄 Nachos With Chicken And Cheese ☛ serving size: 1 nacho = 7 g; Calories = 15

🥄 Nachos With Chicken Cheese And Sour Cream ☛ serving size: 1 nacho = 7 g; Calories = 15

🥄 Nachos With Chili ☛ serving size: 1 nacho = 7 g; Calories = 18

🥄 Nachos With Meat And Cheese ☛ serving size: 1 nacho = 7 g; Calories = 17

🥄 Nachos With Meat Cheese And Sour Cream ☛ serving size: 1 nacho = 7 g; Calories = 15

🥄 Noodle Pudding ☛ serving size: 1 cup = 144 g; Calories = 301

🥄 Noodles With Vegetables In Tomato-Based Sauce Diet Frozen Meal ☛ serving size: 1 meal (10 oz) = 284 g; Calories = 187

🥄 Pad Thai Meatless ☛ serving size: 1 cup = 200 g; Calories = 328

Pad Thai Nfs ☛ serving size: 1 cup = 200 g; Calories = 306

Pad Thai With Chicken ☛ serving size: 1 cup = 200 g; Calories = 306

Pad Thai With Meat ☛ serving size: 1 cup = 200 g; Calories = 316

Pad Thai With Seafood ☛ serving size: 1 cup = 200 g; Calories = 290

Paella Nfs ☛ serving size: 1 cup = 240 g; Calories = 401

Paella With Meat Valenciana Style ☛ serving size: 1 cup, with bone (yield after bone removed) = 137 g; Calories = 370

Paella With Seafood ☛ serving size: 1 cup = 240 g; Calories = 341

Pasta Meat-Filled With Gravy Canned ☛ serving size: 1 cup = 250 g; Calories = 328

Pasta Mix Classic Beef Unprepared ☛ serving size: 1 package = 122 g; Calories = 432

Pasta Mix Classic Cheeseburger Macaroni Unprepared ☛ serving size: 1 package = 123 g; Calories = 429

Pasta Mix Italian Four Cheese Lasagna Unprepared ☛ serving size: 1 package = 117 g; Calories = 415

Pasta Mix Italian Lasagna Unprepared ☛ serving size: 1 package = 141 g; Calories = 502

Pasta Whole Grain With Cream Sauce And Added Vegetables Home Recipe ☛ serving size: 1 cup = 250 g; Calories = 335

Pasta Whole Grain With Cream Sauce And Added Vegetables Ready-To-Heat ☛ serving size: 1 cup = 250 g; Calories = 368

Pasta Whole Grain With Cream Sauce And Added Vegetables Restaurant ☛ serving size: 1 cup = 250 g; Calories = 460

Pasta Whole Grain With Cream Sauce And Meat Home Recipe ☞ serving size: 1 cup = 250 g; Calories = 395

Pasta Whole Grain With Cream Sauce And Meat Ready-To-Heat ☞ serving size: 1 cup = 250 g; Calories = 428

Pasta Whole Grain With Cream Sauce And Meat Restaurant ☞ serving size: 1 cup = 250 g; Calories = 518

Pasta Whole Grain With Cream Sauce And Poultry Home Recipe ☞ serving size: 1 cup = 250 g; Calories = 375

Pasta Whole Grain With Cream Sauce And Poultry Ready-To-Heat ☞ serving size: 1 cup = 250 g; Calories = 408

Pasta Whole Grain With Cream Sauce And Poultry Restaurant ☞ serving size: 1 cup = 250 g; Calories = 498

Pasta Whole Grain With Cream Sauce And Seafood Home Recipe ☞ serving size: 1 cup = 250 g; Calories = 365

Pasta Whole Grain With Cream Sauce And Seafood Ready-To-Heat ☞ serving size: 1 cup = 250 g; Calories = 398

Pasta Whole Grain With Cream Sauce And Seafood Restaurant ☞ serving size: 1 cup = 250 g; Calories = 488

Pasta Whole Grain With Cream Sauce Home Recipe ☞ serving size: 1 cup = 250 g; Calories = 370

Pasta Whole Grain With Cream Sauce Meat And Added Vegetables Home Recipe ☞ serving size: 1 cup = 250 g; Calories = 368

Pasta Whole Grain With Cream Sauce Meat And Added Vegetables Ready-To-Heat ☞ serving size: 1 cup = 250 g; Calories = 400

Pasta Whole Grain With Cream Sauce Meat And Added Vegetables Restaurant ☞ serving size: 1 cup = 250 g; Calories = 490

Pasta Whole Grain With Cream Sauce Poultry And Added Vegetables Home Recipe ☞ serving size: 1 cup = 250 g; Calories = 348

Pasta Whole Grain With Cream Sauce Poultry And Added Vegetables Ready-To-Heat ☛ serving size: 1 cup = 250 g; Calories = 380

Pasta Whole Grain With Cream Sauce Poultry And Added Vegetables Restaurant ☛ serving size: 1 cup = 250 g; Calories = 473

Pasta Whole Grain With Cream Sauce Ready-To-Heat ☛ serving size: 1 cup = 250 g; Calories = 403

Pasta Whole Grain With Cream Sauce Restaurant ☛ serving size: 1 cup = 250 g; Calories = 493

Pasta Whole Grain With Cream Sauce Seafood And Added Vegetables Home Recipe ☛ serving size: 1 cup = 250 g; Calories = 335

Pasta Whole Grain With Cream Sauce Seafood And Added Vegetables Ready-To-Heat ☛ serving size: 1 cup = 250 g; Calories = 370

Pasta Whole Grain With Cream Sauce Seafood And Added Vegetables Restaurant ☛ serving size: 1 cup = 250 g; Calories = 463

Pasta Whole Grain With Tomato-Based Sauce And Added Vegetables Home Recipe ☛ serving size: 1 cup = 250 g; Calories = 245

Pasta Whole Grain With Tomato-Based Sauce And Added Vegetables Ready-To-Heat ☛ serving size: 1 cup = 250 g; Calories = 280

Pasta Whole Grain With Tomato-Based Sauce And Added Vegetables Restaurant ☛ serving size: 1 cup = 250 g; Calories = 380

Pasta Whole Grain With Tomato-Based Sauce And Meat Home Recipe ☛ serving size: 1 cup = 250 g; Calories = 300

Pasta Whole Grain With Tomato-Based Sauce And Meat Ready-To-Heat ☛ serving size: 1 cup = 250 g; Calories = 335

Pasta Whole Grain With Tomato-Based Sauce And Meat Restaurant ☛ serving size: 1 cup = 250 g; Calories = 430

Pasta Whole Grain With Tomato-Based Sauce And Poultry Home Recipe ☛ serving size: 1 cup = 250 g; Calories = 280

Pasta Whole Grain With Tomato-Based Sauce And Poultry Ready-To-Heat ☛ serving size: 1 cup = 250 g; Calories = 315

Pasta Whole Grain With Tomato-Based Sauce And Poultry Restaurant ☛ serving size: 1 cup = 250 g; Calories = 413

Pasta Whole Grain With Tomato-Based Sauce And Seafood Home Recipe ☛ serving size: 1 cup = 250 g; Calories = 270

Pasta Whole Grain With Tomato-Based Sauce And Seafood Ready-To-Heat ☛ serving size: 1 cup = 250 g; Calories = 303

Pasta Whole Grain With Tomato-Based Sauce And Seafood Restaurant ☛ serving size: 1 cup = 250 g; Calories = 403

Pasta Whole Grain With Tomato-Based Sauce Home Recipe ☛ serving size: 1 cup = 250 g; Calories = 253

Pasta Whole Grain With Tomato-Based Sauce Meat And Added Vegetables Home Recipe ☛ serving size: 1 cup = 250 g; Calories = 295

Pasta Whole Grain With Tomato-Based Sauce Meat And Added Vegetables Ready-To-Heat ☛ serving size: 1 cup = 250 g; Calories = 328

Pasta Whole Grain With Tomato-Based Sauce Meat And Added Vegetables Restaurant ☛ serving size: 1 cup = 250 g; Calories = 425

Pasta Whole Grain With Tomato-Based Sauce Poultry And Added Vegetables Home Recipe ☛ serving size: 1 cup = 250 g; Calories = 275

Pasta Whole Grain With Tomato-Based Sauce Poultry And Added Vegetables Ready-To-Heat ☛ serving size: 1 cup = 250 g; Calories = 310

Pasta Whole Grain With Tomato-Based Sauce Poultry And Added Vegetables Restaurant ☛ serving size: 1 cup = 250 g; Calories = 408

Pasta Whole Grain With Tomato-Based Sauce Ready-To-Heat ☛ serving size: 1 cup = 250 g; Calories = 288

Pasta Whole Grain With Tomato-Based Sauce Restaurant ☛ serving size: 1 cup = 250 g; Calories = 388

Pasta Whole Grain With Tomato-Based Sauce Seafood And Added Vegetables Home Recipe ☛ serving size: 1 cup = 250 g; Calories = 263

Pasta Whole Grain With Tomato-Based Sauce Seafood And Added Vegetables Ready-To-Heat ☛ serving size: 1 cup = 250 g; Calories = 298

Pasta Whole Grain With Tomato-Based Sauce Seafood And Added Vegetables Restaurant ☛ serving size: 1 cup = 250 g; Calories = 395

Pasta With Cream Sauce And Added Vegetables From Home Recipe ☛ serving size: 1 cup = 250 g; Calories = 348

Pasta With Cream Sauce And Added Vegetables Ready-To-Heat ☛ serving size: 1 cup = 250 g; Calories = 380

Pasta With Cream Sauce And Added Vegetables Restaurant ☛ serving size: 1 cup = 250 g; Calories = 473

Pasta With Cream Sauce And Meat Home Recipe ☛ serving size: 1 cup = 250 g; Calories = 408

Pasta With Cream Sauce And Meat Ready-To-Heat ☛ serving size: 1 cup = 250 g; Calories = 440

Pasta With Cream Sauce And Meat Restaurant ☛ serving size: 1 cup = 250 g; Calories = 528

Pasta With Cream Sauce And Poultry Home Recipe ☛ serving size: 1 cup = 250 g; Calories = 388

Pasta With Cream Sauce And Poultry Ready-To-Heat ☛ serving size: 1 cup = 250 g; Calories = 420

Pasta With Cream Sauce And Poultry Restaurant ☛ serving size: 1 cup = 250 g; Calories = 510

Pasta With Cream Sauce And Seafood Home Recipe ☛ serving size: 1 cup = 250 g; Calories = 375

Pasta With Cream Sauce And Seafood Ready-To-Heat ☛ serving size: 1 cup = 250 g; Calories = 408

Pasta With Cream Sauce And Seafood Restaurant ☛ serving size: 1 cup = 250 g; Calories = 498

Pasta With Cream Sauce Home Recipe ☛ serving size: 1 cup = 250 g; Calories = 383

Pasta With Cream Sauce Meat And Added Vegetables Home Recipe ☛ serving size: 1 cup = 250 g; Calories = 380

Pasta With Cream Sauce Meat And Added Vegetables Ready-To-Heat ☛ serving size: 1 cup = 250 g; Calories = 410

Pasta With Cream Sauce Meat And Added Vegetables Restaurant ☛ serving size: 1 cup = 250 g; Calories = 503

Pasta With Cream Sauce Poultry And Added Vegetables Home Recipe ☛ serving size: 1 cup = 250 g; Calories = 360

Pasta With Cream Sauce Poultry And Added Vegetables Ready-To-Heat ☛ serving size: 1 cup = 250 g; Calories = 393

Pasta With Cream Sauce Poultry And Added Vegetables Restaurant ☛ serving size: 1 cup = 250 g; Calories = 483

Pasta With Cream Sauce Ready-To-Heat ☛ serving size: 1 cup = 250 g; Calories = 415

Pasta With Cream Sauce Restaurant ☛ serving size: 1 cup = 250 g; Calories = 505

Pasta With Cream Sauce Seafood And Added Vegetables Home Recipe ☛ serving size: 1 cup = 250 g; Calories = 348

Pasta With Cream Sauce Seafood And Added Vegetables Ready-To-Heat ☛ serving size: 1 cup = 250 g; Calories = 380

Pasta With Cream Sauce Seafood And Added Vegetables Restaurant ☛ serving size: 1 cup = 250 g; Calories = 473

Pasta With Sauce And Meat From School Lunch ☛ serving size: 1 cup = 250 g; Calories = 293

Pasta With Sauce Meatless School Lunch ☛ serving size: 1 cup = 250 g; Calories = 255

Pasta With Sauce Nfs ☛ serving size: 1 cup = 250 g; Calories = 313

Pasta With Sliced Franks In Tomato Sauce Canned Entree ☛ serving size: 1 serving (1 cup) = 252 g; Calories = 227

Pasta With Tomato Sauce No Meat Canned ☛ serving size: 1 serving (1 nlea serving) = 252 g; Calories = 179

Pasta With Tomato-Based Sauce And Added Vegetables Home Recipe ☛ serving size: 1 cup = 250 g; Calories = 258

Pasta With Tomato-Based Sauce And Added Vegetables Ready-To-Heat ☛ serving size: 1 cup = 250 g; Calories = 293

Pasta With Tomato-Based Sauce And Added Vegetables Restaurant ☛ serving size: 1 cup = 250 g; Calories = 390

Pasta With Tomato-Based Sauce And Beans Or Lentils ☛ serving size: 1 cup = 227 g; Calories = 284

Pasta With Tomato-Based Sauce And Cheese ☛ serving size: 1 cup = 250 g; Calories = 295

Pasta With Tomato-Based Sauce And Meat Home Recipe ☛ serving size: 1 cup = 250 g; Calories = 313

Pasta With Tomato-Based Sauce And Meat Ready-To-Heat ☛ serving size: 1 cup = 250 g; Calories = 345

Pasta With Tomato-Based Sauce And Meat Restaurant ☛ serving size: 1 cup = 250 g; Calories = 443

Pasta With Tomato-Based Sauce And Poultry Home Recipe ☛ serving size: 1 cup = 250 g; Calories = 293

🔑 Pasta With Tomato-Based Sauce And Poultry Ready-To-Heat ☛ serving size: 1 cup = 250 g; Calories = 328

🔑 Pasta With Tomato-Based Sauce And Poultry Restaurant ☛ serving size: 1 cup = 250 g; Calories = 423

🔑 Pasta With Tomato-Based Sauce And Seafood Home Recipe ☛ serving size: 1 cup = 250 g; Calories = 280

🔑 Pasta With Tomato-Based Sauce And Seafood Ready-To-Heat ☛ serving size: 1 cup = 250 g; Calories = 315

🔑 Pasta With Tomato-Based Sauce And Seafood Restaurant ☛ serving size: 1 cup = 250 g; Calories = 413

🔑 Pasta With Tomato-Based Sauce Cheese And Meat ☛ serving size: 1 cannelloni = 86 g; Calories = 128

🔑 Pasta With Tomato-Based Sauce Home Recipe ☛ serving size: 1 cup = 250 g; Calories = 265

🔑 Pasta With Tomato-Based Sauce Meat And Added Vegetables Home Recipe ☛ serving size: 1 cup = 250 g; Calories = 308

🔑 Pasta With Tomato-Based Sauce Meat And Added Vegetables Ready-To-Heat ☛ serving size: 1 cup = 250 g; Calories = 340

🔑 Pasta With Tomato-Based Sauce Meat And Added Vegetables Restaurant ☛ serving size: 1 cup = 250 g; Calories = 435

🔑 Pasta With Tomato-Based Sauce Poultry And Added Vegetables Home Recipe ☛ serving size: 1 cup = 250 g; Calories = 288

🔑 Pasta With Tomato-Based Sauce Poultry And Added Vegetables Ready-To-Heat ☛ serving size: 1 cup = 250 g; Calories = 320

🔑 Pasta With Tomato-Based Sauce Poultry And Added Vegetables Restaurant ☛ serving size: 1 cup = 250 g; Calories = 418

🔑 Pasta With Tomato-Based Sauce Ready-To-Heat ☛ serving size: 1 cup = 250 g; Calories = 300

Pasta With Tomato-Based Sauce Restaurant ☞ serving size: 1 cup = 250 g; Calories = 398

Pasta With Tomato-Based Sauce Seafood And Added Vegetables Home Recipe ☞ serving size: 1 cup = 250 g; Calories = 275

Pasta With Tomato-Based Sauce Seafood And Added Vegetables Ready-To-Heat ☞ serving size: 1 cup = 250 g; Calories = 310

Pasta With Tomato-Based Sauce Seafood And Added Vegetables Restaurant ☞ serving size: 1 cup = 250 g; Calories = 408

Pasta With Vegetables No Sauce Or Dressing ☞ serving size: 1 cup = 150 g; Calories = 215

Pastry Egg And Cheese Filled ☞ serving size: 1 kolache = 142 g; Calories = 487

Pastry Filled With Potatoes And Peas Fried ☞ serving size: 1 miniature samosa = 9 g; Calories = 28

Pastry Meat / Poultry-Filled ☞ serving size: 1 kolache = 85 g; Calories = 287

Pizza Rolls Frozen Unprepared ☞ serving size: 1 serving 6 rolls = 80 g; Calories = 262

Pork And Onions With Soy-Based Sauce ☞ serving size: 1 cup = 256 g; Calories = 376

Pork And Vegetables Excluding Carrots Broccoli And Dark- Green Leafy; No Potatoes Soy-Based Sauce ☞ serving size: 1 cup = 217 g; Calories = 315

Pork And Vegetables Hawaiian Style ☞ serving size: 1 cup = 252 g; Calories = 227

Pork And Vegetables Including Carrots Broccoli And/or Dark- Green Leafy; No Potatoes Soy-Based Sauce ☞ serving size: 1 cup = 217 g; Calories = 308

Pork And Watercress With Soy-Based Sauce ☞ serving size: 1 cup = 162 g; Calories = 232

Pork Chow Mein Or Chop Suey No Noodles ☞ serving size: 1 cup = 220 g; Calories = 216

Pork Chow Mein Or Chop Suey With Noodles ☞ serving size: 1 cup = 220 g; Calories = 317

Pork Egg Foo Yung ☞ serving size: 1 patty = 86 g; Calories = 126

Pork Or Ham With Soy-Based Sauce ☞ serving size: 1 cup = 244 g; Calories = 456

Pork Rice And Vegetables Excluding Carrots Broccoli And Dark-Green Leafy; Soy-Based Sauce ☞ serving size: 1 cup = 217 g; Calories = 313

Pork Rice And Vegetables Including Carrots Broccoli And/or Dark-Green Leafy; Soy-Based Sauce ☞ serving size: 1 cup = 217 g; Calories = 308

Pork Tofu And Vegetables Excluding Carrots Broccoli And Dark-Green Leafy; No Potatoes Soy-Based Sauce ☞ serving size: 1 cup = 217 g; Calories = 247

Pork Tofu And Vegetables Including Carrots Broccoli And/or Dark-Green Leafy; No Potatoes Soy-Base Sauce ☞ serving size: 1 cup = 217 g; Calories = 245

Potato And Ham Fritters Puerto Rican Style ☞ serving size: 1 fritter (2-3/4" x 2-1/2" x 1") = 70 g; Calories = 137

Potato From Puerto Rican Beef Stew With Gravy ☞ serving size: 1 small = 122 g; Calories = 90

Potato From Puerto Rican Chicken Fricassee With Sauce ☞ serving size: 1 small = 123 g; Calories = 89

Potato From Puerto Rican Style Stuffed Pot Roast With Gravy ☞ serving size: 1 small = 103 g; Calories = 76

Potato Mashed From Dry Mix Made With Milk ☛ serving size: 1 cup = 250 g; Calories = 283

Potato Mashed From Dry Mix Made With Milk With Cheese ☛ serving size: 1 cup = 250 g; Calories = 360

Potato Mashed From Dry Mix Made With Milk With Gravy ☛ serving size: 1 cup = 250 g; Calories = 250

Potato Mashed From Dry Mix Nfs ☛ serving size: 1 cup = 250 g; Calories = 283

Potato Mashed From Fast Food With Gravy ☛ serving size: 1 cup = 250 g; Calories = 203

Potato Mashed From Fresh Made With Milk ☛ serving size: 1 cup = 250 g; Calories = 278

Potato Mashed From Fresh Made With Milk With Cheese ☛ serving size: 1 cup = 250 g; Calories = 358

Potato Mashed From Fresh Made With Milk With Gravy ☛ serving size: 1 cup = 250 g; Calories = 248

Potato Mashed From Fresh Nfs ☛ serving size: 1 cup = 250 g; Calories = 278

Potato Mashed From Restaurant ☛ serving size: 1 cup = 250 g; Calories = 335

Potato Mashed From Restaurant With Gravy ☛ serving size: 1 cup = 250 g; Calories = 293

Potato Mashed From School Lunch ☛ serving size: 1 cup = 250 g; Calories = 190

Potato Mashed Nfs ☛ serving size: 1 cup = 250 g; Calories = 278

Potato Mashed Ready-To-Heat With Cheese ☛ serving size: 1 cup = 250 g; Calories = 345

Potato Mashed Ready-To-Heat With Gravy ☞ serving size: 1 cup = 250 g; Calories = 235

Potato Pancake ☞ serving size: 1 miniature/bite size pancake = 10 g; Calories = 19

Potato Pudding ☞ serving size: 1 cup = 228 g; Calories = 287

Potato Salad From Restaurant ☞ serving size: 1 cup = 275 g; Calories = 476

Potato Salad German Style ☞ serving size: 1 cup = 175 g; Calories = 182

Potato Salad Made With Any Type Of Fat Free Dressing ☞ serving size: 1 cup = 275 g; Calories = 223

Potato Salad Made With Creamy Dressing ☞ serving size: 1 cup = 275 g; Calories = 385

Potato Salad Made With Italian Dressing ☞ serving size: 1 cup = 275 g; Calories = 297

Potato Salad Made With Light Creamy Dressing ☞ serving size: 1 cup = 275 g; Calories = 261

Potato Salad Made With Light Italian Dressing ☞ serving size: 1 cup = 275 g; Calories = 234

Potato Salad Made With Light Mayonnaise ☞ serving size: 1 cup = 275 g; Calories = 289

Potato Salad Made With Light Mayonnaise-Type Salad Dressing ☞ serving size: 1 cup = 275 g; Calories = 289

Potato Salad Made With Mayonnaise ☞ serving size: 1 cup = 275 g; Calories = 462

Potato Salad Made With Mayonnaise-Type Salad Dressing ☞ serving size: 1 cup = 275 g; Calories = 294

Potato Salad With Egg ☞ serving size: 1/2 cup = 125 g; Calories =

196

Potato Salad With Egg From Restaurant ☛ serving size: 1 cup = 275 g; Calories = 470

Potato Salad With Egg Made With Any Type Of Fat Free Dressing ☛ serving size: 1 cup = 275 g; Calories = 245

Potato Salad With Egg Made With Creamy Dressing ☛ serving size: 1 cup = 275 g; Calories = 391

Potato Salad With Egg Made With Italian Dressing ☛ serving size: 1 cup = 275 g; Calories = 314

Potato Salad With Egg Made With Light Creamy Dressing ☛ serving size: 1 cup = 275 g; Calories = 281

Potato Salad With Egg Made With Light Italian Dressing ☛ serving size: 1 cup = 275 g; Calories = 259

Potato Salad With Egg Made With Light Mayonnaise ☛ serving size: 1 cup = 275 g; Calories = 305

Potato Salad With Egg Made With Light Mayonnaise-Type Salad Dressing ☛ serving size: 1 cup = 275 g; Calories = 305

Potato Salad With Egg Made With Mayonnaise-Type Salad Dressing ☛ serving size: 1 cup = 275 g; Calories = 308

Potato Scalloped From Dry Mix ☛ serving size: 1 cup = 250 g; Calories = 418

Potato Scalloped From Dry Mix With Meat ☛ serving size: 1 cup = 250 g; Calories = 418

Potato Scalloped From Fast Food Or Restaurant ☛ serving size: 1 cup = 250 g; Calories = 503

Potato Scalloped From Fresh ☛ serving size: 1 cup = 250 g; Calories = 415

Potato Scalloped From Fresh With Meat ☛ serving size: 1 cup =

250 g; Calories = 433

Potato Scalloped Nfs ☞ serving size: 1 cup = 250 g; Calories = 415

Potato Scalloped Ready-To-Heat ☞ serving size: 1 cup = 250 g; Calories = 438

Potato Scalloped Ready-To-Heat With Meat ☞ serving size: 1 cup = 250 g; Calories = 453

Potsticker Or Wonton Pork And Vegetable Frozen Unprepared ☞ serving size: 5 pieces 1 serving = 145 g; Calories = 197

Puffs Fried Crab Meat And Cream Cheese Filled ☞ serving size: 1 puff = 23 g; Calories = 73

Pulled Pork In Barbecue Sauce ☞ serving size: 1 cup = 249 g; Calories = 418

Pupusa Bean-Filled ☞ serving size: 1 pupusa (about 5" dia) = 126 g; Calories = 228

Quesadilla Just Cheese From Fast Food ☞ serving size: 1 slice or wedge = 18 g; Calories = 62

Quesadilla Just Cheese Meatless ☞ serving size: 1 slice or wedge = 18 g; Calories = 62

Quesadilla With Meat ☞ serving size: 1 slice or wedge = 20 g; Calories = 65

Quesadilla With Vegetables ☞ serving size: 1 slice or wedge = 20 g; Calories = 61

Quesadilla With Vegetables And Chicken ☞ serving size: 1 slice or wedge = 20 g; Calories = 63

Quesadilla With Vegetables And Meat ☞ serving size: 1 slice or wedge = 20 g; Calories = 63

Quiche With Meat Poultry Or Fish ☞ serving size: 1 piece (1/8 of 9" dia) = 192 g; Calories = 741

Ravioli Cheese And Spinach Filled With Tomato Sauce ☛ serving size: 1 piece = 38 g; Calories = 45

Ravioli Cheese And Spinach-Filled No Sauce ☛ serving size: 1 piece = 15 g; Calories = 23

Ravioli Cheese And Spinach-Filled With Cream Sauce ☛ serving size: 1 piece = 38 g; Calories = 55

Ravioli Cheese With Tomato Sauce Frozen Not Prepared Includes Regular And Light Entrees ☛ serving size: 1 cup = 159 g; Calories = 177

Ravioli Cheese-Filled Canned ☛ serving size: 1 cup = 242 g; Calories = 186

Ravioli Cheese-Filled No Sauce ☛ serving size: 1 piece = 15 g; Calories = 27

Ravioli Cheese-Filled With Cream Sauce ☛ serving size: 1 piece = 38 g; Calories = 62

Ravioli Cheese-Filled With Meat Sauce ☛ serving size: 1 piece = 35 g; Calories = 49

Ravioli Cheese-Filled With Tomato Sauce ☛ serving size: 1 piece = 38 g; Calories = 37

Ravioli Cheese-Filled With Tomato Sauce Diet Frozen Meal ☛ serving size: 1 meal (9 oz) = 255 g; Calories = 286

Ravioli Meat-Filled No Sauce ☛ serving size: 1 piece = 15 g; Calories = 28

Ravioli Meat-Filled With Cream Sauce ☛ serving size: 1 piece = 35 g; Calories = 61

Ravioli Meat-Filled With Tomato Sauce Or Meat Sauce ☛ serving size: 1 piece = 35 g; Calories = 52

Ravioli Meat-Filled With Tomato Sauce Or Meat Sauce Canned ☛ serving size: 1 cup = 262 g; Calories = 254

Ravioli Ns As To Filling No Sauce ☞ serving size: 1 piece = 15 g; Calories = 28

Ravioli Ns As To Filling With Cream Sauce ☞ serving size: 1 piece = 38 g; Calories = 65

Ravioli Ns As To Filling With Tomato Sauce ☞ serving size: 1 piece = 38 g; Calories = 53

Red Beans And Rice ☞ serving size: 1 cup = 224 g; Calories = 408

Rice And Vermicelli Mix Beef Flavor Prepared With 80% Margarine ☞ serving size: 1 cup = 247 g; Calories = 319

Rice And Vermicelli Mix Beef Flavor Unprepared ☞ serving size: 1/ 3 cup = 61 g; Calories = 219

Rice And Vermicelli Mix Chicken Flavor Prepared With 80% Margarine ☞ serving size: 1 cup = 233 g; Calories = 317

Rice And Vermicelli Mix Chicken Flavor Unprepared ☞ serving size: 1/ 3 cup = 56 g; Calories = 199

Rice And Vermicelli Mix Rice Pilaf Flavor Prepared With 80% Margarine ☞ serving size: 1 cup = 238 g; Calories = 352

Rice And Vermicelli Mix Rice Pilaf Flavor Unprepared ☞ serving size: 1/ 3 cup = 68 g; Calories = 244

Rice Bowl With Chicken Frozen Entree Prepared (Includes Fried Teriyaki And Sweet And Sour Varieties) ☞ serving size: 1 bowl = 340 g; Calories = 428

Rice Brown With Beans ☞ serving size: 1 cup = 239 g; Calories = 361

Rice Brown With Beans And Tomatoes ☞ serving size: 1 cup = 239 g; Calories = 292

Rice Brown With Carrots And Dark Green Vegetables Fat Added In Cooking ☞ serving size: 1 cup = 189 g; Calories = 223

Rice Brown With Carrots And Dark Green Vegetables Fat Not Added In Cooking ☞ serving size: 1 cup = 186 g; Calories = 193

Rice Brown With Carrots And Dark Green Vegetables Ns As To Fat Added In Cooking ☞ serving size: 1 cup = 189 g; Calories = 223

Rice Brown With Carrots And Tomatoes And/or Tomato-Based Sauce Fat Added In Cooking ☞ serving size: 1 cup = 229 g; Calories = 254

Rice Brown With Carrots And Tomatoes And/or Tomato-Based Sauce Fat Not Added In Cooking ☞ serving size: 1 cup = 225 g; Calories = 218

Rice Brown With Carrots And Tomatoes And/or Tomato-Based Sauce Ns As To Fat Added In Cooking ☞ serving size: 1 cup = 229 g; Calories = 254

Rice Brown With Carrots Dark Green Vegetables And Tomatoes And/or Tomato-Based Sauce Fat Added In Cooking ☞ serving size: 1 cup = 186 g; Calories = 210

Rice Brown With Carrots Dark Green Vegetables And Tomatoes And/or Tomato-Based Sauce Fat Not Added In Cooking ☞ serving size: 1 cup = 220 g; Calories = 220

Rice Brown With Carrots Dark Green Vegetables And Tomatoes And/or Tomato-Based Sauce Ns As To Fat Added In Cooking ☞ serving size: 1 cup = 224 g; Calories = 253

Rice Brown With Carrots Fat Added In Cooking ☞ serving size: 1 cup = 189 g; Calories = 223

Rice Brown With Carrots Fat Not Added In Cooking ☞ serving size: 1 cup = 186 g; Calories = 193

Rice Brown With Carrots Ns As To Fat Added In Cooking ☞ serving size: 1 cup = 189 g; Calories = 223

Rice Brown With Cheese And/or Cream Based Sauce Fat Added In Cooking ☞ serving size: 1 cup = 282 g; Calories = 440

Rice Brown With Cheese And/or Cream Based Sauce Fat Not Added In Cooking ☞ serving size: 1 cup = 277 g; Calories = 399

Rice Brown With Cheese And/or Cream Based Sauce Ns As To Fat Added In Cooking ☞ serving size: 1 cup = 282 g; Calories = 440

Rice Brown With Corn Fat Added In Cooking ☞ serving size: 1 cup = 191 g; Calories = 248

Rice Brown With Corn Fat Not Added In Cooking ☞ serving size: 1 cup = 188 g; Calories = 220

Rice Brown With Corn Ns As To Fat Added In Cooking ☞ serving size: 1 cup = 191 g; Calories = 248

Rice Brown With Dark Green Vegetables And Tomatoes And/or Tomato-Based Sauce Fat Added In Cooking ☞ serving size: 1 cup = 229 g; Calories = 254

Rice Brown With Dark Green Vegetables And Tomatoes And/or Tomato-Based Sauce Fat Not Added In Cooking ☞ serving size: 1 cup = 229 g; Calories = 222

Rice Brown With Dark Green Vegetables And Tomatoes And/or Tomato-Based Sauce Ns As To Fat Added In Cooking ☞ serving size: 1 cup = 229 g; Calories = 254

Rice Brown With Dark Green Vegetables Fat Added In Cooking ☞ serving size: 1 cup = 189 g; Calories = 223

Rice Brown With Dark Green Vegetables Fat Not Added In Cooking ☞ serving size: 1 cup = 186 g; Calories = 193

Rice Brown With Dark Green Vegetables Ns As To Fat Added In Cooking ☞ serving size: 1 cup = 189 g; Calories = 223

Rice Brown With Gravy Fat Added In Cooking ☞ serving size: 1 cup = 237 g; Calories = 270

Rice Brown With Gravy Fat Not Added In Cooking ☛ serving size: 1 cup = 237 g; Calories = 239

Rice Brown With Gravy Ns As To Fat Added In Cooking ☛ serving size: 1 cup = 237 g; Calories = 270

Rice Brown With Other Vegetables Fat Added In Cooking ☛ serving size: 1 cup = 190 g; Calories = 224

Rice Brown With Other Vegetables Fat Not Added In Cooking ☛ serving size: 1 cup = 186 g; Calories = 193

Rice Brown With Other Vegetables Ns As To Fat Added In Cooking ☛ serving size: 1 cup = 190 g; Calories = 224

Rice Brown With Peas And Carrots Fat Added In Cooking ☛ serving size: 1 cup = 190 g; Calories = 228

Rice Brown With Peas And Carrots Fat Not Added In Cooking ☛ serving size: 1 cup = 187 g; Calories = 198

Rice Brown With Peas And Carrots Ns As To Fat Added In Cooking ☛ serving size: 1 cup = 190 g; Calories = 228

Rice Brown With Peas Fat Added In Cooking ☛ serving size: 1 cup = 190 g; Calories = 243

Rice Brown With Peas Fat Not Added In Cooking ☛ serving size: 1 cup = 187 g; Calories = 213

Rice Brown With Peas Ns As To Fat Added In Cooking ☛ serving size: 1 cup = 190 g; Calories = 243

Rice Brown With Soy-Based Sauce Fat Added In Cooking ☛ serving size: 1 cup = 237 g; Calories = 268

Rice Brown With Soy-Based Sauce Fat Not Added In Cooking ☛ serving size: 1 cup = 237 g; Calories = 239

Rice Brown With Soy-Based Sauce Ns As To Fat Added In Cooking ☛ serving size: 1 cup = 237 g; Calories = 268

Rice Brown With Tomatoes And/or Tomato Based Sauce Fat Added In Cooking ☛ serving size: 1 cup = 243 g; Calories = 253

Rice Brown With Tomatoes And/or Tomato Based Sauce Fat Not Added In Cooking ☛ serving size: 1 cup = 243 g; Calories = 224

Rice Brown With Tomatoes And/or Tomato Based Sauce Ns As To Fat Added In Cooking ☛ serving size: 1 cup = 243 g; Calories = 253

Rice Brown With Vegetables And Gravy Fat Added In Cooking ☛ serving size: 1 cup = 292 g; Calories = 307

Rice Brown With Vegetables And Gravy Fat Not Added In Cooking ☛ serving size: 1 cup = 288 g; Calories = 271

Rice Brown With Vegetables And Gravy Ns As To Fat Added In Cooking ☛ serving size: 1 cup = 292 g; Calories = 307

Rice Brown With Vegetables Cheese And/or Cream Based Sauce Fat Added In Cooking ☛ serving size: 1 cup = 293 g; Calories = 410

Rice Brown With Vegetables Cheese And/or Cream Based Sauce Fat Not Added In Cooking ☛ serving size: 1 cup = 289 g; Calories = 376

Rice Brown With Vegetables Cheese And/or Cream Based Sauce Ns As To Fat Added In Cooking ☛ serving size: 1 cup = 293 g; Calories = 410

Rice Brown With Vegetables Soy-Based Sauce Fat Added In Cooking ☛ serving size: 1 cup = 290 g; Calories = 305

Rice Brown With Vegetables Soy-Based Sauce Fat Not Added In Cooking ☛ serving size: 1 cup = 286 g; Calories = 269

Rice Brown With Vegetables Soy-Based Sauce Ns As To Fat Added In Cooking ☛ serving size: 1 cup = 290 g; Calories = 305

Rice Cooked With Coconut Milk ☛ serving size: 1 cup = 200 g; Calories = 534

Rice Croquette ☛ serving size: 1 croquette (1-1/2" dia, 2" high) = 62 g; Calories = 96

Rice Dessert Or Salad With Fruit ☛ serving size: 1 cup = 155 g; Calories = 240

Rice Dressing ☛ serving size: 1 cup = 167 g; Calories = 184

Rice Fried With Beef ☛ serving size: 1 cup = 198 g; Calories = 352

Rice Fried With Chicken ☛ serving size: 1 cup = 198 g; Calories = 343

Rice Fried With Pork ☛ serving size: 1 cup = 198 g; Calories = 354

Rice Fried With Shrimp ☛ serving size: 1 cup = 198 g; Calories = 329

Rice Meal Fritter Puerto Rican Style ☛ serving size: 1 cruller (3" x 2" x 1/2") = 30 g; Calories = 93

Rice Mix Cheese Flavor Dry Mix Unprepared ☛ serving size: 1/4 cup dry rice mix = 57 g; Calories = 206

Rice Mix White And Wild Flavored Unprepared ☛ serving size: 2 oz (1/4 c dry rice mix and 4 tsp seasoning mix) = 57 g; Calories = 81

Rice White With Carrots And Dark Green Vegetables Fat Added In Cooking ☛ serving size: 1 cup = 172 g; Calories = 210

Rice White With Carrots And Dark Green Vegetables Fat Not Added In Cooking ☛ serving size: 1 cup = 172 g; Calories = 182

Rice White With Carrots And Dark Green Vegetables Ns As To Fat Added In Cooking ☛ serving size: 1 cup = 172 g; Calories = 210

Rice White With Carrots And Tomatoes And/or Tomato-Based Sauce Fat Added In Cooking ☛ serving size: 1 cup = 172 g; Calories = 196

Rice White With Carrots And Tomatoes And/or Tomato-Based

Sauce Fat Not Added In Cooking ☞ serving size: 1 cup = 172 g; Calories = 169

Rice White With Carrots And Tomatoes And/or Tomato-Based Sauce Ns As To Fat Added In Cooking ☞ serving size: 1 cup = 172 g; Calories = 196

Rice White With Carrots Dark Green Vegetables And Tomatoes And/or Tomato-Based Sauce Fat Added In Cooking ☞ serving size: 1 cup = 172 g; Calories = 201

Rice White With Carrots Dark Green Vegetables And Tomatoes And/or Tomato-Based Sauce Fat Not Added In Cooking ☞ serving size: 1 cup = 172 g; Calories = 174

Rice White With Carrots Dark Green Vegetables And Tomatoes And/or Tomato-Based Sauce Ns As To Fat Added In Cooking ☞ serving size: 1 cup = 172 g; Calories = 201

Rice White With Carrots Fat Added In Cooking ☞ serving size: 1 cup = 160 g; Calories = 197

Rice White With Carrots Fat Not Added In Cooking ☞ serving size: 1 cup = 160 g; Calories = 170

Rice White With Carrots Ns As To Fat Added In Cooking ☞ serving size: 1 cup = 160 g; Calories = 197

Rice White With Cheese And/or Cream Based Sauce Fat Added In Cooking ☞ serving size: 1 cup = 204 g; Calories = 339

Rice White With Cheese And/or Cream Based Sauce Fat Not Added In Cooking ☞ serving size: 1 cup = 204 g; Calories = 310

Rice White With Cheese And/or Cream Based Sauce Ns As To Fat Added In Cooking ☞ serving size: 1 cup = 204 g; Calories = 339

Rice White With Corn Fat Added In Cooking ☞ serving size: 1 cup = 161 g; Calories = 221

Rice White With Corn Fat Not Added In Cooking ☞ serving size: 1 cup = 161 g; Calories = 195

Rice White With Corn Ns As To Fat Added In Cooking ☞ serving size: 1 cup = 161 g; Calories = 221

Rice White With Dark Green Vegetables And Tomatoes And/or Tomato-Based Sauce Fat Added In Cooking ☞ serving size: 1 cup = 172 g; Calories = 196

Rice White With Dark Green Vegetables And Tomatoes And/or Tomato-Based Sauce Fat Not Added In Cooking ☞ serving size: 1 cup = 172 g; Calories = 169

Rice White With Dark Green Vegetables And Tomatoes And/or Tomato-Based Sauce Ns As To Fat Added In Cooking ☞ serving size: 1 cup = 172 g; Calories = 196

Rice White With Dark Green Vegetables Fat Added In Cooking ☞ serving size: 1 cup = 172 g; Calories = 210

Rice White With Dark Green Vegetables Fat Not Added In Cooking ☞ serving size: 1 cup = 172 g; Calories = 182

Rice White With Dark Green Vegetables Ns As To Fat Added In Cooking ☞ serving size: 1 cup = 172 g; Calories = 210

Rice White With Gravy Fat Added In Cooking ☞ serving size: 1 cup = 237 g; Calories = 277

Rice White With Gravy Fat Not Added In Cooking ☞ serving size: 1 cup = 237 g; Calories = 242

Rice White With Gravy Ns As To Fat Added In Cooking ☞ serving size: 1 cup = 237 g; Calories = 277

Rice White With Lentils Fat Added In Cooking ☞ serving size: 1 cup = 207 g; Calories = 308

Rice White With Lentils Fat Not Added In Cooking ☞ serving size: 1 cup = 198 g; Calories = 228

Rice White With Lentils Ns As To Fat Added In Cooking ☞ serving size: 1 cup = 207 g; Calories = 308

Rice White With Other Vegetables Fat Added In Cooking ☞ serving size: 1 cup = 172 g; Calories = 212

Rice White With Other Vegetables Fat Not Added In Cooking ☞ serving size: 1 cup = 172 g; Calories = 182

Rice White With Other Vegetables Ns As To Fat Added In Cooking ☞ serving size: 1 cup = 172 g; Calories = 212

Rice White With Peas And Carrots Fat Added In Cooking ☞ serving size: 1 cup = 160 g; Calories = 200

Rice White With Peas And Carrots Fat Not Added In Cooking ☞ serving size: 1 cup = 160 g; Calories = 174

Rice White With Peas And Carrots Ns As To Fat Added In Cooking ☞ serving size: 1 cup = 160 g; Calories = 200

Rice White With Peas Fat Added In Cooking ☞ serving size: 1 cup = 160 g; Calories = 214

Rice White With Peas Fat Not Added In Cooking ☞ serving size: 1 cup = 160 g; Calories = 189

Rice White With Peas Ns As To Fat Added In Cooking ☞ serving size: 1 cup = 160 g; Calories = 214

Rice White With Soy-Based Sauce Fat Added In Cooking ☞ serving size: 1 cup = 237 g; Calories = 275

Rice White With Soy-Based Sauce Fat Not Added In Cooking ☞ serving size: 1 cup = 237 g; Calories = 242

Rice White With Soy-Based Sauce Ns As To Fat Added In Cooking ☞ serving size: 1 cup = 237 g; Calories = 275

Rice White With Tomatoes And/or Tomato-Based Sauce Fat Added In Cooking ☞ serving size: 1 cup = 209 g; Calories = 222

Rice White With Tomatoes And/or Tomato-Based Sauce Fat Not Added In Cooking ☛ serving size: 1 cup = 206 g; Calories = 188

Rice White With Tomatoes And/or Tomato-Based Sauce Ns As To Fat Added In Cooking ☛ serving size: 1 cup = 209 g; Calories = 222

Rice White With Vegetables And Gravy Fat Added In Cooking ☛ serving size: 1 cup = 260 g; Calories = 276

Rice White With Vegetables And Gravy Fat Not Added In Cooking ☛ serving size: 1 cup = 256 g; Calories = 243

Rice White With Vegetables And Gravy Ns As To Fat Added In Cooking ☛ serving size: 1 cup = 260 g; Calories = 276

Rice White With Vegetables Cheese And/or Cream Based Sauce Fat Added In Cooking ☛ serving size: 1 cup = 262 g; Calories = 383

Rice White With Vegetables Cheese And/or Cream Based Sauce Fat Not Added In Cooking ☛ serving size: 1 cup = 258 g; Calories = 346

Rice White With Vegetables Cheese And/or Cream Based Sauce Ns As To Fat Added In Cooking ☛ serving size: 1 cup = 261 g; Calories = 381

Rice White With Vegetables Soy-Based Sauce Fat Added In Cooking ☛ serving size: 1 cup = 258 g; Calories = 274

Rice White With Vegetables Soy-Based Sauce Fat Not Added In Cooking ☛ serving size: 1 cup = 255 g; Calories = 240

Rice White With Vegetables Soy-Based Sauce Ns As To Fat Added In Cooking ☛ serving size: 1 cup = 258 g; Calories = 274

Rice With Beans ☛ serving size: 1 cup = 239 g; Calories = 373

Rice With Beans And Beef ☛ serving size: 1 cup = 239 g; Calories = 414

Rice With Beans And Chicken ☛ serving size: 1 cup = 239 g; Calories = 378

Rice With Beans And Pork ☞ serving size: 1 cup = 239 g; Calories = 404

Rice With Beans And Tomatoes ☞ serving size: 1 cup = 239 g; Calories = 296

Rice With Broccoli Cheese Sauce Frozen Side Dish ☞ serving size: 1 side dish (4.5 oz) = 128 g; Calories = 152

Rice With Chicken Puerto Rican Style ☞ serving size: 1 cup, with bone (yield after bone removed) = 157 g; Calories = 466

Rice With Green Beans Water Chestnuts In Sherry Mushroom Sauce Frozen Side Dish ☞ serving size: 1 side dish (10 oz) = 284 g; Calories = 276

Rice With Onions Puerto Rican Style ☞ serving size: 1 cup = 165 g; Calories = 286

Rice With Raisins ☞ serving size: 1 cup = 185 g; Calories = 300

Rice With Spanish Sausage Puerto Rican Style ☞ serving size: 1 cup = 180 g; Calories = 567

Rice With Squid Puerto Rican Style ☞ serving size: 1 cup = 160 g; Calories = 414

Rice With Stewed Beans Puerto Rican Style ☞ serving size: 1 cup = 188 g; Calories = 258

Rice With Vienna Sausage Puerto Rican Style ☞ serving size: 1 cup = 180 g; Calories = 482

Rigatoni With Meat Sauce And Cheese Diet Frozen Meal ☞ serving size: 1 meal (9.75 oz) = 276 g; Calories = 251

Roll With Meat And/or Shrimp Vegetables And Rice Paper Not Fried ☞ serving size: 1 roll (4-1/4" x 1-1/2" dia) = 71 g; Calories = 79

Salisbury Steak With Gravy Frozen ☞ serving size: 1 patty = 63 g; Calories = 94

🦐 Sausage Egg And Cheese Breakfast Biscuit ☛ serving size: 1 biscuit = 126 g; Calories = 408

🦐 Seafood Paella Puerto Rican Style ☛ serving size: 1 cup = 230 g; Calories = 331

🦐 Seaweed Prepared With Soy Sauce ☛ serving size: 1 cup = 96 g; Calories = 41

🦐 Shellfish Mixture And Vegetables Excluding Carrots Broccoli And Dark-Green Leafy; No Potatoes Soy-Based Sauce ☛ serving size: 1 cup = 217 g; Calories = 256

🦐 Shellfish Mixture And Vegetables Including Carrots Broccoli And/or Dark-Green Leafy; No Potatoes Soy-Based Sauce ☛ serving size: 1 cup = 217 g; Calories = 254

🦐 Shrimp And Noodles With Soy-Based Sauce ☛ serving size: 1 cup = 224 g; Calories = 311

🦐 Shrimp And Vegetables Excluding Carrots Broccoli And Dark-Green Leafy; No Potatoes Soy-Based Sauce ☛ serving size: 1 cup = 217 g; Calories = 247

🦐 Shrimp And Vegetables Including Carrots Broccoli And/or Dark-Green Leafy; No Potatoes Soy-Based Sauce ☛ serving size: 1 cup = 217 g; Calories = 245

🦐 Shrimp Chow Mein Or Chop Suey No Noodles ☛ serving size: 1 cup = 220 g; Calories = 152

🦐 Shrimp Chow Mein Or Chop Suey With Noodles ☛ serving size: 1 cup = 220 g; Calories = 260

🦐 Shrimp Egg Foo Yung ☛ serving size: 1 cup = 175 g; Calories = 215

🦐 Shrimp Teriyaki ☛ serving size: 1 cup = 201 g; Calories = 241

🦐 Soft Taco With Chicken And Beans ☛ serving size: 1 small taco or tostada = 112 g; Calories = 223

Soft Taco With Chicken Beans And Sour Cream ☛ serving size: 1 small taco or tostada = 127 g; Calories = 253

Soft Taco With Fish ☛ serving size: 1 small taco or tostada = 94 g; Calories = 187

Soft Taco With Meat ☛ serving size: 1 small taco or tostada = 103 g; Calories = 228

Soft Taco With Meat And Beans ☛ serving size: 1 small taco or tostada = 117 g; Calories = 235

Soft Taco With Meat And Sour Cream From Fast Food ☛ serving size: 1 small taco or tostada = 117 g; Calories = 234

Soft Taco With Meat Beans And Sour Cream ☛ serving size: 1 small taco or tostada = 132 g; Calories = 267

Somen Salad With Noodles Lettuce Egg Fish And Pork ☛ serving size: 1 cup = 160 g; Calories = 219

Spaghetti And Meatballs Dinner NFS Frozen Meal ☛ serving size: 1 meal (12.5 oz) = 354 g; Calories = 397

Spaghetti And Meatballs With Tomato Sauce Sliced Apples Bread Frozen Meal ☛ serving size: 1 meal (11.5 oz) = 326 g; Calories = 424

Spaghetti With Corned Beef Puerto Rican Style ☛ serving size: 1 cup = 215 g; Calories = 540

Spaghetti With Meat And Mushroom Sauce Diet Frozen Meal ☛ serving size: 1 meal (11.5 oz) = 326 g; Calories = 375

Spaghetti With Meat Sauce Diet Frozen Meal ☛ serving size: 1 meal (10.5 oz) = 298 g; Calories = 334

Spaghetti With Meat Sauce Frozen Entree ☛ serving size: 1 serving = 283 g; Calories = 255

Spaghetti With Meatballs In Tomato Sauce Canned ☛ serving size: 1 cup = 246 g; Calories = 246

Spanakopitta ☛ serving size: 1 cubic inch = 12 g; Calories = 25

Spanish Rice Fat Added In Cooking ☛ serving size: 1 cup = 243 g; Calories = 277

Spanish Rice Fat Not Added In Cooking ☛ serving size: 1 cup = 243 g; Calories = 245

Spanish Rice Mix Dry Mix Prepared (With Canola/vegetable Oil Blend Or Diced Tomatoes And Margarine) ☛ serving size: 1 cup = 198 g; Calories = 248

Spanish Rice Mix Dry Mix Unprepared ☛ serving size: 1/2 cup = 70 g; Calories = 254

Spanish Rice Ns As To Fat Added In Cooking ☛ serving size: 1 cup = 243 g; Calories = 277

Spanish Rice With Ground Beef ☛ serving size: 1 cup = 230 g; Calories = 373

Spinach Quiche Meatless ☛ serving size: 1 piece (1/8 of 9" dia) = 143 g; Calories = 423

Steak Teriyaki ☛ serving size: 1 cup = 244 g; Calories = 483

Stewed Potatoes ☛ serving size: 1 cup = 250 g; Calories = 285

Stewed Potatoes Puerto Rican Style ☛ serving size: 1 small = 123 g; Calories = 140

Stewed Potatoes With Tomatoes ☛ serving size: 1 cup = 250 g; Calories = 230

Stewed Rice Puerto Rican Style ☛ serving size: 1 cup = 170 g; Calories = 377

Stir Fried Beef And Vegetables In Soy Sauce ☛ serving size: 1 cup = 162 g; Calories = 151

Stuffed Shells Cheese- And Spinach- Filled No Sauce ☛ serving size: 1 shell (jumbo) = 60 g; Calories = 113

Stuffed Shells Cheese-Filled No Sauce ☛ serving size: 1 shell (jumbo) = 60 g; Calories = 126

Stuffed Shells Cheese-Filled With Meat Sauce ☛ serving size: 1 shell (jumbo) = 85 g; Calories = 137

Stuffed Shells Cheese-Filled With Tomato Sauce Meatless ☛ serving size: 1 shell (jumbo) = 85 g; Calories = 127

Stuffed Shells With Chicken With Tomato Sauce ☛ serving size: 1 shell (jumbo) = 83 g; Calories = 113

Stuffed Shells With Fish And/or Shellfish With Tomato Sauce ☛ serving size: 1 shell (jumbo) = 83 g; Calories = 96

Sushi Nfs ☛ serving size: 1 piece = 30 g; Calories = 28

Sushi Roll Avocado ☛ serving size: 1 piece = 30 g; Calories = 28

Sushi Roll California ☛ serving size: 1 piece = 30 g; Calories = 28

Sushi Roll Eel ☛ serving size: 1 piece = 30 g; Calories = 38

Sushi Roll Salmon ☛ serving size: 1 piece = 30 g; Calories = 31

Sushi Roll Shrimp ☛ serving size: 1 piece = 30 g; Calories = 30

Sushi Roll Tuna ☛ serving size: 1 piece = 30 g; Calories = 29

Sushi Roll Vegetable ☛ serving size: 1 piece = 22 g; Calories = 20

Sushi Topped With Crab ☛ serving size: 1 piece = 35 g; Calories = 33

Sushi Topped With Eel ☛ serving size: 1 piece = 35 g; Calories = 50

Sushi Topped With Egg ☛ serving size: 1 piece = 50 g; Calories = 58

Sushi Topped With Salmon ☛ serving size: 1 piece = 35 g; Calories = 38

Sushi Topped With Shrimp ☛ serving size: 1 piece = 35 g; Calories = 36

Sushi Topped With Tuna ☛ serving size: 1 piece = 35 g; Calories = 35

Sweet And Sour Pork ☛ serving size: 1 cup = 226 g; Calories = 438

Sweet And Sour Pork With Rice ☛ serving size: 1 cup = 244 g; Calories = 449

Sweet And Sour Shrimp ☛ serving size: 1 cup = 176 g; Calories = 296

Sweet Bread Dough Filled With Meat Steamed ☛ serving size: 1 manapua = 93 g; Calories = 253

Tabbouleh ☛ serving size: 1 cup = 160 g; Calories = 197

Taco Or Tostada Salad Meatless ☛ serving size: 1 small taco salad = 234 g; Calories = 377

Taco Or Tostada Salad Meatless With Sour Cream ☛ serving size: 1 small taco salad = 266 g; Calories = 442

Taco Or Tostada Salad With Chicken ☛ serving size: 1 small taco salad = 240 g; Calories = 398

Taco Or Tostada Salad With Chicken And Sour Cream ☛ serving size: 1 small taco salad = 273 g; Calories = 464

Taco Or Tostada Salad With Meat ☛ serving size: 1 small taco salad = 237 g; Calories = 422

Taco Or Tostada Salad With Meat And Sour Cream ☛ serving size: 1 small taco salad = 264 g; Calories = 475

Taco Or Tostada With Beans ☛ serving size: 1 small taco or tostada = 125 g; Calories = 253

Taco Or Tostada With Beans And Sour Cream ☛ serving size: 1 small taco or tostada = 140 g; Calories = 281

Taco Or Tostada With Chicken ☛ serving size: 1 small taco or tostada = 80 g; Calories = 204

Taco Or Tostada With Chicken And Beans ☛ serving size: 1 small taco or tostada = 103 g; Calories = 230

Taco Or Tostada With Chicken And Sour Cream ☛ serving size: 1 small taco or tostada = 96 g; Calories = 235

Taco Or Tostada With Chicken Beans And Sour Cream ☛ serving size: 1 small taco or tostada = 118 g; Calories = 258

Taco Or Tostada With Fish ☛ serving size: 1 miniature taco = 20 g; Calories = 46

Taco Or Tostada With Meat ☛ serving size: 1 miniature taco = 22 g; Calories = 54

Taco Or Tostada With Meat And Beans ☛ serving size: 1 small taco or tostada = 109 g; Calories = 242

Taco Or Tostada With Meat And Beans From Fast Food ☛ serving size: 1 small taco or tostada = 109 g; Calories = 239

Taco Or Tostada With Meat And Sour Cream ☛ serving size: 1 small taco or tostada = 109 g; Calories = 265

Taco Or Tostada With Meat Beans And Sour Cream ☛ serving size: 1 small taco or tostada = 124 g; Calories = 273

Taco With Crab Meat Puerto Rican Style ☛ serving size: 1 taco (4-1/2" dia) = 121 g; Calories = 264

Tamal In A Leaf Puerto Rican Style ☛ serving size: 1 tamal (6" x 2" x 1/2") = 41 g; Calories = 63

Tamale Casserole Puerto Rican Style ☛ serving size: 1 cup = 237 g; Calories = 372

Tamale Casserole With Meat ☛ serving size: 1 cup = 244 g; Calories = 390

Tamale Meatless With Sauce Puerto Rican Or Caribbean Style ☛ serving size: 1 tamale = 72 g; Calories = 325

Tamale Plain Meatless No Sauce Puerto Rican Style Or Carribean Style ☛ serving size: 1 tamale = 36 g; Calories = 78

Tamale With Chicken ☛ serving size: 1 small tamale = 84 g; Calories = 186

Taquito Or Flauta With Cheese ☛ serving size: 1 small taquito = 36 g; Calories = 97

Taquitos Frozen Beef And Cheese Oven-Heated ☛ serving size: 1 piece = 42 g; Calories = 121

Taquitos Frozen Chicken And Cheese Oven-Heated ☛ serving size: 1 piece = 42 g; Calories = 119

Tofu And Vegetables Excluding Carrots Broccoli And Dark-Green Leafy; No Potatoes With Soy-Based Sauce ☛ serving size: 1 cup = 217 g; Calories = 195

Tofu And Vegetables Including Carrots Broccoli And/or Dark-Green Leafy; No Potatoes With Soy-Based Sauce ☛ serving size: 1 cup = 217 g; Calories = 193

Tortellini Cheese-Filled Meatless With Tomato Sauce ☛ serving size: 1 cup = 250 g; Calories = 373

Tortellini Cheese-Filled Meatless With Tomato Sauce Canned ☛ serving size: 1 cup = 247 g; Calories = 225

Tortellini Cheese-Filled Meatless With Vegetables And Vinaigrette Dressing ☛ serving size: 1 cup = 169 g; Calories = 375

Tortellini Cheese-Filled Meatless With Vinaigrette Dressing ☛ serving size: 1 cup = 169 g; Calories = 333

Tortellini Cheese-Filled No Sauce ☛ serving size: 1 cup = 150 g; Calories = 354

Tortellini Cheese-Filled With Cream Sauce ☛ serving size: 1 cup = 250 g; Calories = 390

Tortellini Meat-Filled No Sauce ☛ serving size: 1 cup = 190 g; Calories = 363

Tortellini Meat-Filled With Tomato Sauce ☛ serving size: 1 cup = 210 g; Calories = 281

Tortellini Meat-Filled With Tomato Sauce Canned ☛ serving size: 1 cup = 233 g; Calories = 212

Tortellini Pasta With Cheese Filling Fresh-Refrigerated As Purchased ☛ serving size: 3/4 cup = 81 g; Calories = 249

Tortellini Spinach-Filled No Sauce ☛ serving size: 1 cup = 122 g; Calories = 228

Tortellini Spinach-Filled With Tomato Sauce ☛ serving size: 1 cup = 200 g; Calories = 240

Turkey Pot Pie Frozen Entree ☛ serving size: 1 package yields = 397 g; Calories = 699

Turkey Stuffing Mashed Potatoes W/gravy Assorted Vegetables Frozen Microwaved ☛ serving size: 1 serving = 385 g; Calories = 493

Turnover Cheese-Filled Tomato-Based Sauce ☛ serving size: 1 hot pockets four cheese pizza = 128 g; Calories = 346

Turnover Cheese-Filled Tomato-Based Sauce Frozen Unprepared ☛ serving size: 1 serving 4.5 oz = 127 g; Calories = 299

Turnover Chicken With Gravy ☛ serving size: 1 turnover = 112 g; Calories = 313

Turnover Chicken- Or Turkey- And Vegetable-Filled Reduced Fat Frozen ☛ serving size: 1 piece turnover 1 serving = 127 g; Calories = 213

Turnover Filled With Egg Meat And Cheese Frozen ☛ serving size: 1 piece turnover 1 serving = 127 g; Calories = 290

Turnover Filled With Ground Beef And Cabbage ☛ serving size: 1 bierock = 215 g; Calories = 510

Turnover Filled With Meat And Vegetable No Potatoes No Gravy ☞ serving size: 1 turnover = 88 g; Calories = 268

Turnover Meat- And Bean-Filled No Gravy ☞ serving size: 1 turnover = 88 g; Calories = 305

Turnover Meat- And Cheese-Filled No Gravy ☞ serving size: 1 turnover = 96 g; Calories = 231

Turnover Meat- And Cheese-Filled Tomato-Based Sauce ☞ serving size: 1 turnover = 73 g; Calories = 185

Turnover Meat- And Cheese-Filled Tomato-Based Sauce Reduced Fat Frozen ☞ serving size: 1 piece turnover 1 serving = 127 g; Calories = 273

Turnover Meat- Potato- And Vegetable-Filled No Gravy ☞ serving size: 1 turnover = 88 g; Calories = 257

Turnover Meat-Filled No Gravy ☞ serving size: 1 turnover = 88 g; Calories = 327

Turnover Meat-Filled With Gravy ☞ serving size: 1 turnover = 152 g; Calories = 379

Vada Fried Dumpling ☞ serving size: 1 vada = 29 g; Calories = 77

Veal Lasagna Diet Frozen Meal ☞ serving size: 1 meal (10.25 oz) = 291 g; Calories = 259

Vegetable Combination Excluding Carrots Broccoli And Dark-Green Leafy; Cooked With Soy-Based Sauce ☞ serving size: 1 cup = 185 g; Calories = 198

Vegetable Combination Including Carrots Broccoli And/or Dark-Green Leafy; Cooked With Soy-Based Sauce ☞ serving size: 1 cup = 185 g; Calories = 194

Vegetables And Cheese In Pastry ☞ serving size: 1 pastry = 103 g; Calories = 325

Vegetables In Pastry ☞ serving size: 1 pastry = 103 g; Calories = 316

Wonton Fried Filled With Meat Poultry Or Seafood ☞ serving size: 1 wonton, any size = 19 g; Calories = 36

Wonton Fried Filled With Meat Poultry Or Seafood And Vegetable ☞ serving size: 1 wonton, any size = 19 g; Calories = 36

Wonton Fried Meatless ☞ serving size: 1 wonton, any size = 19 g; Calories = 36

Yat Ga Mein With Meat Fish Or Poultry ☞ serving size: 1 cup = 205 g; Calories = 277

Yellow Rice With Seasoning Dry Packet Mix Unprepared ☞ serving size: 1 serving (2 oz) = 57 g; Calories = 196

Zucchini Lasagna Diet Frozen Meal ☞ serving size: 1 lean cuisine meal (11 oz) = 312 g; Calories = 309

21

RESTAURANT FOODS

🍽 Applebees 9 Oz House Sirloin Steak ☛ serving size: 1 serving = 157 g; Calories = 297

🍽 Applebees Chicken Tenders From Kids Menu ☛ serving size: 1 piece = 35 g; Calories = 104

🍽 Applebees Chicken Tenders Platter ☛ serving size: 1 serving = 209 g; Calories = 621

🍽 Applebees Chili ☛ serving size: 1 cup = 136 g; Calories = 214

🍽 Applebees Coleslaw ☛ serving size: 1 serving = 76 g; Calories = 91

🍽 Applebees Double Crunch Shrimp ☛ serving size: 1 serving = 206 g; Calories = 665

🍽 Applebees Fish Hand Battered ☛ serving size: 1 serving = 250 g; Calories = 505

🍽 Applebees French Fries ☛ serving size: 1 serving = 164 g; Calories = 476

🍽 Applebees Kraft Macaroni & Cheese From Kids Menu ☛ serving size: 1 cup = 124 g; Calories = 177

Applebees Mozzarella Sticks ☞ serving size: 1 piece = 32 g; Calories = 101

Carrabbas Italian Grill Cheese Ravioli With Marinara Sauce ☞ serving size: 1 serving varied from 8 to 10 ravioli per serving = 365 g; Calories = 569

Carrabbas Italian Grill Chicken Parmesan Without Cavatappi Pasta ☞ serving size: 1 serving = 339 g; Calories = 698

Carrabbas Italian Grill Lasagne ☞ serving size: 1 serving = 437 g; Calories = 835

Carrabbas Italian Grill Spaghetti With Meat Sauce ☞ serving size: 1 serving = 537 g; Calories = 655

Carrabbas Italian Grill Spaghetti With Pomodoro Sauce ☞ serving size: 1 serving = 489 g; Calories = 509

Cracker Barrel Chicken Tenderloin Platter Fried ☞ serving size: 1 serving = 175 g; Calories = 513

Cracker Barrel Chicken Tenderloin Platter Fried From Kids Menu ☞ serving size: 1 serving = 103 g; Calories = 303

Cracker Barrel Coleslaw ☞ serving size: 1 serving = 167 g; Calories = 292

Cracker Barrel Country Fried Shrimp Platter ☞ serving size: 1 serving = 149 g; Calories = 428

Cracker Barrel Farm Raised Catfish Platter ☞ serving size: 1 serving = 178 g; Calories = 474

Cracker Barrel Grilled Sirloin Steak ☞ serving size: 1 steak = 151 g; Calories = 307

Cracker Barrel Macaroni N Cheese ☞ serving size: 1 serving = 175 g; Calories = 340

Cracker Barrel Macaroni N Cheese Plate From Kids Menu ☛ serving size: 1 serving = 257 g; Calories = 493

Cracker Barrel Onion Rings Thick-Cut ☛ serving size: 1 serving = 261 g; Calories = 854

Cracker Barrel Steak Fries ☛ serving size: 1 serving = 198 g; Calories = 505

Dennys Chicken Nuggets Star Shaped From Kids Menu ☛ serving size: 1 serving 4 pieces in serving = 67 g; Calories = 253

Dennys Chicken Strips ☛ serving size: 1 serving = 194 g; Calories = 572

Dennys Coleslaw ☛ serving size: 1 serving = 91 g; Calories = 167

Dennys Fish Fillet Battered Or Breaded Fried ☛ serving size: 1 serving = 201 g; Calories = 470

Dennys French Fries ☛ serving size: 1 serving = 165 g; Calories = 465

Dennys Golden Fried Shrimp ☛ serving size: 1 piece = 16 g; Calories = 51

Dennys Hash Browns ☛ serving size: 1 serving = 124 g; Calories = 244

Dennys Macaroni & Cheese From Kids Menu ☛ serving size: 1 serving = 180 g; Calories = 270

Dennys Mozzarella Cheese Sticks ☛ serving size: 1 serving = 228 g; Calories = 739

Dennys Onion Rings ☛ serving size: 1 serving = 166 g; Calories = 639

Dennys Spaghetti And Meatballs ☛ serving size: 1 serving = 565 g; Calories = 961

Dennys Top Sirloin Steak ☞ serving size: 1 steak = 107 g; Calories = 195

French Fries ☞ serving size: 10 strip = 69 g; Calories = 111

Fried Onion Rings ☞ serving size: 1 serving = 350 g; Calories = 1246

Hash Browns ☞ serving size: 1 cup = 156 g; Calories = 413

Olive Garden Cheese Ravioli With Marinara Sauce ☞ serving size: 1 serving varied from 7-9 ravioli per serving = 454 g; Calories = 722

Olive Garden Chicken Parmigiana Without Pasta ☞ serving size: 1 serving = 304 g; Calories = 641

Olive Garden Lasagna Classico ☞ serving size: 1 serving = 422 g; Calories = 777

Olive Garden Spaghetti With Meat Sauce ☞ serving size: 1 serving = 525 g; Calories = 635

Olive Garden Spaghetti With Pomodoro Sauce ☞ serving size: 1 serving = 478 g; Calories = 488

On The Border Cheese Enchilada ☞ serving size: 1 serving serving size varied from 1 to 3 enchiladas = 250 g; Calories = 678

On The Border Cheese Quesadilla ☞ serving size: 1 serving 1 quesadilla = 203 g; Calories = 800

On The Border Mexican Rice ☞ serving size: 1 cup = 114 g; Calories = 222

On The Border Refried Beans ☞ serving size: 1 cup = 135 g; Calories = 194

On The Border Soft Taco With Ground Beef Cheese And Lettuce ☞ serving size: 1 serving varied from 2-3 tacos per serving = 324 g; Calories = 742

Onion Rings ☞ serving size: 1 cup = 48 g; Calories = 133

Restaurant Chinese Beef And Vegetables ☛ serving size: 1 order = 574 g; Calories = 603

Restaurant Chinese Chicken And Vegetables ☛ serving size: 1 order = 693 g; Calories = 658

Restaurant Chinese Chicken Chow Mein ☛ serving size: 1 order = 604 g; Calories = 513

Restaurant Chinese Egg Rolls Assorted ☛ serving size: 1 piece = 89 g; Calories = 223

Restaurant Chinese Fried Rice Without Meat ☛ serving size: 1 cup = 137 g; Calories = 238

Restaurant Chinese General Tsos Chicken ☛ serving size: 1 order = 535 g; Calories = 1578

Restaurant Chinese Kung Pao Chicken ☛ serving size: 1 order = 604 g; Calories = 779

Restaurant Chinese Lemon Chicken ☛ serving size: 1 order = 623 g; Calories = 1570

Restaurant Chinese Orange Chicken ☛ serving size: 1 order = 648 g; Calories = 1698

Restaurant Chinese Sesame Chicken ☛ serving size: 1 order = 547 g; Calories = 1603

Restaurant Chinese Shrimp And Vegetables ☛ serving size: 1 order = 601 g; Calories = 469

Restaurant Chinese Sweet And Sour Chicken ☛ serving size: 1 order = 706 g; Calories = 1765

Restaurant Chinese Sweet And Sour Pork ☛ serving size: 1 order = 609 g; Calories = 1644

Restaurant Chinese Vegetable Chow Mein Without Meat Or Noodles ☛ serving size: 1 order = 777 g; Calories = 334

🏠 Restaurant Chinese Vegetable Lo Mein Without Meat ☛ serving size: 1 order = 741 g; Calories = 897

🏠 Restaurant Family Style Chicken Fingers From Kids Menu ☛ serving size: 1 serving = 114 g; Calories = 350

🏠 Restaurant Family Style Chicken Tenders ☛ serving size: 1 serving = 201 g; Calories = 607

🏠 Restaurant Family Style Chili With Meat And Beans ☛ serving size: 1 cup = 136 g; Calories = 214

🏠 Restaurant Family Style Coleslaw ☛ serving size: 1 serving = 108 g; Calories = 172

🏠 Restaurant Family Style Fish Fillet Battered Or Breaded Fried ☛ serving size: 1 serving = 226 g; Calories = 495

🏠 Restaurant Family Style French Fries ☛ serving size: 1 serving = 170 g; Calories = 491

🏠 Restaurant Family Style Fried Mozzarella Sticks ☛ serving size: 1 serving = 245 g; Calories = 796

🏠 Restaurant Family Style Hash Browns ☛ serving size: 1 cup = 94 g; Calories = 185

🏠 Restaurant Family Style Macaroni & Cheese From Kids Menu ☛ serving size: 1 cup = 136 g; Calories = 205

🏠 Restaurant Family Style Onion Rings ☛ serving size: 1 serving = 259 g; Calories = 922

🏠 Restaurant Family Style Shrimp Breaded And Fried ☛ serving size: 1 serving = 169 g; Calories = 521

🏠 Restaurant Family Style Sirloin Steak ☛ serving size: 1 serving = 166 g; Calories = 324

🏠 Restaurant Family Style Spaghetti And Meatballs ☛ serving size: 1 cup = 134 g; Calories = 228

Restaurant Italian Cheese Ravioli With Marinara Sauce ☛ serving size: 1 serving serving size varied by diameter and count of raviloi = 427 g; Calories = 658

Restaurant Italian Chicken Parmesan Without Pasta ☛ serving size: 1 serving = 301 g; Calories = 614

Restaurant Italian Lasagna With Meat ☛ serving size: 1 serving = 457 g; Calories = 846

Restaurant Italian Spaghetti With Meat Sauce ☛ serving size: 1 serving = 554 g; Calories = 670

Restaurant Italian Spaghetti With Pomodoro Sauce (No Meat) ☛ serving size: 1 serving = 510 g; Calories = 530

Restaurant Latino Arepa (Unleavened Cornmeal Bread) ☛ serving size: 1 piece = 98 g; Calories = 215

Restaurant Latino Arroz Con Frijoles Negros (Rice And Black Beans) ☛ serving size: 1 serving = 461 g; Calories = 696

Restaurant Latino Arroz Con Grandules (Rice And Pigeonpeas) ☛ serving size: 1 serving = 653 g; Calories = 1189

Restaurant Latino Arroz Con Habichuelas Colorados (Rice And Red Beans) ☛ serving size: 1 serving = 590 g; Calories = 838

Restaurant Latino Arroz Con Leche (Rice Pudding) ☛ serving size: 1 serving = 283 g; Calories = 413

Restaurant Latino Black Bean Soup ☛ serving size: 1 cup = 246 g; Calories = 253

Restaurant Latino Bunuelos (Fried Yeast Bread) ☛ serving size: 1 piece = 70 g; Calories = 323

Restaurant Latino Chicken And Rice Entree Prepared ☛ serving size: 1 cup = 141 g; Calories = 245

Restaurant Latino Empanadas Beef Prepared ☛ serving size: 1 piece = 89 g; Calories = 298

Restaurant Latino Pupusas Con Frijoles (Pupusas Bean) ☛ serving size: 1 piece = 126 g; Calories = 289

Restaurant Latino Pupusas Con Queso (Pupusas Cheese) ☛ serving size: 1 piece = 117 g; Calories = 300

Restaurant Latino Pupusas Del Cerdo (Pupusas Pork) ☛ serving size: 1 piece = 122 g; Calories = 283

Restaurant Latino Tamale Corn ☛ serving size: 1 piece = 166 g; Calories = 309

Restaurant Latino Tamale Pork ☛ serving size: 1 piece = 142 g; Calories = 247

Restaurant Latino Tripe Soup ☛ serving size: 1 cup = 200 g; Calories = 148

Restaurant Mexican Cheese Enchilada ☛ serving size: 1 serving serving size varied from 1 to 3 enchiladas = 244 g; Calories = 666

Restaurant Mexican Cheese Quesadilla ☛ serving size: 1 serving serving size varied on diameter and count of quesadila = 205 g; Calories = 754

Restaurant Mexican Cheese Tamales ☛ serving size: 1 serving serving size varied from 1 to 3 tamales = 302 g; Calories = 652

Restaurant Mexican Refried Beans ☛ serving size: 1 cup = 148 g; Calories = 231

Restaurant Mexican Soft Taco With Ground Beef Cheese And Lettuce ☛ serving size: 1 serving varied from 1 to 3 tacos per serving = 281 g; Calories = 615

Restaurant Mexican Spanish Rice ☛ serving size: 1 cup = 116 g; Calories = 215

TGI Fridays Chicken Fingers ☞ serving size: 1 serving = 225 g; Calories = 731

TGI Fridays Chicken Fingers From Kids Menu ☞ serving size: 1 piece = 41 g; Calories = 135

TGI Fridays Classic Sirloin Steak (10 Oz) ☞ serving size: 1 serving = 176 g; Calories = 345

TGI Fridays French Fries ☞ serving size: 1 serving = 184 g; Calories = 545

TGI Fridays Fridays Shrimp Breaded ☞ serving size: 1 serving = 175 g; Calories = 529

TGI Fridays Fried Mozzarella ☞ serving size: 1 piece = 35 g; Calories = 117

TGI Fridays Macaroni & Cheese From Kids Menu ☞ serving size: 1 cup = 144 g; Calories = 174

22

SNACKS

Bean Chips ☛ serving size: 1 chip = 3 g; Calories = 14

Breadsticks Hard Reduced Sodium ☛ serving size: 1 snack size stick = 2 g; Calories = 9

Breadsticks Hard Whole Wheat ☛ serving size: 1 snack size stick = 2 g; Calories = 8

Breakfast Bar Cereal Crust With Fruit Filling Lowfat ☛ serving size: 1 bar = 37 g; Calories = 140

Breakfast Bar Corn Flake Crust With Fruit ☛ serving size: 1 oz = 28.4 g; Calories = 107

Breakfast Bar Nfs ☛ serving size: 1 bar = 43 g; Calories = 162

Breakfast Bars Oats Sugar Raisins Coconut (Include Granola Bar) ☛ serving size: 1 bar = 43 g; Calories = 200

Cereal Or Granola Bar With Rice Cereal ☛ serving size: 1 bar = 28 g; Calories = 116

Cheese Flavored Corn Snacks ☛ serving size: 1 piece = 2 g; Calories = 11

Cheese Flavored Corn Snacks (Cheetos) ☞ serving size: 1 piece = 2 g; Calories = 11

Cheese Puffs And Twists Corn Based Baked Low Fat ☞ serving size: 1 oz = 28.4 g; Calories = 123

Corn Chips Flavored ☞ serving size: 1 chip = 1 g; Calories = 5

Corn Chips Flavored (Fritos) ☞ serving size: 1 chip = 1 g; Calories = 5

Corn Chips Plain ☞ serving size: 1 chip = 1 g; Calories = 5

Corn Chips Plain (Fritos) ☞ serving size: 1 chip = 1 g; Calories = 5

Corn Chips Reduced Sodium ☞ serving size: 1 chip = 1 g; Calories = 6

Crackers Breakfast Biscuit ☞ serving size: 1 biscuit, nfs = 15 g; Calories = 64

Crackers Flatbread ☞ serving size: 1 flatbread = 10 g; Calories = 41

Crackers Rice And Nuts ☞ serving size: 1 cracker = 3 g; Calories = 13

Crackers Saltine Reduced Sodium ☞ serving size: 1 cracker = 3 g; Calories = 13

Crackers Sandwich Cheese Filled (Ritz) ☞ serving size: 1 sandwich = 7 g; Calories = 34

Crackers Sandwich Peanut Butter Filled (Ritz) ☞ serving size: 1 sandwich = 7 g; Calories = 34

Crackers Wheat ☞ serving size: 1 cracker = 3 g; Calories = 13

Crackers Wheat Flavored (Wheat Thins) ☞ serving size: 1 cracker = 3 g; Calories = 13

Crackers Wheat Plain (Wheat Thins) ☞ serving size: 1 cracker = 3 g; Calories = 13

Crackers Woven Wheat ☞ serving size: 1 cracker = 5 g; Calories = 22

Crackers Woven Wheat Flavored (Triscuit) ☞ serving size: 1 cracker = 5 g; Calories = 22

Crackers Woven Wheat Plain (Triscuit) ☞ serving size: 1 cracker = 5 g; Calories = 22

Extruded Corn Chips ☞ serving size: 1 cup, crushed = 88 g; Calories = 490

Formulated Bar High Fiber Chewy Oats And Chocolate ☞ serving size: 1 bar = 40 g; Calories = 156

Formulated Bar Luna Bar Nutz Over Chocolate ☞ serving size: 1 bar = 48 g; Calories = 193

Formulated Bar Mars Snackfood Us Cocoavia Chocolate Almond Snack Bar ☞ serving size: 1 bar = 22 g; Calories = 76

Formulated Bar Mars Snackfood Us Cocoavia Chocolate Blueberry Snack Bar ☞ serving size: 1 bar = 22 g; Calories = 72

Formulated Bar Mars Snackfood Us Snickers Marathon Chewy Chocolate Peanut Bar ☞ serving size: 1 bar = 55 g; Calories = 218

Formulated Bar Mars Snackfood Us Snickers Marathon Energy Bar All Flavors ☞ serving size: 1 bar = 55 g; Calories = 212

Formulated Bar Mars Snackfood Us Snickers Marathon Honey Nut Oat Bar ☞ serving size: 1 bar = 55 g; Calories = 210

Formulated Bar Mars Snackfood Us Snickers Marathon Multigrain Crunch Bar ☞ serving size: 1 bar = 55 g; Calories = 232

Formulated Bar Mars Snackfood Us Snickers Marathon Protein Performance Bar Caramel Nut Rush ☞ serving size: 1 bar = 80 g; Calories = 332

Formulated Bar Power Bar Chocolate ☛ serving size: 1 bar = 68 g; Calories = 247

Formulated Bar Slim-Fast Optima Meal Bar Milk Chocolate Peanut ☛ serving size: 1 bar = 55 g; Calories = 212

Formulated Bar Zone Perfect Classic Crunch Bar Mixed Flavors ☛ serving size: 1 bar = 50 g; Calories = 213

Granola Bar Soft Milk Chocolate Coated Peanut Butter ☛ serving size: 1 oz = 28.4 g; Calories = 152

Microwave Popcorn ☛ serving size: 1 oz = 28.4 g; Calories = 114

Milk And Cereal Bar ☛ serving size: 1 bar = 25 g; Calories = 103

Nutrition Bar (Clif Kids Organic Zbar) ☛ serving size: 1 bar = 36 g; Calories = 147

Nutrition Bar (Tiger's Milk) ☛ serving size: 1 bar = 35 g; Calories = 148

Nutrition Bar (Zone Perfect Classic Crunch) ☛ serving size: 1 bar = 50 g; Calories = 211

Nutrition Bar Or Meal Replacement Bar Nfs ☛ serving size: 1 bar = 34 g; Calories = 144

Popcorn Air-Popped Unbuttered ☛ serving size: 1 cup, popped = 8 g; Calories = 31

Popcorn Air-Popped With Added Butter Or Margarine ☛ serving size: 1 cup, popped = 11 g; Calories = 47

Popcorn Caramel Coated ☛ serving size: 1 cup = 35 g; Calories = 150

Popcorn Caramel Coated With Nuts ☛ serving size: 1 cup = 42 g; Calories = 167

Popcorn Chips Other Flavors ☛ serving size: 1 chip = 1 g; Calories = 4

Popcorn Chips Plain ☛ serving size: 1 chip = 1 g; Calories = 4

Popcorn Chips Sweet Flavors ☛ serving size: 1 chip = 1 g; Calories = 5

Popcorn Microwave Butter Flavored ☛ serving size: 1 regular microwave bag = 85 g; Calories = 457

Popcorn Microwave Butter Flavored Light ☛ serving size: 1 regular microwave bag = 85 g; Calories = 358

Popcorn Microwave Cheese Flavored ☛ serving size: 1 regular microwave bag = 85 g; Calories = 456

Popcorn Microwave Kettle Corn ☛ serving size: 1 regular microwave bag = 85 g; Calories = 439

Popcorn Microwave Kettle Corn Light ☛ serving size: 1 regular microwave bag = 85 g; Calories = 359

Popcorn Microwave Low Fat And Sodium ☛ serving size: 1 oz = 28.4 g; Calories = 122

Popcorn Microwave Low Sodium ☛ serving size: 1 regular microwave bag = 85 g; Calories = 422

Popcorn Microwave Nfs ☛ serving size: 1 regular microwave bag = 85 g; Calories = 457

Popcorn Microwave Other Flavored ☛ serving size: 1 regular microwave bag = 85 g; Calories = 456

Popcorn Microwave Plain ☛ serving size: 1 regular microwave bag = 85 g; Calories = 457

Popcorn Microwave Plain Light ☛ serving size: 1 regular microwave bag = 85 g; Calories = 358

Popcorn Microwave Regular (Butter) Flavor Made With Palm Oil ☛ serving size: 1 cup = 7.9 g; Calories = 42

Popcorn Microwave Unsalted ☛ serving size: 1 regular microwave bag = 85 g; Calories = 422

Popcorn Movie Theater Unbuttered ☛ serving size: 1 kids size order = 66 g; Calories = 398

Popcorn Movie Theater With Added Butter ☛ serving size: 1 kids size order = 84 g; Calories = 551

Popcorn Nfs ☛ serving size: 1 regular microwave bag = 85 g; Calories = 457

Popcorn Popped In Oil Unbuttered ☛ serving size: 1 cup, popped = 11 g; Calories = 55

Popcorn Popped In Oil With Added Butter Or Margarine ☛ serving size: 1 cup, popped = 14 g; Calories = 73

Popcorn Ready-To-Eat Packaged Butter Flavored ☛ serving size: 1 cup = 14 g; Calories = 74

Popcorn Ready-To-Eat Packaged Butter Flavored Light ☛ serving size: 1 cup = 8 g; Calories = 35

Popcorn Ready-To-Eat Packaged Cheese Flavored Light ☛ serving size: 1 cup = 8 g; Calories = 35

Popcorn Ready-To-Eat Packaged Kettle Corn Light ☛ serving size: 1 cup = 8 g; Calories = 35

Popcorn Ready-To-Eat Packaged Low Sodium ☛ serving size: 1 cup = 11 g; Calories = 54

Popcorn Ready-To-Eat Packaged Nfs ☛ serving size: 1 cup = 14 g; Calories = 74

Popcorn Ready-To-Eat Packaged Plain ☛ serving size: 1 cup = 11 g; Calories = 53

Popcorn Ready-To-Eat Packaged Plain Light ☛ serving size: 1 cup = 8 g; Calories = 35

⚬ Popcorn Ready-To-Eat Packaged Unsalted ☛ serving size: 1 cup = 11 g; Calories = 54

⚬ Popcorn Ready-To-Eat-Packaged Kettle Corn ☛ serving size: 1 cup = 14 g; Calories = 74

⚬ Popcorn Sugar Syrup/caramel Fat-Free ☛ serving size: 1 oz = 28.4 g; Calories = 108

⚬ Potato Chips Baked Flavored ☛ serving size: 1 chip = 2 g; Calories = 9

⚬ Potato Chips Fat Free ☛ serving size: 1 chip = 1 g; Calories = 5

⚬ Potato Chips Lightly Salted ☛ serving size: 1 chip = 2 g; Calories = 11

⚬ Potato Chips Popped Flavored ☛ serving size: 1 chip = 1 g; Calories = 5

⚬ Potato Chips Reduced Fat ☛ serving size: 1 chip = 2 g; Calories = 10

⚬ Potato Chips Restructured Flavored ☛ serving size: 1 chip = 2 g; Calories = 11

⚬ Potato Chips Restructured Lightly Salted ☛ serving size: 1 chip = 2 g; Calories = 11

⚬ Potato Chips Restructured Plain ☛ serving size: 1 chip = 2 g; Calories = 11

⚬ Potato Chips Unsalted ☛ serving size: 1 chip = 2 g; Calories = 11

⚬ Potato Chips Without Salt Reduced Fat ☛ serving size: 1 oz = 28.4 g; Calories = 138

⚬ Potato Sticks Flavored ☛ serving size: 10 sticks = 3 g; Calories = 16

⚬ Potato Sticks Fry Shaped ☛ serving size: 10 sticks = 3 g; Calories = 16

Pretzel Chips Hard Flavored ☛ serving size: 1 pretzel chip/crisp/thin = 3 g; Calories = 11

Pretzel Chips Hard Gluten Free ☛ serving size: 1 pretzel chip/crisp/thin = 3 g; Calories = 11

Pretzel Chips Hard Plain ☛ serving size: 1 pretzel chip/crisp/thin = 3 g; Calories = 11

Pretzels Hard Coated Gluten Free ☛ serving size: 1 miniature/bite size = 4 g; Calories = 18

Pretzels Hard Flavored ☛ serving size: 1 miniature/bite size = 2 g; Calories = 8

Pretzels Hard Flavored Gluten Free ☛ serving size: 1 pretzel stick = 1 g; Calories = 4

Pretzels Hard Multigrain ☛ serving size: 1 miniature/bite size = 2 g; Calories = 8

Pretzels Hard Peanut Butter Filled ☛ serving size: 1 miniature/bite size = 3 g; Calories = 14

Pretzels Hard Plain Lightly Salted ☛ serving size: 1 miniature/bite size = 2 g; Calories = 8

Pretzels Hard White Chocolate Coated ☛ serving size: 1 miniature/bite size = 4 g; Calories = 18

Pretzels Hard Yogurt Coated ☛ serving size: 1 miniature/bite size = 4 g; Calories = 17

Pretzels Soft Filled With Cheese ☛ serving size: 1 medium/regular = 99 g; Calories = 335

Pretzels Soft From Frozen Cinnamon Sugar Coated ☛ serving size: 1 medium/regular = 71 g; Calories = 263

Pretzels Soft From Frozen Coated Or Flavored ☛ serving size: 1 medium/regular = 71 g; Calories = 259

Pretzels Soft From Frozen Nfs ☞ serving size: 1 medium/regular = 71 g; Calories = 242

Pretzels Soft From Frozen Salted ☞ serving size: 1 medium/regular = 71 g; Calories = 239

Pretzels Soft From Frozen Topped With Cheese ☞ serving size: 1 medium/regular = 71 g; Calories = 240

Pretzels Soft From Frozen Topped With Meat ☞ serving size: 1 medium/regular = 71 g; Calories = 249

Pretzels Soft From School Lunch ☞ serving size: 1 medium/regular = 71 g; Calories = 241

Pretzels Soft Gluten Free ☞ serving size: 1 medium/regular = 95 g; Calories = 282

Pretzels Soft Gluten Free Cinnamon Sugar Coated ☞ serving size: 1 medium/regular = 95 g; Calories = 319

Pretzels Soft Gluten Free Coated Or Flavored ☞ serving size: 1 medium/regular = 95 g; Calories = 310

Pretzels Soft Multigrain ☞ serving size: 1 small = 62 g; Calories = 206

Pretzels Soft Nfs ☞ serving size: 1 bite size/nugget = 14 g; Calories = 48

Pretzels Soft Ready-To-Eat Cinnamon Sugar Coated ☞ serving size: 1 bite size/nugget = 14 g; Calories = 52

Pretzels Soft Ready-To-Eat Coated Or Flavored ☞ serving size: 1 bite size/nugget = 14 g; Calories = 51

Pretzels Soft Ready-To-Eat Nfs ☞ serving size: 1 bite size/nugget = 14 g; Calories = 48

Pretzels Soft Ready-To-Eat Salted Buttered ☞ serving size: 1 bite size/nugget = 14 g; Calories = 48

🍘 Pretzels Soft Ready-To-Eat Salted No Butter ☛ serving size: 1 bite size/nugget = 14 g; Calories = 47

🍘 Pretzels Soft Ready-To-Eat Topped With Cheese ☛ serving size: 1 bite size/nugget = 14 g; Calories = 47

🍘 Pretzels Soft Ready-To-Eat Topped With Meat ☛ serving size: 1 bite size/nugget = 14 g; Calories = 49

🍘 Pretzels Soft Ready-To-Eat Unsalted Buttered ☛ serving size: 1 bite size/nugget = 14 g; Calories = 49

🍘 Rice And Wheat Cereal Bar ☛ serving size: 1 bar = 22 g; Calories = 90

🍘 Rice Cake Cracker (Include Hain Mini Rice Cakes) ☛ serving size: 1 cubic inch = 4.2 g; Calories = 17

🍘 Rice Paper ☛ serving size: 1 small paper (6-3/8" dia) = 5 g; Calories = 17

🍘 Snack Mix ☛ serving size: 1 cup = 60 g; Calories = 301

🍘 Snack Mix Plain (Chex Mix) ☛ serving size: 1 cup = 60 g; Calories = 257

🍘 Snack Mixed Berry Bar ☛ serving size: 1 bar = 38 g; Calories = 146

🍘 Snack Potato Chips Made From Dried Potatoes Plain ☛ serving size: 1 oz = 28 g; Calories = 153

🍘 Snack Pretzel Hard Chocolate Coated ☛ serving size: 1 serving = 28 g; Calories = 131

🍘 Snacks Bagel Chips Plain ☛ serving size: 1 oz = 28.4 g; Calories = 128

🍘 Snacks Banana Chips ☛ serving size: 1 oz = 28.4 g; Calories = 147

🍘 Snacks Beef Jerky Chopped And Formed ☛ serving size: 1 oz = 28.4 g; Calories = 116

Snacks Beef Sticks Smoked ☛ serving size: 1 oz = 28.4 g; Calories = 156

Snacks Brown Rice Chips ☛ serving size: 1 cake = 9 g; Calories = 35

Snacks Candy Bits Yogurt Covered With Vitamin C ☛ serving size: 1 package = 20 g; Calories = 83

Snacks Candy Rolls Yogurt-Covered Fruit Flavored With High Vitamin C ☛ serving size: 1 roll = 23 g; Calories = 83

Snacks Clif Bar Mixed Flavors ☛ serving size: 1 bar = 68 g; Calories = 235

Snacks Corn Cakes ☛ serving size: 1 cake = 9 g; Calories = 35

Snacks Corn Cakes Very Low Sodium ☛ serving size: 1 cake = 9 g; Calories = 35

Snacks Corn-Based Extruded Chips Barbecue-Flavor ☛ serving size: 1 oz = 28.4 g; Calories = 149

Snacks Corn-Based Extruded Chips Barbecue-Flavor Made With Enriched Masa Flour ☛ serving size: 1 oz = 28.4 g; Calories = 149

Snacks Corn-Based Extruded Chips Plain ☛ serving size: 1 oz = 28 g; Calories = 151

Snacks Corn-Based Extruded Cones Plain ☛ serving size: 1 oz = 28.4 g; Calories = 145

Snacks Corn-Based Extruded Onion-Flavor ☛ serving size: 1 oz = 28.4 g; Calories = 142

Snacks Corn-Based Extruded Puffs Or Twists Cheese-Flavor ☛ serving size: 1 oz = 28.4 g; Calories = 161

Snacks Corn-Based Extruded Puffs Or Twists Cheese-Flavor Unenriched ☛ serving size: 1 oz = 28.4 g; Calories = 159

Snacks Cornnuts Barbecue-Flavor ☛ serving size: 1 oz = 28.4 g; Calories = 124

Snacks Crisped Rice Bar Almond ☞ serving size: 1 bar (1 oz) = 28 g; Calories = 128

Snacks Crisped Rice Bar Chocolate Chip ☞ serving size: 1 bar (1 oz) = 28 g; Calories = 113

Snacks Farley Candy Farley Fruit Snacks With Vitamins A C And E ☞ serving size: 1 pouch = 26 g; Calories = 89

Snacks Fritolay Sunchips Multigrain French Onion Flavor ☞ serving size: 1 oz = 28.4 g; Calories = 141

Snacks Fritolay Sunchips Multigrain Snack Harvest Cheddar Flavor ☞ serving size: 1 oz = 28.4 g; Calories = 139

Snacks Fritolay Sunchips Multigrain Snack Original Flavor ☞ serving size: 1 oz = 28.4 g; Calories = 139

Snacks Fruit Leather Pieces With Vitamin C ☞ serving size: 1 serving = 21 g; Calories = 78

Snacks General Mills Betty Crocker Fruit Roll Ups Berry Flavored With Vitamin C ☞ serving size: 2 rolls = 28 g; Calories = 104

Snacks Granola Bar Chewy Reduced Sugar All Flavors ☞ serving size: 1 bar = 24 g; Calories = 99

Snacks Granola Bar General Mills Nature Valley Chewy Trail Mix ☞ serving size: 1 bar = 35 g; Calories = 145

Snacks Granola Bar General Mills Nature Valley Sweet&salty Nut Peanut ☞ serving size: 1 bar = 35 g; Calories = 171

Snacks Granola Bar General Mills Nature Valley With Yogurt Coating ☞ serving size: 1 bar = 35 g; Calories = 148

Snacks Granola Bar Kashi Golean Chewy Mixed Flavors ☞ serving size: 1 bar = 78 g; Calories = 304

Snacks Granola Bar Kashi Golean Crunchy Mixed Flavors ☞ serving size: 1 bar = 47 g; Calories = 185

Snacks Granola Bar Kashi Tlc Bar Chewy Mixed Flavors ☛ serving size: 1 bar = 35 g; Calories = 150

Snacks Granola Bar Kashi Tlc Bar Crunchy Mixed Flavors ☛ serving size: 2 bar = 40 g; Calories = 178

Snacks Granola Bar Quaker Chewy 90 Calorie Bar ☛ serving size: 1 bar = 24 g; Calories = 98

Snacks Granola Bar Quaker Dipps All Flavors ☛ serving size: 1 bar = 31 g; Calories = 149

Snacks Granola Bar With Coconut Chocolate Coated ☛ serving size: 1 oz = 28.4 g; Calories = 151

Snacks Granola Bars Hard Almond ☛ serving size: 1 oz = 28.4 g; Calories = 141

Snacks Granola Bars Hard Chocolate Chip ☛ serving size: 1 oz = 28.4 g; Calories = 124

Snacks Granola Bars Hard Peanut Butter ☛ serving size: 1 oz = 28.4 g; Calories = 137

Snacks Granola Bars Hard Plain ☛ serving size: 1 bar = 21 g; Calories = 99

Snacks Granola Bars Quaker Oatmeal To Go All Flavors ☛ serving size: 1 bar = 60 g; Calories = 233

Snacks Granola Bars Soft Almond Confectioners Coating ☛ serving size: 1 bar = 35 g; Calories = 159

Snacks Granola Bars Soft Coated Milk Chocolate Coating Chocolate Chip ☛ serving size: 1 bar (1.25 oz) = 35 g; Calories = 163

Snacks Granola Bars Soft Coated Milk Chocolate Coating Peanut Butter ☛ serving size: 1 oz = 28.4 g; Calories = 144

Snacks Granola Bars Soft Uncoated Chocolate Chip ☛ serving size: 1 bar (1.5 oz) = 43 g; Calories = 180

Snacks Granola Bars Soft Uncoated Chocolate Chip Graham And Marshmallow ☛ serving size: 1 bar (1 oz) = 28 g; Calories = 120

Snacks Granola Bars Soft Uncoated Nut And Raisin ☛ serving size: 1 bar (1 oz) = 28 g; Calories = 127

Snacks Granola Bars Soft Uncoated Peanut Butter ☛ serving size: 1 bar (1 oz) = 28 g; Calories = 119

Snacks Granola Bars Soft Uncoated Peanut Butter And Chocolate Chip ☛ serving size: 1 bar (1 oz) = 28 g; Calories = 121

Snacks Granola Bars Soft Uncoated Plain ☛ serving size: 1 bar (1 oz) = 28 g; Calories = 124

Snacks Granola Bars Soft Uncoated Raisin ☛ serving size: 1 bar (1.5 oz) = 43 g; Calories = 193

Snacks Granola Bites Mixed Flavors ☛ serving size: 1 package = 20 g; Calories = 90

Snacks Kellogg Kelloggs Low Fat Granola Bar Crunchy Almond/brown Sugar ☛ serving size: 1 bar = 37 g; Calories = 144

Snacks Kellogg Kelloggs Rice Krispies Treats Squares ☛ serving size: 1 serving = 22 g; Calories = 92

Snacks Kraft Cornnuts Plain ☛ serving size: 1 oz = 28.4 g; Calories = 127

Snacks M&m Mars Combos Snacks Cheddar Cheese Pretzel ☛ serving size: 1 oz = 28.4 g; Calories = 132

Snacks M&m Mars Kudos Whole Grain Bar Chocolate Chip ☛ serving size: 1 bar = 28 g; Calories = 118

Snacks M&m Mars Kudos Whole Grain Bar M&Ms Milk Chocolate ☛ serving size: 1 bar = 24 g; Calories = 100

Snacks M&m Mars Kudos Whole Grain Bars Peanut Butter ☛ serving size: 1 bar = 28 g; Calories = 130

Snacks Nutri-Grain Fruit And Nut Bar ☛ serving size: 1 bar = 32 g; Calories = 129

Snacks Oriental Mix Rice-Based ☛ serving size: 1 oz = 28.4 g; Calories = 144

Snacks Pita Chips Salted ☛ serving size: 1 oz = 28.4 g; Calories = 130

Snacks Plantain Chips Salted ☛ serving size: 1 oz = 28.4 g; Calories = 151

Snacks Popcorn Air-Popped ☛ serving size: 1 cup = 8 g; Calories = 31

Snacks Popcorn Air-Popped (Unsalted) ☛ serving size: 1 cup = 8 g; Calories = 31

Snacks Popcorn Cakes ☛ serving size: 1 cake = 10 g; Calories = 38

Snacks Popcorn Caramel-Coated With Peanuts ☛ serving size: 1 oz (approx 2/3 cup) = 28.4 g; Calories = 114

Snacks Popcorn Caramel-Coated Without Peanuts ☛ serving size: 1 oz = 28.4 g; Calories = 122

Snacks Popcorn Cheese-Flavor ☛ serving size: 1 cup = 11 g; Calories = 58

Snacks Popcorn Home-Prepared Oil-Popped Unsalted ☛ serving size: 1 cup = 8 g; Calories = 40

Snacks Popcorn Microwave Low Fat ☛ serving size: 1 oz = 28.4 g; Calories = 120

Snacks Popcorn Microwave Regular (Butter) Flavor Made With Partially Hydrogenated Oil ☛ serving size: 1 cup = 7.9 g; Calories = 44

Snacks Popcorn Oil-Popped Microwave Regular Flavor No Trans Fat ☛ serving size: 1 cup = 11 g; Calories = 64

Snacks Popcorn Oil-Popped White Popcorn Salt Added ☞ serving size: 1 cup = 11 g; Calories = 55

Snacks Pork Skins Barbecue-Flavor ☞ serving size: 1 oz = 28.4 g; Calories = 153

Snacks Pork Skins Plain ☞ serving size: 1 oz = 28.4 g; Calories = 155

Snacks Potato Chips Barbecue-Flavor ☞ serving size: 1 oz = 28.4 g; Calories = 138

Snacks Potato Chips Cheese-Flavor ☞ serving size: 1 oz = 28.4 g; Calories = 141

Snacks Potato Chips Fat Free Salted ☞ serving size: 1 oz = 28.4 g; Calories = 108

Snacks Potato Chips Fat-Free Made With Olestra ☞ serving size: 1 oz = 28.4 g; Calories = 78

Snacks Potato Chips Lightly Salted ☞ serving size: pieces = 28 g; Calories = 157

Snacks Potato Chips Made From Dried Potatoes (Preformed) Multigrain ☞ serving size: 1 oz = 28.4 g; Calories = 143

Snacks Potato Chips Made From Dried Potatoes Cheese-Flavor ☞ serving size: 1 oz = 28.4 g; Calories = 157

Snacks Potato Chips Made From Dried Potatoes Fat-Free Made With Olestra ☞ serving size: 1 oz = 28.4 g; Calories = 72

Snacks Potato Chips Made From Dried Potatoes Reduced Fat ☞ serving size: 1 oz = 28.4 g; Calories = 143

Snacks Potato Chips Made From Dried Potatoes Sour-Cream And Onion-Flavor ☞ serving size: 1 oz = 28.4 g; Calories = 155

Snacks Potato Chips Plain Made With Partially Hydrogenated Soybean Oil Salted ☞ serving size: 1 oz = 28.4 g; Calories = 152

Snacks Potato Chips Plain Made With Partially Hydrogenated Soybean Oil Unsalted ☛ serving size: 1 oz = 28.4 g; Calories = 152

Snacks Potato Chips Plain Salted ☛ serving size: 1 oz = 28 g; Calories = 149

Snacks Potato Chips Plain Unsalted ☛ serving size: 1 oz = 28.4 g; Calories = 152

Snacks Potato Chips Reduced Fat ☛ serving size: 1 oz = 28.4 g; Calories = 134

Snacks Potato Chips Sour-Cream-And-Onion-Flavor ☛ serving size: 1 oz = 28.4 g; Calories = 151

Snacks Potato Chips White Restructured Baked ☛ serving size: 1 cup = 34 g; Calories = 160

Snacks Potato Sticks ☛ serving size: 1 oz = 28.4 g; Calories = 148

Snacks Pretzels Hard Confectioners Coating Chocolate-Flavor ☛ serving size: 1 oz = 28.4 g; Calories = 130

Snacks Pretzels Hard Plain Made With Enriched Flour Unsalted ☛ serving size: 1 oz = 28.4 g; Calories = 108

Snacks Pretzels Hard Plain Made With Unenriched Flour Salted ☛ serving size: 1 oz = 28.4 g; Calories = 108

Snacks Pretzels Hard Plain Made With Unenriched Flour Unsalted ☛ serving size: 1 oz = 28.4 g; Calories = 108

Snacks Pretzels Hard Plain Salted ☛ serving size: 1 oz = 28.4 g; Calories = 109

Snacks Pretzels Hard Whole-Wheat Including Both Salted And Unsalted ☛ serving size: 1 oz = 28.4 g; Calories = 103

Snacks Rice Cakes Brown Rice Buckwheat ☛ serving size: 1 cake = 9 g; Calories = 34

Snacks Rice Cakes Brown Rice Buckwheat Unsalted ☞ serving size: 1 cake = 9 g; Calories = 34

Snacks Rice Cakes Brown Rice Corn ☞ serving size: 1 cake = 9 g; Calories = 35

Snacks Rice Cakes Brown Rice Multigrain ☞ serving size: 1 cake = 9 g; Calories = 35

Snacks Rice Cakes Brown Rice Multigrain Unsalted ☞ serving size: 1 cake = 9 g; Calories = 35

Snacks Rice Cakes Brown Rice Plain Unsalted ☞ serving size: 1 cake = 9 g; Calories = 35

Snacks Rice Cakes Brown Rice Rye ☞ serving size: 1 cake = 9 g; Calories = 35

Snacks Rice Cakes Brown Rice Sesame Seed ☞ serving size: 1 cake = 9 g; Calories = 35

Snacks Rice Cakes Brown Rice Sesame Seed Unsalted ☞ serving size: 1 cake = 9 g; Calories = 35

Snacks Rice Cracker Brown Rice Plain ☞ serving size: 1 cake = 9 g; Calories = 35

Snacks Sesame Sticks Wheat-Based Salted ☞ serving size: 1 oz = 28.4 g; Calories = 154

Snacks Sesame Sticks Wheat-Based Unsalted ☞ serving size: 1 oz = 28.4 g; Calories = 154

Snacks Sunkist Sunkist Fruit Roll Strawberry With Vitamins A C And E ☞ serving size: 1 roll = 21 g; Calories = 72

Snacks Sweet Potato Chips Unsalted ☞ serving size: 1 oz = 28.4 g; Calories = 151

Snacks Taro Chips ☞ serving size: 1 oz = 28.4 g; Calories = 141

Snacks Tortilla Chips Light (Baked With Less Oil) ☛ serving size: 1 cup, crushed = 63 g; Calories = 293

Snacks Tortilla Chips Low Fat Made With Olestra Nacho Cheese ☛ serving size: 1 oz = 28.4 g; Calories = 90

Snacks Tortilla Chips Low Fat Unsalted ☛ serving size: 1 oz = 28.4 g; Calories = 118

Snacks Tortilla Chips Nacho Cheese ☛ serving size: 1 oz = 28.4 g; Calories = 147

Snacks Tortilla Chips Nacho-Flavor Made With Enriched Masa Flour ☛ serving size: 1 oz = 28.4 g; Calories = 145

Snacks Tortilla Chips Nacho-Flavor Reduced Fat ☛ serving size: 1 oz = 28.4 g; Calories = 126

Snacks Tortilla Chips Plain White Corn Salted ☛ serving size: 1 oz = 28.4 g; Calories = 134

Snacks Tortilla Chips Ranch-Flavor ☛ serving size: 1 oz = 28.4 g; Calories = 142

Snacks Tortilla Chips Taco-Flavor ☛ serving size: 1 oz = 28.4 g; Calories = 136

Snacks Tortilla Chips Unsalted White Corn ☛ serving size: 1 cup = 26 g; Calories = 131

Snacks Trail Mix Regular ☛ serving size: 1 cup = 150 g; Calories = 693

Snacks Trail Mix Regular Unsalted ☛ serving size: 1 cup = 150 g; Calories = 693

Snacks Trail Mix Regular With Chocolate Chips Unsalted Nuts And Seeds ☛ serving size: 1 cup = 146 g; Calories = 707

Snacks Trail Mix Tropical ☛ serving size: 1 cup = 140 g; Calories = 619

Snacks Vegetable Chips Hain Celestial Group Terra Chips ☛ serving size: 1 oz = 28.4 g; Calories = 147

Snacks Vegetable Chips Made From Garden Vegetables ☛ serving size: 1 oz = 28.4 g; Calories = 134

Snacks Yucca (Cassava) Chips Salted ☛ serving size: 1 oz = 28.4 g; Calories = 146

Snickers Marathon Double Chocolate Nut Bar ☛ serving size: 1 bar = 55 g; Calories = 207

Soft Pretzels ☛ serving size: 1 large = 143 g; Calories = 493

Soft Pretzels (Salted) ☛ serving size: 1 large = 143 g; Calories = 483

Soychips ☛ serving size: 1 oz = 28.4 g; Calories = 109

Sweet Potato Chips ☛ serving size: 1 chip = 2 g; Calories = 11

Tortilla Chips Cool Ranch Flavor (Doritos) ☛ serving size: 1 chip = 3 g; Calories = 14

Tortilla Chips Low Fat Baked Without Fat ☛ serving size: 1 oz = 28.4 g; Calories = 127

Tortilla Chips Popped ☛ serving size: 1 chip = 2 g; Calories = 9

Tortilla Chips Reduced Fat Flavored ☛ serving size: 1 chip = 2 g; Calories = 8

Tortilla Chips Reduced Fat Plain ☛ serving size: 1 chip = 2 g; Calories = 8

Tortilla Chips Reduced Sodium ☛ serving size: 1 chip = 2 g; Calories = 10

Tortilla Chips Yellow Plain Salted ☛ serving size: 1 oz = 28.4 g; Calories = 141

Trail Mix ☛ serving size: 1 cup = 146 g; Calories = 707

Vegetable Chips ☛ serving size: 1 chip = 2 g; Calories = 10

23

SOUPS AND SAUCES

Alfredo Sauce ☛ serving size: 1 cup = 260 g; Calories = 382

Alfredo Sauce With Added Vegetables ☛ serving size: 1 cup = 260 g; Calories = 307

Alfredo Sauce With Meat ☛ serving size: 1 cup = 260 g; Calories = 437

Alfredo Sauce With Meat And Added Vegetables ☛ serving size: 1 cup = 260 g; Calories = 377

Alfredo Sauce With Poultry ☛ serving size: 1 cup = 260 g; Calories = 395

Alfredo Sauce With Poultry And Added Vegetables ☛ serving size: 1 cup = 260 g; Calories = 333

Alfredo Sauce With Seafood ☛ serving size: 1 cup = 260 g; Calories = 369

Alfredo Sauce With Seafood And Added Vegetables ☛ serving size: 1 cup = 260 g; Calories = 309

Artichoke Dip ☛ serving size: 1 tablespoon = 15 g; Calories = 50

Asparagus Soup Cream Of Ns As To Made With Milk Or Water ☛ serving size: 1 cup = 248 g; Calories = 149

Asparagus Soup Cream Of Prepared With Milk ☛ serving size: 1 cup = 248 g; Calories = 149

Asparagus Soup Cream Of Prepared With Water ☛ serving size: 1 cup = 244 g; Calories = 85

Bacon Soup Cream Of Prepared With Water ☛ serving size: 1 cup = 244 g; Calories = 112

Barbecue Sauce ☛ serving size: 1 tbsp = 17 g; Calories = 29

Barley Soup Sweet With Or Without Nuts Asian Style ☛ serving size: 1 cup = 244 g; Calories = 149

Bean And Ham Soup Home Recipe ☛ serving size: 1 cup = 247 g; Calories = 203

Bean Soup Home Recipe ☛ serving size: 1 cup = 247 g; Calories = 161

Bean Soup Mixed Beans Home Recipe Canned Or Ready-To-Serve ☛ serving size: 1 cup = 238 g; Calories = 150

Bean Soup Nfs ☛ serving size: 1 cup = 253 g; Calories = 172

Bean Soup With Macaroni Home Recipe Canned Or Ready-To-Serve ☛ serving size: 1 cup = 253 g; Calories = 228

Bean With Bacon Or Ham Soup Canned Or Ready-To-Serve ☛ serving size: 1 cup = 253 g; Calories = 172

Beef And Rice Soup Puerto Rican Style ☛ serving size: 1 cup = 250 g; Calories = 148

Beef Broth From Bouillon ☛ serving size: 1 cup (8 fl oz) = 241 g; Calories = 29

Beef Broth With Tomato Home Recipe ☛ serving size: 1 cup = 237 g; Calories = 116

Beef Noodle Soup Canned Or Ready-To-Serve ☛ serving size: 1 cup = 244 g; Calories = 83

Beef Noodle Soup Home Recipe ☛ serving size: 1 cup = 244 g; Calories = 171

Beef Noodle Soup Puerto Rican Style ☛ serving size: 1 cup = 250 g; Calories = 148

Beef Stock ☛ serving size: 1 cup = 240 g; Calories = 31

Beef Vegetable Soup Home Recipe Mexican Style ☛ serving size: 1 cup = 239 g; Calories = 167

Beer Cheese Soup Made With Milk ☛ serving size: 1 cup = 245 g; Calories = 470

Bird's Nest Soup ☛ serving size: 1 cup = 244 g; Calories = 112

Black Bean Sauce ☛ serving size: 1 cup = 275 g; Calories = 600

Black Bean Soup ☛ serving size: 1 cup = 247 g; Calories = 114

Borscht ☛ serving size: 1 cup = 245 g; Calories = 101

Broccoli Cheese Soup Prepared With Milk Home Recipe Canned Or Ready-To-Serve ☛ serving size: 1 cup = 239 g; Calories = 165

Broccoli Soup Prepared With Milk Home Recipe Canned Or Ready-To-Serve ☛ serving size: 1 cup = 237 g; Calories = 164

Broccoli Soup Prepared With Water Home Recipe Canned Or Ready-To-Serve ☛ serving size: 1 cup = 239 g; Calories = 105

Brown Nut Gravy Meatless ☛ serving size: 1 tablespoon = 15 g; Calories = 19

Cabbage Soup Home Recipe Canned Or Ready-To-Serve ☛ serving size: 1 cup = 245 g; Calories = 93

Cabbage With Meat Soup Home Recipe Canned Or Ready-To-Serve ☛ serving size: 1 cup = 245 g; Calories = 113

Campbells Beef Barley Soup ☞ serving size: 1 cup = 206 g; Calories = 115

Campbells Chunky Classic Chicken Noodle Soup ☞ serving size: 1 cup = 243 g; Calories = 114

Campbells Chunky New England Clam Chowder ☞ serving size: 1 cup = 251 g; Calories = 203

Campbells Chunky Soups Old Fashioned Vegetable Beef Soup ☞ serving size: 1 cup = 247 g; Calories = 121

Campbells Cream Of Mushroom Soup Condensed ☞ serving size: 1/2 cup condensed = 129 g; Calories = 105

Campbells Red And White Chicken Noodle Soup Condensed ☞ serving size: 1/2 cup = 123 g; Calories = 58

Campbells Tomato Soup Condensed ☞ serving size: 1/2 cup condensed = 124 g; Calories = 88

Canned Minestrone ☞ serving size: 1 cup = 240 g; Calories = 127

Canned Pizza Sauce ☞ serving size: 1/4 cup = 63 g; Calories = 34

Carrot Soup Cream Of Prepared With Milk Home Recipe Canned Or Ready-To-Serve ☞ serving size: 1 cup = 237 g; Calories = 76

Carrot With Rice Soup Cream Of Prepared With Milk Home Recipe Canned Or Ready-To-Serve ☞ serving size: 1 cup = 245 g; Calories = 135

Celery Soup Cream Of Prepared With Milk Home Recipe Canned Or Ready-To-Serve ☞ serving size: 1 cup = 248 g; Calories = 151

Celery Soup Cream Of Prepared With Water Home Recipe Canned Or Ready-To-Serve ☞ serving size: 1 cup = 244 g; Calories = 90

Cheddar Cheese Soup Home Recipe Canned Or Ready-To-Serve ☞ serving size: 1 cup = 251 g; Calories = 168

Cheese Dip ☛ serving size: 1 tablespoon = 15 g; Calories = 24

Cheese Fondue ☛ serving size: 1 tablespoon = 13 g; Calories = 36

Cheese Sauce ☛ serving size: 1 cup = 243 g; Calories = 389

Cheese Sauce Made With Lowfat Cheese ☛ serving size: 1 cup = 243 g; Calories = 304

Chicken Or Turkey And Corn Hominy Soup Home Recipe Mexican Style ☛ serving size: 1 cup = 238 g; Calories = 179

Chicken Or Turkey Broth With Tomato Home Recipe ☛ serving size: 1 cup = 237 g; Calories = 114

Chicken Or Turkey Corn Soup With Noodles Home Recipe ☛ serving size: 1 cup = 251 g; Calories = 156

Chicken Or Turkey Mushroom Soup Cream Of Prepared With Milk ☛ serving size: 1 cup = 248 g; Calories = 186

Chicken Or Turkey Noodle Soup Canned Or Ready-To-Serve ☛ serving size: 1 cup = 241 g; Calories = 58

Chicken Or Turkey Noodle Soup Cream Of Home Recipe Canned Or Ready-To-Serve ☛ serving size: 1 cup = 245 g; Calories = 120

Chicken Or Turkey Noodle Soup Home Recipe ☛ serving size: 1 cup = 241 g; Calories = 147

Chicken Or Turkey Rice Soup Canned Or Ready-To-Serve ☛ serving size: 1 cup = 241 g; Calories = 82

Chicken Or Turkey Rice Soup Home Recipe ☛ serving size: 1 cup = 231 g; Calories = 143

Chicken Or Turkey Rice Soup Reduced Sodium Canned Prepared With Milk ☛ serving size: 1 cup = 245 g; Calories = 118

Chicken Or Turkey Rice Soup Reduced Sodium Canned Prepared With Water Or Ready-To-Serve ☛ serving size: 1 cup = 241 g; Calories = 55

Chicken Or Turkey Soup Cream Of Canned Reduced Sodium Made With Milk ☛ serving size: 1 cup = 248 g; Calories = 134

Chicken Or Turkey Soup Cream Of Canned Reduced Sodium Made With Water ☛ serving size: 1 cup = 244 g; Calories = 71

Chicken Or Turkey Soup Cream Of Canned Reduced Sodium Ns As To Made With Milk Or Water ☛ serving size: 1 cup = 244 g; Calories = 71

Chicken Or Turkey Soup Cream Of Ns As To Prepared With Milk Or Water ☛ serving size: 1 cup = 244 g; Calories = 112

Chicken Or Turkey Soup Cream Of Prepared With Milk ☛ serving size: 1 cup = 248 g; Calories = 174

Chicken Or Turkey Soup Cream Of Prepared With Water ☛ serving size: 1 cup = 244 g; Calories = 112

Chicken Or Turkey Soup With Vegetables And Fruit Asian Style ☛ serving size: 1 cup = 234 g; Calories = 91

Chicken Or Turkey Soup With Vegetables Broccoli Carrots Celery Potatoes And Onions Asian Style ☛ serving size: 1 cup = 228 g; Calories = 112

Chicken Or Turkey Vegetable Soup Home Recipe ☛ serving size: 1 cup = 239 g; Calories = 115

Chicken Or Turkey Vegetable Soup With Rice Home Recipe Mexican Style ☛ serving size: 1 cup = 242 g; Calories = 186

Chicken Rice Soup Puerto Rican Style ☛ serving size: 1 cup = 220 g; Calories = 169

Chicken Soup With Noodles And Potatoes Puerto Rican Style ☛ serving size: 1 cup = 220 g; Calories = 163

Chicken Stock ☛ serving size: 1 cup = 240 g; Calories = 86

Chipotle Dip Light ☛ serving size: 1 tablespoon = 15 g; Calories = 29

Chipotle Dip Regular ☛ serving size: 1 tablespoon = 15 g; Calories = 64

Chipotle Dip Yogurt Based ☛ serving size: 1 tablespoon = 15 g; Calories = 28

Chutney ☛ serving size: 1 tablespoon = 17 g; Calories = 26

Clam Chowder New England Prepared With Milk ☛ serving size: 1 cup = 248 g; Calories = 151

Clam Chowder Ns As To Manhattan Or New England Style ☛ serving size: 1 cup = 244 g; Calories = 149

Cocktail Sauce ☛ serving size: 1 cup = 273 g; Calories = 339

Codfish Rice And Vegetable Soup Puerto Rican Style ☛ serving size: 1 cup = 245 g; Calories = 167

Codfish Soup With Noodles Puerto Rican Style ☛ serving size: 1 cup = 245 g; Calories = 176

Corn Soup Cream Of Prepared With Milk ☛ serving size: 1 cup = 248 g; Calories = 104

Corn Soup Cream Of Prepared With Water ☛ serving size: 1 cup = 244 g; Calories = 159

Crab Soup Cream Of Prepared With Milk ☛ serving size: 1 cup = 248 g; Calories = 127

Crab Soup Ns As To Tomato-Base Or Cream Style ☛ serving size: 1 cup = 244 g; Calories = 124

Crab Soup Tomato-Base ☛ serving size: 1 cup = 244 g; Calories = 95

Cream Of Asparagus Soup ☛ serving size: 1 cup (8 fl oz) = 244 g; Calories = 85

Cream Of Chicken Soup ☛ serving size: 1 cup = 244 g; Calories = 117

Cream Of Mushroom Soup ☛ serving size: 1 serving 1 cup = 248 g; Calories = 97

Dark-Green Leafy Vegetable Soup Meatless Asian Style ☛ serving size: 1 cup = 226 g; Calories = 109

Dark-Green Leafy Vegetable Soup With Meat Asian Style ☛ serving size: 1 cup = 228 g; Calories = 176

Dill Dip Light ☛ serving size: 1 tablespoon = 15 g; Calories = 30

Dill Dip Regular ☛ serving size: 1 tablespoon = 15 g; Calories = 64

Dill Dip Yogurt Based ☛ serving size: 1 tablespoon = 15 g; Calories = 29

Dip Bean Original Flavor ☛ serving size: 2 tbsp = 36 g; Calories = 43

Dip Fritos Bean Original Flavor ☛ serving size: 2 tbsp = 36 g; Calories = 43

Dip Nfs ☛ serving size: 1 tablespoon = 15 g; Calories = 65

Dip Salsa Con Queso Cheese And Salsa- Medium ☛ serving size: 2 tbsp = 30 g; Calories = 43

Dip Tostitos Salsa Con Queso Medium ☛ serving size: 2 tbsp = 30 g; Calories = 40

Duck Sauce ☛ serving size: 1 cup = 290 g; Calories = 711

Duck Soup ☛ serving size: 1 cup = 244 g; Calories = 183

Eggplant Dip ☛ serving size: 1 tablespoon = 15 g; Calories = 25

Enchilada Sauce Green ☛ serving size: 1 cup = 250 g; Calories = 70

Fish And Vegetable Soup No Potatoes Mexican Style ☛ serving size: 1 cup = 250 g; Calories = 98

Fish Broth ☛ serving size: 1 cup = 244 g; Calories = 39

Fish Chowder ☛ serving size: 1 cup = 244 g; Calories = 276

Fish Soup With Potatoes Mexican Style ☛ serving size: 1 cup = 241 g; Calories = 111

Fish Stock ☛ serving size: 1 cup = 233 g; Calories = 37

Flour And Water Gravy ☛ serving size: 1 cup = 240 g; Calories = 192

Garbanzo Bean Or Chickpea Soup Home Recipe Canned Or Ready-To-Serve ☛ serving size: 1 cup = 253 g; Calories = 180

Garlic Cooked ☛ serving size: 1 clove = 2 g; Calories = 3

Garlic Egg Soup Puerto Rican Style ☛ serving size: 1 cup = 202 g; Calories = 164

Garlic Sauce ☛ serving size: 1 cup = 228 g; Calories = 246

Gazpacho ☛ serving size: 1 cup = 244 g; Calories = 90

Gravy Au Jus Canned ☛ serving size: 1/4 cup = 59 g; Calories = 9

Gravy Au Jus Dry ☛ serving size: 1 tsp = 3 g; Calories = 9

Gravy Beef Canned Ready-To-Serve ☛ serving size: 1 cup = 233 g; Calories = 124

Gravy Beef Or Meat Fat Free ☛ serving size: 1 cup = 227 g; Calories = 93

Gravy Beef Or Meat Home Recipe ☛ serving size: 1 cup = 233 g; Calories = 247

Gravy Brown Dry ☛ serving size: 1 tbsp = 6 g; Calories = 22

Gravy Brown Instant Dry ☛ serving size: 1 serving = 6.7 g; Calories = 26

Gravy Campbells Chicken ☞ serving size: 1/4 cup = 56 g; Calories = 29

Gravy Chicken Canned Or Bottled Ready-To-Serve ☞ serving size: 1/4 cup = 57 g; Calories = 27

Gravy Chicken Dry ☞ serving size: 1 tbsp = 8 g; Calories = 31

Gravy Giblet ☞ serving size: 1 cup = 238 g; Calories = 145

Gravy Heinz Home Style Classic Chicken ☞ serving size: 1/4 cup = 58 g; Calories = 27

Gravy Heinz Home Style Savory Beef ☞ serving size: 1 serving 1/4 cup 2 oz = 57 g; Calories = 22

Gravy Instant Beef Dry ☞ serving size: 1 serving = 6.7 g; Calories = 25

Gravy Instant Turkey Dry ☞ serving size: 1 serving = 6.7 g; Calories = 27

Gravy Meat Or Poultry Low Sodium Prepared ☞ serving size: 1 cup = 236 g; Calories = 125

Gravy Meat Or Poultry With Wine ☞ serving size: 1 cup = 236 g; Calories = 87

Gravy Meat With Fruit ☞ serving size: 1 cup = 238 g; Calories = 119

Gravy Meat-Based From Puerto-Rican Style Beef Stew ☞ serving size: 1 cup = 208 g; Calories = 171

Gravy Meat-Based From Puerto-Rican Style Stuffed Pot Roast ☞ serving size: 1 cup = 272 g; Calories = 666

Gravy Mushroom ☞ serving size: 1 cup = 238 g; Calories = 64

Gravy Mushroom Canned ☞ serving size: 1 cup = 238 g; Calories = 119

Gravy Mushroom Dry Powder ☛ serving size: 1 cup (8 fl oz) = 21 g; Calories = 69

Gravy Onion Dry Mix ☛ serving size: 1 cup (8 fl oz) = 24 g; Calories = 77

Gravy Or Sauce Made With Soy Sauce Stock Or Bouillon Cornstarch ☛ serving size: 1 cup = 233 g; Calories = 105

Gravy Or Sauce Poultry-Based From Puerto Rican-Style Chicken Fricasse ☛ serving size: 1 cup = 240 g; Calories = 509

Gravy Pork Dry Powder ☛ serving size: 1 serving = 6.7 g; Calories = 25

Gravy Poultry Fat Free ☛ serving size: 1 cup = 227 g; Calories = 102

Gravy Poultry Home Recipe ☛ serving size: 1 cup = 238 g; Calories = 250

Gravy Redeye ☛ serving size: 1 cup = 242 g; Calories = 107

Gravy Turkey Canned Ready-To-Serve ☛ serving size: 1 cup = 238 g; Calories = 121

Gravy Turkey Dry ☛ serving size: 1 serving = 7 g; Calories = 26

Gravy Unspecified Type Dry ☛ serving size: 1 cup (8 fl oz) = 25 g; Calories = 86

Guacamole Nfs ☛ serving size: 1 tablespoon = 15 g; Calories = 23

Guacamole With Tomatoes ☛ serving size: 1 tablespoon = 15 g; Calories = 22

Ham Noodle And Vegetable Soup Puerto Rican Style ☛ serving size: 1 cup = 250 g; Calories = 150

Ham Rice And Potato Soup Puerto Rican Style ☛ serving size: 1 cup = 240 g; Calories = 134

Hoisin Sauce ☛ serving size: 1 tbsp = 16 g; Calories = 35

Hollandaise Sauce ☛ serving size: 1 cup = 257 g; Calories = 1295

Honey Mustard Dip ☛ serving size: 1 tablespoon = 15 g; Calories = 40

Hot Sauce ☛ serving size: 1 tsp = 4.7 g; Calories = 1

Hummus Flavored ☛ serving size: 1 tablespoon = 15 g; Calories = 39

Hummus Plain ☛ serving size: 1 tablespoon = 15 g; Calories = 39

Instant Soup Noodle ☛ serving size: 1 cup = 240 g; Calories = 60

Instant Soup Noodle With Egg Shrimp Or Chicken ☛ serving size: 1 cup = 240 g; Calories = 161

Italian Wedding Soup ☛ serving size: 1 cup = 244 g; Calories = 168

Lamb Pasta And Vegetable Soup Puerto Rican Style ☛ serving size: 1 cup = 250 g; Calories = 225

Layer Dip ☛ serving size: 1 tablespoon = 15 g; Calories = 22

Leek Soup Cream Of Prepared With Milk ☛ serving size: 1 cup = 248 g; Calories = 171

Lemon-Butter Sauce ☛ serving size: 1 cup = 228 g; Calories = 1420

Lentil Soup Home Recipe Canned Or Ready-To-Serve ☛ serving size: 1 cup = 248 g; Calories = 159

Lima Bean Soup Home Recipe Canned Or Ready-To-Serve ☛ serving size: 1 cup = 253 g; Calories = 147

Lobster Bisque ☛ serving size: 1 cup = 248 g; Calories = 129

Lobster Sauce ☛ serving size: 1 cup = 234 g; Calories = 342

Low Sodium Minestrone ☛ serving size: 1 cup = 245 g; Calories = 123

Manhattan Clam Chowder ☛ serving size: 1 cup (8 fl oz) = 240 g; Calories = 134

Manhattan Clam Chowder (Prepared With Equal Part Water) ☛ serving size: 1 serving 1 cup = 249 g; Calories = 75

Matzo Ball Soup ☛ serving size: 1 cup = 241 g; Calories = 145

Meat And Corn Hominy Soup Home Recipe Mexican Style ☛ serving size: 1 cup = 238 g; Calories = 214

Meatball Soup Home Recipe Mexican Style ☛ serving size: 1 cup = 237 g; Calories = 256

Menudo Soup Canned Prepared With Water Or Ready-To-Serve ☛ serving size: 1 cup = 241 g; Calories = 96

Menudo Soup Home Recipe ☛ serving size: 1 cup = 241 g; Calories = 118

Mexican Style Chicken Broth Soup Stock ☛ serving size: 1 cup = 242 g; Calories = 119

Milk Gravy Quick Gravy ☛ serving size: 1 cup = 250 g; Calories = 340

Minestrone ☛ serving size: 1 cup (8 fl oz) = 241 g; Calories = 82

Minestrone Soup Canned Prepared With Water Or Ready-To-Serve ☛ serving size: 1 cup = 241 g; Calories = 82

Minestrone Soup Home Recipe ☛ serving size: 1 cup = 235 g; Calories = 143

Miso Sauce ☛ serving size: 1 cup = 240 g; Calories = 372

Mole Poblano Sauce ☛ serving size: 1 cup = 265 g; Calories = 376

Mole Verde Sauce ☛ serving size: 1 cup = 265 g; Calories = 220

Mushroom Barley Soup ☛ serving size: 1 cup (8 fl oz) = 244 g; Calories = 73

Mushroom Soup Cream Of Canned Reduced Sodium Ns As To Made With Milk Or Water ☛ serving size: 1 cup = 246 g; Calories = 64

Mushroom Soup Cream Of Canned Reduced Sodium Prepared With Milk ☛ serving size: 1 cup = 248 g; Calories = 127

Mushroom Soup Cream Of Canned Reduced Sodium Prepared With Water ☛ serving size: 1 cup = 244 g; Calories = 63

Mushroom Soup Cream Of Ns As To Made With Milk Or Water ☛ serving size: 1 cup = 246 g; Calories = 160

Mushroom Soup Cream Of Prepared With Milk ☛ serving size: 1 cup = 248 g; Calories = 161

Mushroom Soup Cream Of Prepared With Water ☛ serving size: 1 cup = 244 g; Calories = 98

Mushroom Soup With Meat Broth Prepared With Water ☛ serving size: 1 cup = 244 g; Calories = 83

Mushroom With Chicken Soup Cream Of Prepared With Milk ☛ serving size: 1 cup = 248 g; Calories = 186

New England Clam Chowder ☛ serving size: 1 serving 1 cup = 248 g; Calories = 87

Noodle And Potato Soup Puerto Rican Style ☛ serving size: 1 cup = 245 g; Calories = 71

Noodle Soup Nfs ☛ serving size: 1 cup = 241 g; Calories = 162

Noodle Soup With Fish Ball Shrimp And Dark Green Leafy Vegetable ☛ serving size: 1 cup = 234 g; Calories = 173

Noodle Soup With Vegetables Asian Style ☛ serving size: 1 cup = 228 g; Calories = 162

Onion Dip Light ☛ serving size: 1 tablespoon = 15 g; Calories = 25

Onion Dip Regular ☛ serving size: 1 tablespoon = 15 g; Calories = 52

Onion Dip Yogurt Based ☞ serving size: 1 tablespoon = 15 g; Calories = 24

Onion Soup Cream Of Prepared With Milk ☞ serving size: 1 cup = 248 g; Calories = 171

Onion Soup French ☞ serving size: 1 cup = 241 g; Calories = 378

Osyter Sauce ☞ serving size: 1 tbsp = 18 g; Calories = 9

Oxtail Soup ☞ serving size: 1 cup = 244 g; Calories = 207

Oyster Sauce ☞ serving size: 1 cup = 256 g; Calories = 325

Oyster Stew ☞ serving size: 1 cup = 245 g; Calories = 196

Pasta Sauce ☞ serving size: 1 serving 1/2 cup = 132 g; Calories = 66

Pea Soup Prepared With Milk ☞ serving size: 1 cup = 254 g; Calories = 226

Pepper Hot Chili Raw ☞ serving size: 1 piece = 11 g; Calories = 4

Pepperpot Soup ☞ serving size: 1 cup = 241 g; Calories = 113

Peppers Hot Cooked From Canned Fat Added In Cooking Ns As To Type Of Fat ☞ serving size: 1 cup, chopped = 141 g; Calories = 59

Peppers Hot Cooked From Canned Fat Not Added In Cooking ☞ serving size: 1 cup, chopped = 136 g; Calories = 30

Peppers Hot Cooked From Canned Ns As To Fat Added In Cooking ☞ serving size: 1 cup, chopped = 141 g; Calories = 59

Peppers Hot Cooked From Fresh Fat Added In Cooking Ns As To Type Of Fat ☞ serving size: 1 cup, chopped = 141 g; Calories = 86

Peppers Hot Cooked From Fresh Fat Not Added In Cooking ☞ serving size: 1 cup, chopped = 136 g; Calories = 56

Peppers Hot Cooked From Fresh Ns As To Fat Added In Cooking ☞ serving size: 1 cup, chopped = 141 g; Calories = 86

Peppers Hot Cooked From Frozen Fat Added In Cooking Ns As To Type Of Fat ☛ serving size: 1 cup, chopped = 141 g; Calories = 86

Peppers Hot Cooked From Frozen Fat Not Added In Cooking ☛ serving size: 1 cup, chopped = 136 g; Calories = 56

Peppers Hot Cooked From Frozen Ns As To Fat Added In Cooking ☛ serving size: 1 cup, chopped = 141 g; Calories = 86

Peppers Hot Cooked Ns As To Form Fat Added In Cooking Ns As To Type Of Fat ☛ serving size: 1 cup, chopped = 141 g; Calories = 86

Peppers Hot Cooked Ns As To Form Fat Not Added In Cooking ☛ serving size: 1 cup, chopped = 136 g; Calories = 56

Peppers Hot Cooked Ns As To Form Ns As To Fat Added In Cooking ☛ serving size: 1 cup, chopped = 141 g; Calories = 86

Pesto ☛ serving size: 1/4 cup = 63 g; Calories = 263

Pesto Sauce ☛ serving size: 1 cup = 232 g; Calories = 1320

Pho ☛ serving size: 1 cup = 244 g; Calories = 215

Pigeon Pea Asopao Asopao De Gandules ☛ serving size: 1 cup = 178 g; Calories = 247

Pimiento ☛ serving size: 1 cup = 192 g; Calories = 54

Pinto Bean Soup Home Recipe Canned Or Ready-To-Serve ☛ serving size: 1 cup = 253 g; Calories = 359

Plantain Soup Puerto Rican Style ☛ serving size: 1 cup = 245 g; Calories = 98

Plum Sauce Asian Style ☛ serving size: 1 cup = 311 g; Calories = 622

Pork Vegetable Soup With Potato Pasta Or Rice Stew Type Chunky Style ☛ serving size: 1 cup = 240 g; Calories = 132

Pork With Vegetable Excluding Carrots Broccoli And/or Dark-

Green Leafy; Soup Asian Style ☛ serving size: 1 cup = 228 g; Calories = 123

Portuguese Bean Soup Home Recipe Canned Or Ready-To-Serve ☛ serving size: 1 cup = 253 g; Calories = 276

Potato And Cheese Soup ☛ serving size: 1 cup = 248 g; Calories = 184

Potato Chowder ☛ serving size: 1 cup = 248 g; Calories = 228

Potato Soup Cream Of Prepared With Milk ☛ serving size: 1 cup = 248 g; Calories = 154

Potato Soup Instant Dry Mix ☛ serving size: 1 serving 1/3 cup = 39 g; Calories = 134

Potato Soup Ns As To Made With Milk Or Water ☛ serving size: 1 cup = 244 g; Calories = 122

Potato Soup Prepared With Water ☛ serving size: 1 cup = 244 g; Calories = 93

Puerto Rican Seasoning With Ham ☛ serving size: 1 cup = 240 g; Calories = 619

Puerto Rican Seasoning With Ham And Tomato Sauce ☛ serving size: 1 cup = 240 g; Calories = 418

Puerto Rican Seasoning Without Ham And Tomato Sauce ☛ serving size: 1 cup = 240 g; Calories = 295

Ranch Dip Light ☛ serving size: 1 tablespoon = 15 g; Calories = 30

Ranch Dip Regular ☛ serving size: 1 tablespoon = 15 g; Calories = 65

Ranch Dip Yogurt Based ☛ serving size: 1 tablespoon = 15 g; Calories = 29

Recaito ☛ serving size: 1 cup = 240 g; Calories = 55

Rice And Potato Soup Puerto Rican Style ☛ serving size: 1 cup = 245 g; Calories = 184

Rice Soup Nfs ☛ serving size: 1 cup = 241 g; Calories = 82

Salmon Soup Cream Style ☛ serving size: 1 cup = 248 g; Calories = 146

Salsa Pico De Gallo ☛ serving size: 1 cup = 240 g; Calories = 41

Salsa Red Homemade ☛ serving size: 1 cup = 234 g; Calories = 131

Sauce Barbecue Bulls-Eye Original ☛ serving size: 1 tbsp = 16 g; Calories = 27

Sauce Barbecue Kc Masterpiece Original ☛ serving size: 1 tbsp = 18 g; Calories = 29

Sauce Barbecue Kraft Original ☛ serving size: 1 tbsp = 16 g; Calories = 28

Sauce Barbecue Open Pit Original ☛ serving size: 1 tbsp = 17 g; Calories = 22

Sauce Barbecue Sweet Baby Rays Original ☛ serving size: 1 tbsp = 18 g; Calories = 35

Sauce Cheese Ready-To-Serve ☛ serving size: 1/4 cup = 63 g; Calories = 110

Sauce Chili Peppers Hot Immature Green Canned ☛ serving size: 1 tbsp = 15 g; Calories = 3

Sauce Cocktail Ready-To-Serve ☛ serving size: 1/4 cup = 60 g; Calories = 77

Sauce Duck Ready-To-Serve ☛ serving size: 2 tbsp = 33 g; Calories = 81

Sauce Enchilada Red Mild Ready To Serve ☛ serving size: 1/4 cup = 56 g; Calories = 17

Sauce Fish Ready-To-Serve ☛ serving size: 1 tbsp = 18 g; Calories = 6

Sauce Homemade White Medium ☛ serving size: 1 cup = 250 g; Calories = 368

Sauce Homemade White Thick ☛ serving size: 1 cup = 250 g; Calories = 465

Sauce Horseradish ☛ serving size: 1 tsp = 5.6 g; Calories = 28

Sauce Hot Chile Sriracha Cha! By Texas Pete ☛ serving size: 1 tsp = 6.9 g; Calories = 8

Sauce Hot Chile Sriracha Tuong Ot Sriracha ☛ serving size: 1 tsp = 6.2 g; Calories = 5

Sauce Pasta Spaghetti/marinara Ready-To-Serve Low Sodium ☛ serving size: 1 serving 1/2 cup = 128 g; Calories = 65

Sauce Peanut Made From Coconut Water Sugar Peanuts ☛ serving size: 1 tbsp = 17 g; Calories = 30

Sauce Peanut Made From Peanut Butter Water Soy Sauce ☛ serving size: 1 tbsp = 18 g; Calories = 46

Sauce Peppers Hot Chili Mature Red Canned ☛ serving size: 1 tbsp = 15 g; Calories = 3

Sauce Pesto Buitoni Pesto With Basil Ready-To-Serve Refrigerated ☛ serving size: 1/4 cup = 63 g; Calories = 263

Sauce Pesto Classico Basil Pesto Ready-To-Serve ☛ serving size: 1/4 cup = 62 g; Calories = 231

Sauce Pesto Mezzetta Napa Valley Bistro Basil Pesto Ready-To-Serve ☛ serving size: 1/4 cup = 60 g; Calories = 298

Sauce Pesto Ready-To-Serve Shelf Stable ☛ serving size: 1/4 cup = 61 g; Calories = 260

Sauce Plum Ready-To-Serve ☛ serving size: 1 tbsp = 19 g; Calories = 35

Sauce Salsa Ready-To-Serve ☛ serving size: 2 tbsp = 36 g; Calories = 10

Sauce Salsa Verde Ready-To-Serve ☛ serving size: 2 tbsp = 30 g; Calories = 11

Sauce Sofrito Prepared From Recipe ☛ serving size: 1/2 cup = 103 g; Calories = 244

Sauce Steak Tomato Based ☛ serving size: 2 tbsp = 34 g; Calories = 32

Sauce Sweet And Sour Ready-To-Serve ☛ serving size: 2 tbsp = 35 g; Calories = 54

Sauce Tartar Ready-To-Serve ☛ serving size: 2 tablespoons = 30 g; Calories = 63

Sauce Teriyaki Ready-To-Serve ☛ serving size: 1 tbsp = 18 g; Calories = 16

Sauce Tomato Chili Sauce Bottled With Salt ☛ serving size: 1 packet = 6 g; Calories = 6

Seafood Dip ☛ serving size: 1 tablespoon = 15 g; Calories = 51

Seafood Soup With Potatoes And Vegetables Excluding Carrots Broccoli And Dark-Green Leafy ☛ serving size: 1 cup = 244 g; Calories = 110

Seafood Soup With Potatoes And Vegetables Including Carrots Broccoli And/or Dark-Green Leafy ☛ serving size: 1 cup = 244 g; Calories = 110

Seafood Soup With Vegetables Excluding Carrots Broccoli And Dark-Green Leafy; No Potatoes ☛ serving size: 1 cup = 244 g; Calories = 103

Seafood Soup With Vegetables Including Carrots Broccoli And/or Dark-Green Leafy; No Potatoes ☛ serving size: 1 cup = 244 g; Calories = 103

Seaweed Soup ☛ serving size: 1 cup = 230 g; Calories = 81

Shav Soup ☛ serving size: 1 cup = 240 g; Calories = 125

Smart Soup French Lentil ☛ serving size: 10 oz 1 pouch = 283 g; Calories = 150

Smart Soup Greek Minestrone ☛ serving size: 10 oz 1 pouch = 283 g; Calories = 113

Smart Soup Indian Bean Masala ☛ serving size: 10 oz 1 pouch = 283 g; Calories = 161

Smart Soup Moroccan Chick Pea ☛ serving size: 10 oz 1 pouch = 283 g; Calories = 144

Smart Soup Santa Fe Corn Chowder ☛ serving size: 10 oz 1 pouch = 283 g; Calories = 156

Smart Soup Thai Coconut Curry ☛ serving size: 10 oz 1 pouch = 283 g; Calories = 102

Smart Soup Vietnamese Carrot Lemongrass ☛ serving size: 10 oz 1 pouch = 283 g; Calories = 125

Sopa De Fideo Aguada Mexican Style Noodle Soup Home Recipe ☛ serving size: 1 cup = 242 g; Calories = 194

Sopa De Tortilla Mexican Style Tortilla Soup Home Recipe ☛ serving size: 1 cup = 240 g; Calories = 281

Sopa Seca De Arroz Home Recipe Mexican Style ☛ serving size: 1 cup = 218 g; Calories = 325

Sopa Seca De Fideo Mexican Style Made With Dry Noodles Home Recipe ☛ serving size: 1 cup = 218 g; Calories = 301

Sopa Seca Mexican Style Nfs ☛ serving size: 1 cup = 218 g; Calories = 305

Soup Bean & Ham Canned Reduced Sodium Prepared With Water Or Ready-To-Serve ☛ serving size: 1 cup = 245 g; Calories = 199

Soup Bean With Bacon Condensed Single Brand ☛ serving size: 1 serving 1/2 cup = 128 g; Calories = 150

Soup Bean With Frankfurters Canned Condensed ☛ serving size: 1 cup (8 fl oz) = 263 g; Calories = 374

Soup Bean With Frankfurters Canned Prepared With Equal Volume Water ☛ serving size: 1 cup (8 fl oz) = 250 g; Calories = 188

Soup Bean With Ham Canned Chunky Ready-To-Serve ☛ serving size: 1 cup (8 fl oz) = 243 g; Calories = 231

Soup Bean With Pork Canned Condensed ☛ serving size: 1/2 cup = 130 g; Calories = 168

Soup Bean With Pork Canned Prepared With Equal Volume Water ☛ serving size: 1 serving 1 cup = 266 g; Calories = 168

Soup Beef And Mushroom Low Sodium Chunk Style ☛ serving size: 1 cup = 251 g; Calories = 173

Soup Beef And Vegetables Canned Ready-To-Serve ☛ serving size: 1 cup = 250 g; Calories = 120

Soup Beef And Vegetables Reduced Sodium Canned Ready-To-Serve ☛ serving size: 1 cup = 245 g; Calories = 103

Soup Beef Barley Ready To Serve ☛ serving size: 1 cup = 208 g; Calories = 108

Soup Beef Broth Bouillon And Consomme Canned Condensed ☛ serving size: 1/2 cup = 124 g; Calories = 14

Soup Beef Broth Cubed Dry ☛ serving size: 1 cube = 3.6 g; Calories = 6

Soup Beef Broth Cubed Prepared With Water ☛ serving size: 1 serving 1 cup = 240 g; Calories = 7

Soup Beef Broth Less/reduced Sodium Ready To Serve ☛ serving size: 1 cup = 219 g; Calories = 13

Soup Beef Broth Or Bouillon Canned Ready-To-Serve ☛ serving size: 1 cup = 240 g; Calories = 17

Soup Beef Broth Or Bouillon Powder Dry ☛ serving size: 1 cube = 3.6 g; Calories = 8

Soup Beef Broth Or Bouillon Powder Prepared With Water ☛ serving size: 1 serving 1 cup = 240 g; Calories = 7

Soup Beef Mushroom Canned Condensed ☛ serving size: 1/2 cup (4 fl oz) = 126 g; Calories = 77

Soup Beef Mushroom Canned Prepared With Equal Volume Water ☛ serving size: 1 cup (8 fl oz) = 244 g; Calories = 73

Soup Beef Noodle Canned Condensed ☛ serving size: 1/2 cup = 125 g; Calories = 84

Soup Beef Noodle Canned Prepared With Equal Volume Water ☛ serving size: 1 cup (8 fl oz) = 244 g; Calories = 83

Soup Beef Stroganoff Canned Chunky Style Ready-To-Serve ☛ serving size: 1 cup = 240 g; Calories = 235

Soup Black Bean Canned Condensed ☛ serving size: 1 cup (8 fl oz) = 257 g; Calories = 234

Soup Bouillon Cubes And Granules Low Sodium Dry ☛ serving size: 1 tsp = 2.6 g; Calories = 11

Soup Broccoli Cheese Canned Condensed Commercial ☛ serving size: 1 serving 1/2 cup = 121 g; Calories = 105

Soup Cheese Canned Condensed ☛ serving size: 1/2 cup = 124 g; Calories = 102

Soup Cheese Canned Prepared With Equal Volume Milk serving size: 1 cup = 251 g; Calories = 231

Soup Cheese Canned Prepared With Equal Volume Water serving size: 1 cup (8 fl oz) = 247 g; Calories = 156

Soup Chicken And Vegetable Canned Ready-To-Serve serving size: 1 cup = 255 g; Calories = 84

Soup Chicken Broth Canned Condensed serving size: 1/2 cup (4 fl oz) = 126 g; Calories = 39

Soup Chicken Broth Canned Prepared With Equal Volume Water serving size: 1 cup (8 fl oz) = 244 g; Calories = 39

Soup Chicken Broth Cubes Dry serving size: 1 cube = 4.8 g; Calories = 10

Soup Chicken Broth Cubes Dry Prepared With Water serving size: 1 cup (8 fl oz) = 243 g; Calories = 12

Soup Chicken Broth Less/reduced Sodium Ready To Serve serving size: 1 cup = 240 g; Calories = 17

Soup Chicken Broth Low Sodium Canned serving size: 1 cup = 240 g; Calories = 38

Soup Chicken Broth Or Bouillon Dry serving size: 1 cube = 4 g; Calories = 11

Soup Chicken Broth Or Bouillon Dry Prepared With Water serving size: 1 cup 8 fl oz = 241 g; Calories = 10

Soup Chicken Broth Ready-To-Serve serving size: 1 cup = 249 g; Calories = 15

Soup Chicken Canned Chunky Ready-To-Serve serving size: 1 cup = 245 g; Calories = 174

Soup Chicken Corn Chowder Chunky Ready-To-Serve Single Brand serving size: 1 serving = 240 g; Calories = 238

Soup Chicken Gumbo Canned Condensed ☛ serving size: 1/2 cup (4 fl oz) = 126 g; Calories = 57

Soup Chicken Gumbo Canned Prepared With Equal Volume Water ☛ serving size: 1 cup = 244 g; Calories = 56

Soup Chicken Mushroom Canned Condensed ☛ serving size: 1/2 cup = 124 g; Calories = 124

Soup Chicken Mushroom Canned Prepared With Equal Volume Water ☛ serving size: 1 cup (8 fl oz) = 244 g; Calories = 132

Soup Chicken Noodle Canned Condensed ☛ serving size: 1/2 cup = 124 g; Calories = 60

Soup Chicken Noodle Canned Prepared With Equal Volume Water ☛ serving size: 1 serving 1 cup = 248 g; Calories = 60

Soup Chicken Noodle Dry Mix ☛ serving size: 1 packet = 74 g; Calories = 279

Soup Chicken Noodle Dry Mix Prepared With Water ☛ serving size: 1 cup = 245 g; Calories = 56

Soup Chicken Noodle Low Sodium Canned Prepared With Equal Volume Water ☛ serving size: 1 serving 1 cup = 248 g; Calories = 62

Soup Chicken Noodle Reduced Sodium Canned Ready-To-Serve ☛ serving size: 1 cup = 245 g; Calories = 101

Soup Chicken Rice Canned Chunky Ready-To-Serve ☛ serving size: 1 cup = 240 g; Calories = 127

Soup Chicken Vegetable Canned Condensed ☛ serving size: 1/2 cup = 121 g; Calories = 74

Soup Chicken Vegetable With Potato And Cheese Chunky Ready-To-Serve ☛ serving size: 1 cup = 245 g; Calories = 159

Soup Chicken With Rice Canned Condensed ☛ serving size: 1/2 cup = 126 g; Calories = 86

Soup Chicken With Rice Canned Prepared With Equal Volume Water ☛ serving size: 1 serving 1 cup = 243 g; Calories = 58

Soup Chili Beef Canned Condensed ☛ serving size: 1 cup (8 fl oz) = 263 g; Calories = 308

Soup Chili Beef Canned Prepared With Equal Volume Water ☛ serving size: 1 cup = 261 g; Calories = 149

Soup Chunky Beef Canned Ready-To-Serve ☛ serving size: 1 cup = 245 g; Calories = 162

Soup Chunky Chicken Noodle Canned Ready-To-Serve ☛ serving size: 1 can = 530 g; Calories = 217

Soup Chunky Vegetable Canned Ready-To-Serve ☛ serving size: 1 cup = 230 g; Calories = 90

Soup Chunky Vegetable Reduced Sodium Canned Ready-To-Serve ☛ serving size: 1 cup = 240 g; Calories = 120

Soup Clam Chowder Manhattan Canned Condensed ☛ serving size: 1/2 cup (4 fl oz) = 126 g; Calories = 77

Soup Clam Chowder New England Canned Condensed ☛ serving size: 1/2 cup = 126 g; Calories = 91

Soup Clam Chowder New England Canned Prepared With Equal Volume Low Fat (2%) Milk ☛ serving size: 1 serving 1 cup = 252 g; Calories = 154

Soup Clam Chowder New England Canned Ready-To-Serve ☛ serving size: 1 cup = 254 g; Calories = 201

Soup Clam Chowder New England Reduced Sodium Canned Ready-To-Serve ☛ serving size: 1 can = 519 g; Calories = 363

Soup Cream Of Asparagus Canned Condensed ☛ serving size: 1/2 cup (4 fl oz) = 126 g; Calories = 87

Soup Cream Of Asparagus Canned Prepared With Equal Volume Milk ☛ serving size: 1 cup (8 fl oz) = 248 g; Calories = 161

Soup Cream Of Celery Canned Condensed ☛ serving size: 1/2 cup = 126 g; Calories = 91

Soup Cream Of Celery Canned Prepared With Equal Volume Milk ☛ serving size: 1 cup (8 fl oz) = 248 g; Calories = 164

Soup Cream Of Celery Canned Prepared With Equal Volume Water ☛ serving size: 1 cup = 248 g; Calories = 92

Soup Cream Of Chicken Canned Condensed ☛ serving size: 1/2 cup (4 fl oz) = 126 g; Calories = 113

Soup Cream Of Chicken Canned Condensed Reduced Sodium ☛ serving size: 1/2 cup = 124 g; Calories = 72

Soup Cream Of Chicken Canned Prepared With Equal Volume Milk ☛ serving size: 1 cup (8 fl oz) = 248 g; Calories = 191

Soup Cream Of Chicken Dry Mix Prepared With Water ☛ serving size: 1 cup 8 fl oz = 261 g; Calories = 107

Soup Cream Of Mushroom Canned Condensed ☛ serving size: 1/2 cup = 126 g; Calories = 100

Soup Cream Of Mushroom Canned Condensed Reduced Sodium ☛ serving size: 1 cup = 251 g; Calories = 131

Soup Cream Of Mushroom Canned Prepared With Equal Volume Low Fat (2%) Milk ☛ serving size: 1 serving 1 cup = 252 g; Calories = 164

Soup Cream Of Mushroom Low Sodium Ready-To-Serve Canned ☛ serving size: 1 cup = 244 g; Calories = 129

Soup Cream Of Nfs ☛ serving size: 1 cup = 244 g; Calories = 142

Soup Cream Of Onion Canned Condensed ☛ serving size: 1/2 cup = 126 g; Calories = 111

Soup Cream Of Onion Canned Prepared With Equal Volume Milk serving size: 1 cup (8 fl oz) = 248 g; Calories = 186

Soup Cream Of Onion Canned Prepared With Equal Volume Water serving size: 1 cup (8 fl oz) = 244 g; Calories = 107

Soup Cream Of Potato Canned Condensed serving size: 1/2 cup = 124 g; Calories = 92

Soup Cream Of Potato Canned Prepared With Equal Volume Milk serving size: 1 cup (8 fl oz) = 248 g; Calories = 149

Soup Cream Of Potato Canned Prepared With Equal Volume Water serving size: 1 cup (8 fl oz) = 244 g; Calories = 73

Soup Cream Of Shrimp Canned Condensed serving size: 1/2 cup = 126 g; Calories = 91

Soup Cream Of Shrimp Canned Prepared With Equal Volume Low Fat (2%) Milk serving size: 1 cup (8 fl oz) = 253 g; Calories = 154

Soup Cream Of Shrimp Canned Prepared With Equal Volume Water serving size: 1 cup = 244 g; Calories = 88

Soup Cream Of Vegetable Dry Powder serving size: 1 packet = 18 g; Calories = 80

Soup Egg Drop Chinese Restaurant serving size: 1 cup = 241 g; Calories = 65

Soup Fruit serving size: 1 cup = 242 g; Calories = 174

Soup Healthy Choice Chicken And Rice Soup Canned serving size: 1 serving 1 cup = 240 g; Calories = 89

Soup Healthy Choice Chicken Noodle Soup Canned serving size: 1 serving 1 cup = 243 g; Calories = 100

Soup Healthy Choice Garden Vegetable Soup Canned serving size: 1 serving 1 cup = 246 g; Calories = 126

Soup Hot And Sour Chinese Restaurant ☞ serving size: 1 cup = 233 g; Calories = 91

Soup Lentil With Ham Canned Ready-To-Serve ☞ serving size: 1 cup (8 fl oz) = 248 g; Calories = 139

Soup Minestrone Canned Condensed ☞ serving size: 1/2 cup (4 fl oz) = 123 g; Calories = 84

Soup Mostly Noodles ☞ serving size: 1 cup = 233 g; Calories = 156

Soup Mostly Noodles Reduced Sodium ☞ serving size: 1 cup = 233 g; Calories = 124

Soup Mushroom Barley Canned Condensed ☞ serving size: 1/2 cup (4 fl oz) = 126 g; Calories = 77

Soup Mushroom With Beef Stock Canned Condensed ☞ serving size: 1/2 cup (4 fl oz) = 126 g; Calories = 86

Soup Mushroom With Beef Stock Canned Prepared With Equal Volume Water ☞ serving size: 1 cup (8 fl oz) = 244 g; Calories = 85

Soup Nfs ☞ serving size: 1 cup = 241 g; Calories = 58

Soup Onion Canned Condensed ☞ serving size: 1/2 cup (4 fl oz) = 123 g; Calories = 57

Soup Onion Dry Mix ☞ serving size: 1 serving 1 tbsp = 7.5 g; Calories = 22

Soup Onion Dry Mix Prepared With Water ☞ serving size: 1 serving 1 cup = 230 g; Calories = 28

Soup Oyster Stew Canned Condensed ☞ serving size: 1/2 cup (4 fl oz) = 123 g; Calories = 59

Soup Oyster Stew Canned Prepared With Equal Volume Milk ☞ serving size: 1 cup (8 fl oz) = 245 g; Calories = 135

Soup Oyster Stew Canned Prepared With Equal Volume Water ☞ serving size: 1 cup (8 fl oz) = 241 g; Calories = 58

Soup Pea Green Canned Condensed ☛ serving size: 1/2 cup = 128 g; Calories = 160

Soup Pea Green Canned Prepared With Equal Volume Milk ☛ serving size: 1 cup (8 fl oz) = 254 g; Calories = 239

Soup Pea Green Canned Prepared With Equal Volume Water ☛ serving size: 1 serving 1 cup = 259 g; Calories = 158

Soup Pea Low Sodium Prepared With Equal Volume Water ☛ serving size: 1 cup = 259 g; Calories = 161

Soup Pea Split With Ham Canned Chunky Ready-To-Serve ☛ serving size: 1 cup = 240 g; Calories = 185

Soup Pea Split With Ham Canned Condensed ☛ serving size: 1/2 cup (4 fl oz) = 135 g; Calories = 190

Soup Pea Split With Ham Canned Prepared With Equal Volume Water ☛ serving size: 1 cup (8 fl oz) = 253 g; Calories = 190

Soup Ramen Noodle Any Flavor Dry ☛ serving size: 1 package without flavor packet = 81 g; Calories = 356

Soup Ramen Noodle Beef Flavor Dry ☛ serving size: 1 package without flavor packet = 82 g; Calories = 362

Soup Ramen Noodle Chicken Flavor Dry ☛ serving size: 1 package without flavor packet = 81 g; Calories = 356

Soup Ramen Noodle Dry Any Flavor Reduced Fat Reduced Sodium ☛ serving size: 1 (2/5) oz dry (half noodle block) = 40 g; Calories = 140

Soup Shark Fin Restaurant-Prepared ☛ serving size: 1 cup = 216 g; Calories = 99

Soup Swanson Beef Broth Lower Sodium ☛ serving size: 1 cup = 213 g; Calories = 13

Soup Swanson Vegetable Broth ☛ serving size: 1 cup = 220 g; Calories = 13

Soup Tomato Beef With Noodle Canned Condensed ☛ serving size: 1 cup (8 fl oz) = 251 g; Calories = 281

Soup Tomato Beef With Noodle Canned Prepared With Equal Volume Water ☛ serving size: 1 cup = 244 g; Calories = 137

Soup Tomato Bisque Canned Condensed ☛ serving size: 1/2 cup (4 fl oz) = 129 g; Calories = 124

Soup Tomato Bisque Canned Prepared With Equal Volume Milk ☛ serving size: 1 cup (8 fl oz) = 251 g; Calories = 198

Soup Tomato Bisque Canned Prepared With Equal Volume Water ☛ serving size: 1 cup (8 fl oz) = 247 g; Calories = 124

Soup Tomato Canned Condensed ☛ serving size: 1 cup = 148 g; Calories = 98

Soup Tomato Canned Condensed Reduced Sodium ☛ serving size: 1 serving 1/2 cup = 121 g; Calories = 79

Soup Tomato Canned Prepared With Equal Volume Low Fat (2%) Milk ☛ serving size: 1 serving 1 cup = 252 g; Calories = 139

Soup Tomato Canned Prepared With Equal Volume Water Commercial ☛ serving size: 1 serving 1 cup = 248 g; Calories = 79

Soup Tomato Dry Mix Prepared With Water ☛ serving size: 1 cup 8 fl oz = 265 g; Calories = 101

Soup Tomato Low Sodium With Water ☛ serving size: 1 serving 1 cup = 248 g; Calories = 74

Soup Tomato Rice Canned Condensed ☛ serving size: 1/2 cup (4 fl oz) = 129 g; Calories = 120

Soup Tomato Rice Canned Prepared With Equal Volume Water ☛ serving size: 1 cup = 247 g; Calories = 116

Soup Turkey Chunky Canned Ready-To-Serve ☛ serving size: 1 cup (8 fl oz) = 236 g; Calories = 135

Soup Turkey Noodle Canned Prepared With Equal Volume Water ☛ serving size: 1 cup = 244 g; Calories = 68

Soup Turkey Vegetable Canned Prepared With Equal Volume Water ☛ serving size: 1 cup (8 fl oz) = 241 g; Calories = 72

Soup Vegetable Beef Canned Condensed ☛ serving size: 1/2 cup = 126 g; Calories = 79

Soup Vegetable Beef Canned Prepared With Equal Volume Water ☛ serving size: 1 cup (8 fl oz) = 244 g; Calories = 76

Soup Vegetable Beef Microwavable Ready-To-Serve Single Brand ☛ serving size: 1 serving = 292 g; Calories = 129

Soup Vegetable Canned Low Sodium Condensed ☛ serving size: 1/2 cup = 126 g; Calories = 82

Soup Vegetable Chicken Canned Prepared With Water Low Sodium ☛ serving size: 1 cup = 241 g; Calories = 166

Soup Vegetable Soup Condensed Low Sodium Prepared With Equal Volume Water ☛ serving size: 1 cup = 253 g; Calories = 84

Soup Vegetable With Beef Broth Canned Condensed ☛ serving size: 1/2 cup = 123 g; Calories = 81

Soup Vegetable With Beef Broth Canned Prepared With Equal Volume Water ☛ serving size: 1 cup (8 fl oz) = 241 g; Calories = 80

Soup Vegetarian Vegetable Canned Condensed ☛ serving size: 1/2 cup = 126 g; Calories = 74

Soup Wonton Chinese Restaurant ☛ serving size: 1 cup = 223 g; Calories = 71

Soupy Rice Mixture With Chicken And Potatoes Puerto Rican Style ☛ serving size: 1 cup = 240 g; Calories = 269

Soupy Rice With Chicken Puerto Rican Style ☛ serving size: 1 cup, with bone (yield after bone removed) = 215 g; Calories = 325

Soybean Soup Miso Broth ☛ serving size: 1 cup = 240 g; Calories = 77

Spaghetti Sauce With Added Vegetables ☛ serving size: 1 cup = 260 g; Calories = 114

Spaghetti Sauce With Meat ☛ serving size: 1 cup = 260 g; Calories = 231

Spaghetti Sauce With Meat And Added Vegetables ☛ serving size: 1 cup = 260 g; Calories = 218

Spaghetti Sauce With Poultry ☛ serving size: 1 cup = 260 g; Calories = 190

Spaghetti Sauce With Poultry And Added Vegetables ☛ serving size: 1 cup = 260 g; Calories = 177

Spaghetti Sauce With Seafood ☛ serving size: 1 cup = 260 g; Calories = 164

Spaghetti Sauce With Seafood And Added Vegetables ☛ serving size: 1 cup = 260 g; Calories = 151

Spanish Vegetable Soup Puerto Rican Style ☛ serving size: 1 cup = 250 g; Calories = 260

Spinach And Artichoke Dip ☛ serving size: 1 tablespoon = 15 g; Calories = 49

Spinach Dip Light ☛ serving size: 1 tablespoon = 15 g; Calories = 25

Spinach Dip Regular ☛ serving size: 1 tablespoon = 15 g; Calories = 52

Spinach Dip Yogurt Based ☛ serving size: 1 tablespoon = 15 g; Calories = 24

Spinach Soup ☛ serving size: 1 cup = 245 g; Calories = 74

Split Pea Soup Canned Reduced Sodium Prepared With Water Or Ready-To Serve ☛ serving size: 1 cup = 253 g; Calories = 180

Split Pea With Ham Soup Canned Reduced Sodium Prepared With Water Or Ready-To-Serve ☛ serving size: 1 cup = 245 g; Calories = 167

Squash Winter Type Soup Home Recipe Canned Or Ready-To-Serve ☛ serving size: 1 cup = 248 g; Calories = 97

Sriracha ☛ serving size: 1 tsp = 6.5 g; Calories = 6

Sweet And Sour Sauce ☛ serving size: 1 cup = 240 g; Calories = 360

Sweet And Sour Soup ☛ serving size: 1 cup = 244 g; Calories = 164

Tabasco Sauce ☛ serving size: 1 tsp = 4.7 g; Calories = 1

Teriyaki Sauce ☛ serving size: 2 tbsp = 36 g; Calories = 32

Tomato Noodle Soup Canned Prepared With Milk ☛ serving size: 1 cup = 248 g; Calories = 174

Tomato Noodle Soup Canned Prepared With Water Or Ready-To-Serve ☛ serving size: 1 cup = 244 g; Calories = 142

Tomato Relish ☛ serving size: 1 cup = 320 g; Calories = 502

Tomato Soup Canned Reduced Sodium Prepared With Milk ☛ serving size: 1 cup = 248 g; Calories = 144

Tomato Soup Canned Reduced Sodium Prepared With Water Or Ready-To-Serve ☛ serving size: 1 cup = 244 g; Calories = 81

Tomato Soup Cream Of Prepared With Milk ☛ serving size: 1 cup = 248 g; Calories = 144

Tomato Soup Nfs ☛ serving size: 1 cup = 244 g; Calories = 81

Tomato Soup Prepared With Water Or Ready-To-Serve ☛ serving size: 1 cup = 244 g; Calories = 81

Tomato Vegetable Soup Prepared With Water ☛ serving size: 1 cup = 241 g; Calories = 80

Turtle And Vegetable Soup ☛ serving size: 1 cup = 244 g; Calories = 103

Tzatziki Dip ☛ serving size: 1 tablespoon = 15 g; Calories = 14

Vegetable Beef Noodle Soup Prepared With Water ☛ serving size: 1 cup = 244 g; Calories = 78

Vegetable Beef Soup Canned Prepared With Milk ☛ serving size: 1 cup = 248 g; Calories = 141

Vegetable Beef Soup Canned Prepared With Water Or Ready-To-Serve ☛ serving size: 1 cup = 244 g; Calories = 78

Vegetable Beef Soup Home Recipe ☛ serving size: 1 cup = 241 g; Calories = 133

Vegetable Beef Soup With Noodles Or Pasta Home Recipe ☛ serving size: 1 cup = 241 g; Calories = 162

Vegetable Beef Soup With Rice Canned Prepared With Water Or Ready-To-Serve ☛ serving size: 1 cup = 244 g; Calories = 78

Vegetable Beef Soup With Rice Home Recipe ☛ serving size: 1 cup = 244 g; Calories = 164

Vegetable Broth ☛ serving size: 1 cup = 221 g; Calories = 11

Vegetable Dip Light ☛ serving size: 1 tablespoon = 15 g; Calories = 30

Vegetable Dip Regular ☛ serving size: 1 tablespoon = 15 g; Calories = 64

Vegetable Dip Yogurt Based ☛ serving size: 1 tablespoon = 15 g; Calories = 29

Vegetable Noodle Soup Canned Prepared With Water Or Ready-To-Serve ☛ serving size: 1 cup = 241 g; Calories = 72

Vegetable Noodle Soup Home Recipe ☛ serving size: 1 cup = 241 g; Calories = 113

Vegetable Soup ☛ serving size: 1 cup = 241 g; Calories = 68

Vegetable Soup Cream Of Prepared With Milk ☛ serving size: 1 cup = 248 g; Calories = 213

Vegetable Soup Home Recipe ☛ serving size: 1 cup = 234 g; Calories = 89

Vegetable Soup Made From Dry Mix ☛ serving size: 1 cup = 253 g; Calories = 101

Vegetable Soup Spanish Style Stew Type ☛ serving size: 1 cup = 227 g; Calories = 198

Vegetable Soup With Chicken Broth Home Recipe Mexican Style ☛ serving size: 1 cup = 232 g; Calories = 142

Vegetarian Vegetable Soup Prepared With Water ☛ serving size: 1 cup = 241 g; Calories = 72

Vodka Sauce With Tomatoes And Cream ☛ serving size: 1 cup = 260 g; Calories = 192

Wasabi ☛ serving size: 1 tablespoon = 20 g; Calories = 58

Watercress Broth With Shrimp ☛ serving size: 1 cup = 245 g; Calories = 118

Welsh Rarebit ☛ serving size: 1 tablespoon = 15 g; Calories = 25

White Sauce Milk Sauce ☛ serving size: 1 cup = 250 g; Calories = 368

Worcestershire Sauce ☛ serving size: 1 tbsp = 17 g; Calories = 13

Yeast Extract Spread ☛ serving size: 1 tsp = 6 g; Calories = 11

Zucchini Soup Cream Of Prepared With Milk ☛ serving size: 1 cup = 248 g; Calories = 57

24

SPICES AND HERBS

🌿 Anise Seeds 🖛 serving size: 1 tsp, whole = 2.1 g; Calories = 7

🌿 Apple Cider Vinegar 🖛 serving size: 1 tbsp = 14.9 g; Calories = 3

🌿 Balsamic Vinegar 🖛 serving size: 1 tbsp = 16 g; Calories = 14

🌿 Basil 🖛 serving size: 5 leaves = 2.5 g; Calories = 1

🌿 Bay Leaves 🖛 serving size: 1 tsp, crumbled = 0.6 g; Calories = 2

🌿 Black Pepper 🖛 serving size: 1 tsp, ground = 2.3 g; Calories = 6

🌿 Capers 🖛 serving size: 1 tbsp, drained = 8.6 g; Calories = 2

🌿 Caraway Seed 🖛 serving size: 1 tsp = 2.1 g; Calories = 7

🌿 Cardamom 🖛 serving size: 1 tsp, ground = 2 g; Calories = 6

🌿 Cayenne Pepper 🖛 serving size: 1 tsp = 1.8 g; Calories = 6

🌿 Celery Seed 🖛 serving size: 1 tsp = 2 g; Calories = 8

🌿 Chili Powder 🖛 serving size: 1 tsp = 2.7 g; Calories = 8

🌿 Cinnamon 🖛 serving size: 1 tsp = 2.6 g; Calories = 6

- Coriander Seed ☛ serving size: 1 tsp = 1.8 g; Calories = 5

- Cumin Seed ☛ serving size: 1 tsp, whole = 2.1 g; Calories = 8

- Curry Powder ☛ serving size: 1 tsp = 2 g; Calories = 7

- Dill ☛ serving size: 5 sprigs = 1 g; Calories = 0

- Dill Seed ☛ serving size: 1 tsp = 2.1 g; Calories = 6

- Distilled Vinegar ☛ serving size: 1 tbsp = 14.9 g; Calories = 3

- Dried Basil ☛ serving size: 1 tsp, leaves = 0.7 g; Calories = 2

- Dried Chervil ☛ serving size: 1 tsp = 0.6 g; Calories = 1

- Dried Coriander ☛ serving size: 1 tsp = 0.6 g; Calories = 2

- Dried Dill Weed ☛ serving size: 1 tsp = 1 g; Calories = 3

- Dried Marjoram ☛ serving size: 1 tsp = 0.6 g; Calories = 2

- Dried Oregano ☛ serving size: 1 tsp, leaves = 1 g; Calories = 3

- Dried Parsley ☛ serving size: 1 tsp = 0.5 g; Calories = 2

- Dried Rosemary ☛ serving size: 1 tsp = 1.2 g; Calories = 4

- Dried Spearmint ☛ serving size: 1 tsp = 0.5 g; Calories = 1

- Dried Tarragon ☛ serving size: 1 tsp, leaves = 0.6 g; Calories = 2

- Fennel Seed ☛ serving size: 1 tsp, whole = 2 g; Calories = 7

- Fenugreek Seed ☛ serving size: 1 tsp = 3.7 g; Calories = 12

- Garlic Powder ☛ serving size: 1 tsp = 3.1 g; Calories = 10

- Ground Allspice ☛ serving size: 1 tsp = 1.9 g; Calories = 5

- Ground Cloves ☛ serving size: 1 tsp = 2.1 g; Calories = 6

- Ground Ginger ☛ serving size: 1 tsp = 1.8 g; Calories = 6

- Ground Mace ☛ serving size: 1 tsp = 1.7 g; Calories = 8

🌿 Ground Mustard Seed ☛ serving size: 1 tsp = 2 g; Calories = 10

🌿 Ground Nutmeg ☛ serving size: 1 tsp = 2.2 g; Calories = 12

🌿 Ground Sage ☛ serving size: 1 tsp = 0.7 g; Calories = 2

🌿 Ground Savory ☛ serving size: 1 tsp = 1.4 g; Calories = 4

🌿 Ground Turmeric ☛ serving size: 1 tsp = 3 g; Calories = 9

🌿 Horseradish ☛ serving size: 1 tsp = 5 g; Calories = 2

🌿 Imitation Vanilla Extract ☛ serving size: 1 tsp = 4.2 g; Calories = 10

🌿 Imitation Vanilla Extract (No Alcohol) ☛ serving size: 1 tsp = 4.2 g; Calories = 2

🌿 Onion Powder ☛ serving size: 1 tsp = 2.4 g; Calories = 8

🌿 Paprika ☛ serving size: 1 tsp = 2.3 g; Calories = 7

🌿 Peppermint ☛ serving size: 2 leaves = 0.1 g; Calories = 0

🌿 Poppy Seeds ☛ serving size: 1 tsp = 2.8 g; Calories = 15

🌿 Poultry Seasoning ☛ serving size: 1 tsp = 1.5 g; Calories = 5

🌿 Pumpkin Pie Spice ☛ serving size: 1 tsp = 1.7 g; Calories = 6

🌿 Red Wine Vinegar ☛ serving size: 1 tbsp = 14.9 g; Calories = 3

🌿 Rosemary ☛ serving size: 1 tsp = 0.7 g; Calories = 1

🌿 Saffron ☛ serving size: 1 tsp = 0.7 g; Calories = 2

🌿 Seasoning Mix Dry Chili Original ☛ serving size: tbsp = 9 g; Calories = 30

🌿 Seasoning Mix Dry Sazon Coriander & Annatto ☛ serving size: 1/4 tsp = 1 g; Calories = 0

🌿 Seasoning Mix Dry Taco Original ☛ serving size: 2 tsp = 5.7 g; Calories = 18

🌿 Spearmint ☛ serving size: 2 leaves = 0.3 g; Calories = 0

- Spices Thyme Dried ☛ serving size: 1 tsp, leaves = 1 g; Calories = 3

- Table Salt ☛ serving size: 1 tsp = 6 g; Calories = 0

- Thyme (Fresh) ☛ serving size: 1 tsp = 0.8 g; Calories = 1

- Vanilla Extract ☛ serving size: 1 tsp = 4.2 g; Calories = 12

- White Pepper ☛ serving size: 1 tsp, ground = 2.4 g; Calories = 7

- Yellow Mustard ☛ serving size: 1 tsp or 1 packet = 5 g; Calories = 3

25

SWEETENERS

❧ Sugar ☛ serving size: 1 serving packet = 2.8 g; Calories = 11

❧ Sugar Brown And Water Syrup ☛ serving size: 1 cup = 242 g; Calories = 748

❧ Sugar Brown Liquid ☛ serving size: 1 cup = 335 g; Calories = 884

❧ Sugar Cinnamon ☛ serving size: 1 cup = 200 g; Calories = 754

❧ Sugar Substitute And Sugar Blend ☛ serving size: 1 teaspoon = 2 g; Calories = 8

❧ Sugar Substitute Liquid Nfs ☛ serving size: 1 teaspoon = 5 g; Calories = 3

❧ Sugar Substitute Powder Nfs ☛ serving size: 1 individual packet = 1 g; Calories = 4

❧ Sugar Substitute Saccharin Liquid ☛ serving size: 1 teaspoon = 5 g; Calories = 0

❧ Sugar Substitute Stevia Liquid ☛ serving size: 1 teaspoon = 5 g; Calories = 3

Sugar Turbinado ☛ serving size: 1 tsp = 4.6 g; Calories = 18

Sugar White And Water Syrup ☛ serving size: 1 cup = 242 g; Calories = 736

Sugar-Coated Almonds ☛ serving size: 1 piece = 3.5 g; Calories = 16

Sugared Pecans Sugar And Egg White Coating ☛ serving size: 1 cup = 79 g; Calories = 442

Sugars Brown ☛ serving size: 1 tsp unpacked = 3 g; Calories = 11

Sugars Maple ☛ serving size: 1 tsp = 3 g; Calories = 11

Sugars Powdered ☛ serving size: 1 cup unsifted = 120 g; Calories = 467

Sweet Chocolate ☛ serving size: 1 oz = 28.4 g; Calories = 144

Sweet Chocolate Coated Fondant ☛ serving size: 1 patty, large = 43 g; Calories = 157

Sweet Potato Paste ☛ serving size: 1 tablespoon = 20 g; Calories = 59

Sweetener Herbal Extract Powder From Stevia Leaf ☛ serving size: 1 package = 1 g; Calories = 0

Sweetener Syrup Agave ☛ serving size: 1 tsp = 6.9 g; Calories = 21

Sweeteners For Baking Brown Contains Sugar And Sucralose ☛ serving size: 1 tbsp = 12.9 g; Calories = 50

Sweeteners For Baking Contains Sugar And Sucralose ☛ serving size: 1 tbsp = 14.5 g; Calories = 58

Sweeteners Sugar Substitute Granulated Brown ☛ serving size: 1 tsp = 0.5 g; Calories = 2

Sweeteners Tabletop Aspartame Equal Packets ☛ serving size: 1 tsp = 3.5 g; Calories = 13

Sweeteners Tabletop Fructose Dry Powder ☛ serving size: 1 cup = 196 g; Calories = 721

Sweeteners Tabletop Fructose Liquid ☛ serving size: 1 serving = 0.1 g; Calories = 0

Sweeteners Tabletop Saccharin (Sodium Saccharin) ☛ serving size: 1 serving 1 packet = 1 g; Calories = 4

Sweeteners Tabletop Sucralose Splenda Packets ☛ serving size: 1 serving 1 packet = 1 g; Calories = 3

Symphony Milk Chocolate Bar ☛ serving size: 1 bar 1.5 oz = 42 g; Calories = 223

Syrup Cane ☛ serving size: 1 serving = 21 g; Calories = 57

Syrup Dietetic ☛ serving size: 1 cup = 240 g; Calories = 125

Syrup Fruit Flavored ☛ serving size: 1 serving = 20 g; Calories = 52

Syrup Maple Canadian ☛ serving size: 60 milliliter = 80 g; Calories = 216

Syrup Nestle Chocolate ☛ serving size: 1 tablespoon = 20 g; Calories = 54

Syrups Chocolate Fudge-Type ☛ serving size: 1 cup = 304 g; Calories = 1064

Syrups Chocolate Hersheys Genuine Chocolate Flavored Lite Syrup ☛ serving size: 2 tbsp = 35 g; Calories = 54

Syrups Chocolate Hersheys Sugar Free Genuine Chocolate Flavored Lite Syrup ☛ serving size: 2 tbsp = 35 g; Calories = 15

Syrups Corn Dark ☛ serving size: 1 cup = 328 g; Calories = 938

Syrups Corn High-Fructose ☛ serving size: 1 cup = 310 g; Calories = 871

Syrups Corn Light ☛ serving size: 1 cup = 341 g; Calories = 965

Syrups Grenadine ☛ serving size: 1 tbsp = 20 g; Calories = 54

Syrups Malt ☛ serving size: 1 cup = 332 g; Calories = 1056

Syrups Maple ☛ serving size: 1 tbsp = 20 g; Calories = 52

Syrups Sorghum ☛ serving size: 1 cup = 330 g; Calories = 957

Syrups Sugar Free ☛ serving size: 1 cup = 240 g; Calories = 122

Syrups Table Blends Corn Refiner And Sugar ☛ serving size: 1 cup = 316 g; Calories = 1008

Syrups Table Blends Pancake ☛ serving size: 1 cup = 314 g; Calories = 735

Syrups Table Blends Pancake Reduced-Calorie ☛ serving size: 1 serving 1/4 cup = 73 g; Calories = 121

Syrups Table Blends Pancake With 2% Maple ☛ serving size: 1 tbsp = 20 g; Calories = 53

Syrups Table Blends Pancake With 2% Maple With Added Potassium ☛ serving size: 1 cup = 315 g; Calories = 835

Syrups Table Blends Pancake With Butter ☛ serving size: 1 serving 1/4 cup = 73 g; Calories = 212

26

VEGETABLES & VEGETABLES PRODUCTS

Acorn Squash ☛ serving size: 1 cup, cubes = 140 g; Calories = 56

Alfalfa Sprouts ☛ serving size: 1 cup = 33 g; Calories = 8

Amaranth Leaves Raw ☛ serving size: 1 cup = 28 g; Calories = 6

Arrowhead Raw ☛ serving size: 1 large = 25 g; Calories = 25

Arrowroot ☛ serving size: 1 cup, sliced = 120 g; Calories = 78

Artichoke Cooked From Canned Ns As To Fat Added In Cooking ☛ serving size: 1 small globe = 103 g; Calories = 63

Artichoke Cooked From Fresh Ns As To Fat Added In Cooking ☛ serving size: 1 small globe = 103 g; Calories = 71

Artichoke Cooked From Frozen Ns As To Fat Added In Cooking ☛ serving size: 1 cup, hearts = 173 g; Calories = 106

Arugula ☛ serving size: 1 leaf = 2 g; Calories = 1

Asparagus ☛ serving size: 1 cup = 134 g; Calories = 27

Asparagus (Cooked) ☛ serving size: 1/2 cup = 90 g; Calories = 20

🥒 Asparagus Cooked From Canned Ns As To Fat Added In Cooking ☛ serving size: 1 cup = 247 g; Calories = 77

🥒 Asparagus Cooked From Fresh Ns As To Fat Added In Cooking ☛ serving size: 1 piece = 3 g; Calories = 1

🥒 Asparagus Cooked From Frozen Fat Added In Cooking Ns As To Type Of Fat ☛ serving size: 1 piece = 3 g; Calories = 1

🥒 Asparagus Cooked From Frozen Ns As To Fat Added In Cooking ☛ serving size: 1 piece = 3 g; Calories = 1

🥒 Baby Carrots ☛ serving size: 1 large = 15 g; Calories = 5

🥒 Baked Acorn Squash ☛ serving size: 1 cup, cubes = 205 g; Calories = 115

🥒 Baked Potato (No Skin) ☛ serving size: 1/2 cup = 61 g; Calories = 57

🥒 Baked Potatoes ☛ serving size: 1 potato large (3 inch to 4-1/4 inch dia) = 299 g; Calories = 275

🥒 Baked Potatoes (With Skin) ☛ serving size: 1 nlea serving = 148 g; Calories = 138

🥒 Baked Red Potatoes ☛ serving size: 1 potato large (3 inch to 4-1/4 inch dia. = 299 g; Calories = 260

🥒 Baked Russet Potatoes ☛ serving size: 1 potato large (3 inch to 4-1/4 inch dia. = 299 g; Calories = 284

🥒 Balsam-Pear (Bitter Gourd) Leafy Tips Cooked Boiled Drained With Salt ☛ serving size: 1 cup = 58 g; Calories = 19

🥒 Bamboo Shoots ☛ serving size: 1 cup (1/2 inch slices) = 151 g; Calories = 41

🥒 Bamboo Shoots (Canned) ☛ serving size: 1 cup (1/8 inch slices) = 131 g; Calories = 25

🥒 Bamboo Shoots (Cooked) ☛ serving size: 1 cup (1/2 inch slices) = 120 g; Calories = 14

Banana Peppers ☛ serving size: 1 cup = 124 g; Calories = 34

Bean Salad Yellow And/or Green String Beans ☛ serving size: 1 cup = 150 g; Calories = 161

Bean Sprouts Cooked Ns As To Form Ns As To Fat Added In Cooking ☛ serving size: 1 cup = 129 g; Calories = 103

Beans Lima Immature Cooked From Canned Ns As To Fat Added In Cooking ☛ serving size: 1 cup = 179 g; Calories = 209

Beans Navy Mature Seeds Sprouted Raw ☛ serving size: 1 cup = 104 g; Calories = 70

Beans Pinto Immature Seeds Frozen Cooked Boiled Drained With Salt ☛ serving size: 1/ 3 package (10 oz) yields = 94 g; Calories = 152

Beans Shellie Canned Solids And Liquids ☛ serving size: 1 cup = 245 g; Calories = 74

Beans Snap Canned All Styles Seasoned Solids And Liquids ☛ serving size: 1/2 cup = 114 g; Calories = 18

Beans String Cooked From Fresh ☛ serving size: 1 cup = 125 g; Calories = 44

Beet Greens Cooked ☛ serving size: 1 cup = 149 g; Calories = 69

Beets (Raw) ☛ serving size: 1 cup = 136 g; Calories = 59

Bitter Melon ☛ serving size: 1 cup (1/2 inch pieces) = 93 g; Calories = 16

Bitter Melon (Cooked) ☛ serving size: 1 cup (1/2 inch pieces) = 124 g; Calories = 24

Bok Choy ☛ serving size: 1 cup, shredded = 70 g; Calories = 9

Borage Raw ☛ serving size: 1 cup (1 inch pieces) = 89 g; Calories = 19

🍃 Breadfruit Cooked Ns As To Fat Added In Cooking 🐾 serving size: 1 cup = 257 g; Calories = 337

🍃 Breadfruit Fried 🐾 serving size: 1 cup = 170 g; Calories = 269

🍃 Broadbeans Immature Seeds Raw 🐾 serving size: 1 cup = 109 g; Calories = 79

🍃 Broccoflower Cooked Ns As To Fat Added In Cooking 🐾 serving size: 1 cup, fresh = 87 g; Calories = 51

🍃 Broccoli 🐾 serving size: 1 cup chopped = 91 g; Calories = 31

🍃 Broccoli (Cooked) 🐾 serving size: 1/2 cup, chopped = 78 g; Calories = 27

🍃 Brussels Sprouts (Cooked) 🐾 serving size: 1 sprout = 21 g; Calories = 8

🍃 Brussels Sprouts (Raw) 🐾 serving size: 1 cup = 88 g; Calories = 38

🍃 Burdock Cooked Ns As To Fat Added In Cooking 🐾 serving size: 1 cup = 130 g; Calories = 150

🍃 Burdock Root Cooked Boiled Drained With Salt 🐾 serving size: 1 cup (1 inch pieces) = 125 g; Calories = 110

🍃 Burdock Root Raw 🐾 serving size: 1 cup (1 inch pieces) = 118 g; Calories = 85

🍃 Butterbur (Fuki) Raw 🐾 serving size: 1 cup = 94 g; Calories = 13

🍃 Butterbur Canned 🐾 serving size: 1 cup, chopped = 124 g; Calories = 4

🍃 Butterhead Lettuce 🐾 serving size: 1 cup, shredded or chopped = 55 g; Calories = 7

🍃 Butternut Squash 🐾 serving size: 1 cup, cubes = 140 g; Calories = 63

🍃 Cabbage 🐾 serving size: 1 cup, chopped = 89 g; Calories = 22

Cabbage Chinese (Pak-Choi) Cooked Boiled Drained With Salt ☛ serving size: 1 cup, shredded = 170 g; Calories = 20

Cabbage Chinese (Pe-Tsai) Cooked Boiled Drained With Salt ☛ serving size: 1 cup, shredded = 119 g; Calories = 17

Cabbage Red Cooked Fat Added In Cooking Ns As To Type Of Fat ☛ serving size: 1 cup = 155 g; Calories = 73

Cabbage Red Cooked Ns As To Fat Added In Cooking ☛ serving size: 1 cup = 155 g; Calories = 73

Cabbage Salad Or Coleslaw Made With Any Type Of Fat Free Dressing ☛ serving size: 1 cup = 219 g; Calories = 90

Cabbage Savoy Cooked Ns As To Fat Added In Cooking ☛ serving size: 1 cup = 150 g; Calories = 72

Cactus Cooked Ns As To Fat Added In Cooking ☛ serving size: 1 cup = 154 g; Calories = 52

Caesar Salad With Romaine No Dressing ☛ serving size: 1 cup = 79 g; Calories = 56

Calabaza Cooked ☛ serving size: 1 cup, cubes = 166 g; Calories = 75

Canned Asparagus ☛ serving size: 1 cup = 242 g; Calories = 46

Canned Green Beans ☛ serving size: 1 cup = 240 g; Calories = 36

Canned Lima Beans ☛ serving size: 1 cup = 248 g; Calories = 176

Canned Mung Bean Sprouts ☛ serving size: 1 cup = 125 g; Calories = 15

Canned Mushrooms ☛ serving size: 1 cup = 156 g; Calories = 39

Canned Pimentos ☛ serving size: 1 tbsp = 12 g; Calories = 3

Canned Pumpkin ☛ serving size: 1 cup = 245 g; Calories = 83

Canned Straw Mushrooms ☛ serving size: 1 cup = 182 g; Calories = 58

🥄 Canned Tomato Paste ☛ serving size: 1/4 cup = 66 g; Calories = 54

🥄 Canned Tomato Puree ☛ serving size: 1 cup = 250 g; Calories = 95

🥄 Cardoon Raw ☛ serving size: 1 cup, shredded = 178 g; Calories = 30

🥄 Carrot Dehydrated ☛ serving size: 1 cup = 74 g; Calories = 252

🥄 Carrot Juice Canned ☛ serving size: 1 cup = 236 g; Calories = 94

🥄 Carrots ☛ serving size: 1 cup chopped = 128 g; Calories = 53

🥄 Cassava ☛ serving size: 1 cup = 206 g; Calories = 330

🥄 Cauliflower ☛ serving size: 1 cup chopped (1/2 inch pieces) = 107 g; Calories = 27

🥄 Cauliflower Frozen Unprepared ☛ serving size: 1/2 cup (1 inch pieces) = 66 g; Calories = 16

🥄 Cauliflower Green Cooked With Salt ☛ serving size: 1/2 cup (1 inch pieces) = 62 g; Calories = 20

🥄 Celeriac ☛ serving size: 1 cup = 156 g; Calories = 66

🥄 Celery ☛ serving size: 1 cup chopped = 101 g; Calories = 14

🥄 Celtuce ☛ serving size: 1 leaf = 8 g; Calories = 1

🥄 Chamnamul Cooked Ns As To Fat Added In Cooking ☛ serving size: 1 cup = 151 g; Calories = 127

🥄 Channa Saag ☛ serving size: 1 cup = 245 g; Calories = 201

🥄 Chantarelle Mushrooms ☛ serving size: 1 cup = 54 g; Calories = 17

🥄 Chard Cooked Ns As To Fat Added In Cooking ☛ serving size: 1 cup, stalk and leaves = 150 g; Calories = 54

🥄 Chard Swiss Cooked Boiled Drained With Salt ☛ serving size: 1 cup, chopped = 175 g; Calories = 35

🥄 Chayote Fruit Cooked Boiled Drained With Salt ☛ serving size: 1 cup (1 inch pieces) = 160 g; Calories = 35

Chayote Fruit Raw ☛ serving size: 1 cup (1 inch pieces) = 132 g; Calories = 25

Chicory Greens ☛ serving size: 1 cup, chopped = 29 g; Calories = 7

Chicory Roots ☛ serving size: 1 root = 60 g; Calories = 43

Chives ☛ serving size: 1 tbsp chopped = 3 g; Calories = 1

Christophine Cooked ☛ serving size: 1 cup = 165 g; Calories = 69

Chrysanthemum ☛ serving size: 1 cup (1 inch pieces) = 25 g; Calories = 6

Chrysanthemum Leaves ☛ serving size: 1 cup, chopped = 51 g; Calories = 12

Cilantro ☛ serving size: 1/4 cup = 4 g; Calories = 1

Citronella (Lemon Grass) ☛ serving size: 1 cup = 67 g; Calories = 66

Cobb Salad No Dressing ☛ serving size: 1 cup = 105 g; Calories = 97

Collards ☛ serving size: 1 cup, chopped = 36 g; Calories = 12

Corn Cooked From Canned ☛ serving size: 1 cup = 169 g; Calories = 140

Corn Cooked From Fresh ☛ serving size: 1 cup = 158 g; Calories = 185

Corn Cooked From Frozen ☛ serving size: 1 cup = 169 g; Calories = 162

Corn Dried Cooked ☛ serving size: 1 oz = 28 g; Calories = 31

Corn Fritter ☛ serving size: 1 cup = 107 g; Calories = 422

Corn White Ns As To Form Cream Style ☛ serving size: 1 cup = 256 g; Calories = 189

Corn Yellow Ns As To Form Cream Style ☛ serving size: 1 cup = 256 g; Calories = 184

🍃 Cornsalad Raw ☛ serving size: 1 cup = 56 g; Calories = 12

🍃 Cowpeas (Blackeyes) Immature Seeds Cooked Boiled Drained With Salt ☛ serving size: 1 cup = 165 g; Calories = 155

🍃 Cowpeas (Blackeyes) Immature Seeds Frozen Cooked Boiled Drained With Salt ☛ serving size: 1 cup = 170 g; Calories = 223

🍃 Cowpeas (Blackeyes) Immature Seeds Frozen Unprepared ☛ serving size: 1 cup = 160 g; Calories = 222

🍃 Cremini Mushrooms ☛ serving size: 1 cup whole = 87 g; Calories = 19

🍃 Cress Cooked ☛ serving size: 1 cup = 140 g; Calories = 62

🍃 Cress Garden Cooked Boiled Drained With Salt ☛ serving size: 1 cup = 135 g; Calories = 31

🍃 Crookneck Summer Squash ☛ serving size: 1 cup sliced = 127 g; Calories = 24

🍃 Cucumber ☛ serving size: 1/2 cup slices = 52 g; Calories = 8

🍃 Dandelion Greens ☛ serving size: 1 cup, chopped = 55 g; Calories = 25

🍃 Dasheen Boiled ☛ serving size: 1 cup, pieces = 142 g; Calories = 200

🍃 Dock Raw ☛ serving size: 1 cup, chopped = 133 g; Calories = 29

🍃 Dried Ancho Peppers ☛ serving size: 1 pepper = 17 g; Calories = 48

🍃 Dried Chives ☛ serving size: 1 tbsp = 0.2 g; Calories = 1

🍃 Dried Fungi Cloud Ears ☛ serving size: 1 cup = 28 g; Calories = 80

🍃 Dried Pasilla Peppers ☛ serving size: 1 pepper = 7 g; Calories = 24

🍃 Dried Shiitake Mushrooms ☛ serving size: 1 mushroom = 3.6 g; Calories = 11

Dried Spirulina Seaweed ☛ serving size: 1 cup = 112 g; Calories = 325

Drumstick Leaves Raw ☛ serving size: 1 cup, chopped = 21 g; Calories = 13

Edamame Frozen Unprepared ☛ serving size: 1 cup = 118 g; Calories = 129

Egg Curry ☛ serving size: 1 cup = 236 g; Calories = 184

Eggplant ☛ serving size: 1 cup, cubes = 82 g; Calories = 21

Endive ☛ serving size: 1/2 cup, chopped = 25 g; Calories = 4

Enoki Mushrooms ☛ serving size: 1 large = 5 g; Calories = 2

Epazote Raw ☛ serving size: 1 tbsp = 0.8 g; Calories = 0

Eppaw Raw ☛ serving size: 1 cup = 100 g; Calories = 150

Escarole Cooked Ns As To Fat Added In Cooking ☛ serving size: 1 cup = 135 g; Calories = 64

Escarole Creamed ☛ serving size: 1 cup = 200 g; Calories = 160

Fennel ☛ serving size: 1 cup, sliced = 87 g; Calories = 27

Fireweed Leaves Raw ☛ serving size: 1 cup, chopped = 23 g; Calories = 24

Flowers Or Blossoms Of Sesbania Squash Or Lily Fat Added In Cooking ☛ serving size: 1 cup = 109 g; Calories = 39

Freeze-Dried Parsley ☛ serving size: 1 tbsp = 0.4 g; Calories = 1

Fufu ☛ serving size: 1 cup, cooked = 240 g; Calories = 374

Garden Cress ☛ serving size: 1 cup = 50 g; Calories = 16

Garlic ☛ serving size: 1 cup = 136 g; Calories = 203

Ginger ☛ serving size: 1 tsp = 2 g; Calories = 2

🥒 Gourd Dishcloth (Towelgourd) Raw ☛ serving size: 1 cup (1 inch pieces) = 95 g; Calories = 19

🥒 Grape Leaves Canned ☛ serving size: 1 leaf = 4 g; Calories = 3

🥒 Grape Leaves Raw ☛ serving size: 1 cup = 14 g; Calories = 13

🥒 Green Banana Cooked In Salt Water ☛ serving size: 1 small = 54 g; Calories = 48

🥒 Green Banana Fried ☛ serving size: 1 slice = 23 g; Calories = 34

🥒 Green Bell Peppers ☛ serving size: 1 cup, chopped = 149 g; Calories = 30

🥒 Green Cauliflower ☛ serving size: 1 cup = 64 g; Calories = 20

🥒 Green Chili Peppers ☛ serving size: 1 cup = 139 g; Calories = 29

🥒 Green Leaf Lettuce ☛ serving size: 1 cup shredded = 36 g; Calories = 5

🥒 Green Plantains Boiled ☛ serving size: 1 slice = 27 g; Calories = 31

🥒 Green Snap Beans (Raw) ☛ serving size: 1 cup 1/2 inch pieces = 100 g; Calories = 31

🥒 Green Tomatoes ☛ serving size: 1 cup = 180 g; Calories = 41

🥒 Homemade Mashed Potatoes With Milk And Butter ☛ serving size: 1 cup = 210 g; Calories = 237

🥒 Hot Green Chili Peppers ☛ serving size: 1 pepper = 45 g; Calories = 18

🥒 Hubbard Squash ☛ serving size: 1 cup, cubes = 116 g; Calories = 46

🥒 Hungarian Peppers ☛ serving size: 1 pepper = 27 g; Calories = 8

🥒 Hyacinth-Beans Immature Seeds Raw ☛ serving size: 1 cup = 80 g; Calories = 37

🥒 Iceberg Lettuce ☛ serving size: 1 cup shredded = 72 g; Calories = 10

Irishmoss Seaweed ☛ serving size: 2 tbsp (1/8 cup) = 10 g; Calories = 5

Jai Monk's Food ☛ serving size: 1 cup = 188 g; Calories = 167

Jalapeno Peppers ☛ serving size: 1 cup, sliced = 90 g; Calories = 26

Jerusalem-Artichokes Raw ☛ serving size: 1 cup slices = 150 g; Calories = 110

Jews Ear ☛ serving size: 1 cup slices = 99 g; Calories = 25

Jute Potherb Raw ☛ serving size: 1 cup = 28 g; Calories = 10

Kale ☛ serving size: 1 cup 1 inch pieces, loosely packed = 16 g; Calories = 6

Kanpyo ☛ serving size: 1 strip = 6.3 g; Calories = 16

Kelp Seaweed ☛ serving size: 2 tbsp (1/8 cup) = 10 g; Calories = 4

Ketchup ☛ serving size: 1 tbsp = 17 g; Calories = 17

Kidney Bean Sprouts ☛ serving size: 1 cup = 184 g; Calories = 53

Kimchi ☛ serving size: 1 cup = 150 g; Calories = 23

Kohlrabi ☛ serving size: 1 cup = 135 g; Calories = 37

Lambsquarter Cooked Ns As To Fat Added In Cooking ☛ serving size: 1 cup = 185 g; Calories = 87

Laver Seaweed ☛ serving size: 10 sheets = 26 g; Calories = 9

Leeks ☛ serving size: 1 cup = 89 g; Calories = 54

Lentil Sprouts ☛ serving size: 1 cup = 77 g; Calories = 82

Lettuce Cooked Ns As To Fat Added In Cooking ☛ serving size: 1 cup = 86 g; Calories = 43

Lima Beans Immature Seeds Raw ☛ serving size: 1 cup = 156 g; Calories = 176

🥬 Lotus Root 🖝 serving size: 10 slices (2-1/2 inch dia) = 81 g; Calories = 60

🥬 Luffa Cooked Ns As To Fat Added In Cooking 🖝 serving size: 1 cup = 183 g; Calories = 84

🥬 Maitake Mushrooms 🖝 serving size: 1 cup diced = 70 g; Calories = 22

🥬 Mashed Sweet Potatoes 🖝 serving size: 1 cup = 255 g; Calories = 258

🥬 Morel Mushrooms 🖝 serving size: 1 cup = 66 g; Calories = 21

🥬 Mountain Yam Hawaii Raw 🖝 serving size: 1/2 cup, cubes = 68 g; Calories = 46

🥬 Mung Bean Sprouts 🖝 serving size: 1 cup = 104 g; Calories = 31

🥬 Mushroom Asian Cooked From Dried 🖝 serving size: 1 cup = 145 g; Calories = 81

🥬 Mustard Greens 🖝 serving size: 1 cup, chopped = 56 g; Calories = 15

🥬 New Zealand Spinach 🖝 serving size: 1 cup, chopped = 56 g; Calories = 8

🥬 Nopales 🖝 serving size: 1 cup, sliced = 86 g; Calories = 14

🥬 Okra 🖝 serving size: 1 cup = 100 g; Calories = 33

🥬 Onion Rings Breaded Par Fried Frozen Unprepared 🖝 serving size: 6 rings = 85 g; Calories = 219

🥬 Onion Rings From Fresh Batter-Dipped Baked Or Fried 🖝 serving size: 10 small rings (1" - 2" dia) = 48 g; Calories = 157

🥬 Onions 🖝 serving size: 1 cup, chopped = 160 g; Calories = 64

🥬 Onions Pearl Cooked Ns As To Form 🖝 serving size: 1 cup = 185 g; Calories = 52

Onions Young Green Tops Only ☛ serving size: 1 tbsp = 6 g; Calories = 2

Oriental Radishes ☛ serving size: 1 cup slices = 116 g; Calories = 21

Oyster Mushrooms ☛ serving size: 1 large = 148 g; Calories = 49

Pak-Choi (Bok Choy) (Cooked) ☛ serving size: 1 cup, shredded = 170 g; Calories = 20

Palak Paneer ☛ serving size: 1 cup = 200 g; Calories = 192

Palm Hearts (Canned) ☛ serving size: 1 cup = 146 g; Calories = 41

Parsley ☛ serving size: 1 cup chopped = 60 g; Calories = 22

Parsnips ☛ serving size: 1 cup slices = 133 g; Calories = 100

Pea Salad ☛ serving size: 1 cup = 214 g; Calories = 383

Pea Sprouts ☛ serving size: 1 cup = 120 g; Calories = 149

Peas ☛ serving size: 1 cup = 145 g; Calories = 118

Peas And Carrots Cooked Ns As To Form Made With Margarine ☛ serving size: 1 cup = 165 g; Calories = 102

Peas Green Cooked From Frozen Ns As To Fat Added In Cooking ☛ serving size: 1 cup = 165 g; Calories = 155

Pepeao Dried ☛ serving size: 1 cup = 24 g; Calories = 72

Pepper Raw Nfs ☛ serving size: 1 piece = 10 g; Calories = 2

Pepper Sweet Red Raw ☛ serving size: 1 piece = 10 g; Calories = 3

Peppers Hot Chili Green Canned Pods Excluding Seeds Solids And Liquids ☛ serving size: 1 pepper = 73 g; Calories = 15

Peppers Hot Chili Red Canned Excluding Seeds Solids And Liquids ☛ serving size: 1 pepper = 73 g; Calories = 15

Peppers Hot Pickled Canned ☛ serving size: 1/4 cup drained = 34 g; Calories = 8

🥒 Peppers Jalapeno Canned Solids And Liquids ☛ serving size: 1 cup, chopped = 136 g; Calories = 37

🥒 Pickled Beets ☛ serving size: 1 cup slices = 227 g; Calories = 148

🥒 Pickles Chowchow With Cauliflower Onion Mustard Sweet ☛ serving size: 1 cup = 245 g; Calories = 297

🥒 Pigeon Peas Cooked From Fresh Ns As To Fat Added In Cooking ☛ serving size: 1 cup = 158 g; Calories = 199

🥒 Pinacbet ☛ serving size: 1 cup = 214 g; Calories = 96

🥒 Plantain Boiled Ns As To Green Or Ripe ☛ serving size: 1 slice = 27 g; Calories = 31

🥒 Poi ☛ serving size: 1 cup = 240 g; Calories = 269

🥒 Poke Greens Cooked Fat Added In Cooking Ns As To Type Of Fat ☛ serving size: 1 cup = 160 g; Calories = 59

🥒 Pokeberry Shoots (Poke) Raw ☛ serving size: 1 cup = 160 g; Calories = 37

🥒 Portobellos (Exposed To Sunlight Or Uv) ☛ serving size: 1 cup sliced = 121 g; Calories = 35

🥒 Portobellos Mushrooms ☛ serving size: 1 cup diced = 86 g; Calories = 19

🥒 Potato Baked Nfs ☛ serving size: 1 small = 230 g; Calories = 214

🥒 Potatoes French Fried All Types Salt Not Added In Processing Frozen Oven-Heated ☛ serving size: 10 strip = 74 g; Calories = 124

🥒 Potatoes Mashed Dehydrated Granules With Milk Dry Form ☛ serving size: 1 cup = 200 g; Calories = 714

🥒 Potatoes Mashed Dehydrated Granules Without Milk Dry Form ☛ serving size: 1 cup = 200 g; Calories = 744

Potatoes Yellow Fleshed Roasted Salt Added In Processing Frozen Unprepared ☛ serving size: 3 oz = 85 g; Calories = 101

Pumpkin Canned With Salt ☛ serving size: 1 cup = 245 g; Calories = 83

Pumpkin Cooked From Canned Fat Not Added In Cooking ☛ serving size: 1 cup = 245 g; Calories = 83

Pumpkin Raw ☛ serving size: 1 cup (1 inch cubes) = 116 g; Calories = 30

Purslane ☛ serving size: 1 cup = 43 g; Calories = 9

Radicchio ☛ serving size: 1 cup, shredded = 40 g; Calories = 9

Radish Daikon Cooked Ns As To Fat Added In Cooking ☛ serving size: 1 cup = 153 g; Calories = 66

Radish Sprouts ☛ serving size: 1 cup = 38 g; Calories = 16

Radishes ☛ serving size: 1 cup slices = 116 g; Calories = 19

Radishes Hawaiian Style Pickled ☛ serving size: 1 cup = 150 g; Calories = 42

Radishes Oriental Cooked Boiled Drained With Salt ☛ serving size: 1 cup slices = 147 g; Calories = 25

Radishes Oriental Dried ☛ serving size: 1 cup = 116 g; Calories = 314

Ratatouille ☛ serving size: 1 cup = 214 g; Calories = 139

Raw Cremini Mushrooms (Exposed To Sunlight Or Uv) ☛ serving size: 1 cup whole = 87 g; Calories = 19

Raw Portobellos (Exposed To Sunlight Or Uv) ☛ serving size: 1 cup diced = 86 g; Calories = 19

Red Cabbage ☛ serving size: 1 cup, chopped = 89 g; Calories = 28

Red Chili Peppers ☛ serving size: 1 pepper = 45 g; Calories = 18

Red Leaf Lettuce ☞ serving size: 1 cup shredded = 28 g; Calories = 4

Romaine Lettuce ☞ serving size: 1 cup shredded = 47 g; Calories = 8

Rutabagas (Neeps Swedes) ☞ serving size: 1 cup, cubes = 140 g; Calories = 52

Salsify (Vegetable Oyster) Raw ☞ serving size: 1 cup slices = 133 g; Calories = 109

Salsify Cooked Ns As To Fat Added In Cooking ☞ serving size: 1 cup = 140 g; Calories = 122

Sambar Vegetable Stew ☞ serving size: 1 cup = 248 g; Calories = 208

Sauerkraut ☞ serving size: 1 cup = 142 g; Calories = 27

Sauteed Green Bell Peppers ☞ serving size: 1 cup chopped = 115 g; Calories = 133

Savoy Cabbage ☞ serving size: 1 cup, shredded = 70 g; Calories = 19

Scallop Squash ☞ serving size: 1 cup slices = 130 g; Calories = 23

Seaweed Agar Raw ☞ serving size: 2 tbsp (1/8 cup) = 10 g; Calories = 3

Seaweed Canadian Cultivated Emi-Tsunomata Dry ☞ serving size: 1/4 cup = 5 g; Calories = 13

Seaweed Canadian Cultivated Emi-Tsunomata Rehydrated ☞ serving size: 1/4 cup = 25 g; Calories = 8

Seaweed Raw ☞ serving size: 1 cup = 80 g; Calories = 30

Serrano Peppers ☞ serving size: 1 cup, chopped = 105 g; Calories = 34

Sesbania Flower Raw ☞ serving size: 1 flower = 3 g; Calories = 1

Shallots ☛ serving size: 1 tbsp chopped = 10 g; Calories = 7

Shiitake Mushrooms ☛ serving size: 1 piece whole = 19 g; Calories = 7

Snow Peas ☛ serving size: 1 cup, chopped = 98 g; Calories = 41

Sour Pickled Cucumber ☛ serving size: 1 cup = 155 g; Calories = 17

Soybean Sprouts ☛ serving size: 1/2 cup = 35 g; Calories = 43

Spaghetti Squash ☛ serving size: 1 cup, cubes = 101 g; Calories = 31

Spinach ☛ serving size: 1 cup = 30 g; Calories = 7

Spinach Cooked From Frozen Ns As To Fat Added In Cooking ☛ serving size: 1 cup, frozen, leaf = 195 g; Calories = 96

Spring Onions ☛ serving size: 1 cup, chopped = 100 g; Calories = 32

Squash Summer Yellow Or Green Cooked From Canned Ns As To Fat Added In Cooking ☛ serving size: 1 cup, slices = 185 g; Calories = 48

Squash Summer Yellow Or Green Cooked From Frozen Ns As To Fat Added In Cooking ☛ serving size: 1 cup, slices = 185 g; Calories = 63

Succotash ☛ serving size: 1 cup = 192 g; Calories = 221

Sweet Onions ☛ serving size: 1 nlea serving = 148 g; Calories = 47

Sweet Pickled Cucumbers ☛ serving size: 1 cup, chopped = 160 g; Calories = 146

Sweet Pickled Relish ☛ serving size: 1 tbsp = 15 g; Calories = 20

Sweet Potato Boiled Ns As To Fat Added In Cooking ☛ serving size: 1 small = 80 g; Calories = 86

Sweet Potato Candied ☛ serving size: 1 piece = 45 g; Calories = 80

🥔 Sweet Potato Nfs ☛ serving size: 1 small = 80 g; Calories = 86

🥔 Swiss Chard ☛ serving size: 1 cup = 36 g; Calories = 7

🥔 Tahitian Taro ☛ serving size: 1 cup slices = 125 g; Calories = 55

🥔 Tannier Cooked ☛ serving size: 1 cup = 190 g; Calories = 291

🥔 Taro ☛ serving size: 1 cup, sliced = 104 g; Calories = 117

🥔 Taro Leaves Raw ☛ serving size: 1 cup = 28 g; Calories = 12

🥔 Taro Shoots Raw ☛ serving size: 1/2 cup slices = 43 g; Calories = 5

🥔 Tomatillos ☛ serving size: 1 medium = 34 g; Calories = 11

🥔 Tomato Aspic ☛ serving size: 1 cup = 227 g; Calories = 64

🥔 Tomato Juice Canned With Salt Added ☛ serving size: 1 cup = 243 g; Calories = 41

🥔 Tomato Juice Canned Without Salt Added ☛ serving size: 1 cup = 243 g; Calories = 41

🥔 Tomato Products Canned Puree With Salt Added ☛ serving size: 1 cup = 250 g; Calories = 95

🥔 Tomato Products Canned Sauce ☛ serving size: 1 cup = 245 g; Calories = 59

🥔 Tomatoes ☛ serving size: 1 cup cherry tomatoes = 149 g; Calories = 27

🥔 Tomatoes Sun-Dried Packed In Oil Drained ☛ serving size: 1 cup = 110 g; Calories = 234

🥔 Turnip Cooked From Fresh Ns As To Fat Added In Cooking ☛ serving size: 1 cup, pieces = 160 g; Calories = 64

🥔 Turnip Cooked From Frozen Ns As To Fat Added In Cooking ☛ serving size: 1 cup, pieces = 160 g; Calories = 66

🥔 Wakame ☛ serving size: 2 tbsp (1/8 cup) = 10 g; Calories = 5

🥒 Wasabi Root ☛ serving size: 1 cup, sliced = 130 g; Calories = 142

🥒 Water Chestnut ☛ serving size: 1 cup = 158 g; Calories = 123

🥒 Waterchestnuts Chinese (Matai) Raw ☛ serving size: 1/2 cup slices = 62 g; Calories = 60

🥒 Waterchestnuts Chinese Canned Solids And Liquids ☛ serving size: 1/2 cup slices = 70 g; Calories = 35

🥒 Watercress ☛ serving size: 1 cup, chopped = 34 g; Calories = 4

🥒 Watercress Cooked Ns As To Fat Added In Cooking ☛ serving size: 1 cup = 142 g; Calories = 43

🥒 Waxgourd (Chinese Preserving Melon) Raw ☛ serving size: 1 cup, cubes = 132 g; Calories = 17

🥒 White Button Mushrooms ☛ serving size: 1 cup, pieces or slices = 70 g; Calories = 15

🥒 Winged Beans Immature Seeds Raw ☛ serving size: 1 cup slices = 44 g; Calories = 22

🥒 Winter Melon Cooked ☛ serving size: 1 cup = 175 g; Calories = 25

🥒 Winter Squash ☛ serving size: 1 cup, cubes = 116 g; Calories = 39

🥒 Witloof Chicory ☛ serving size: 1 head = 53 g; Calories = 9

🥒 Yam ☛ serving size: 1 cup, cubes = 150 g; Calories = 177

🥒 Yambean (Jicama) Raw ☛ serving size: 1 cup slices = 120 g; Calories = 46

🥒 Yardlong Bean Raw ☛ serving size: 1 cup slices = 91 g; Calories = 43

🥒 Yautia ☛ serving size: 1 cup, sliced = 135 g; Calories = 132

🥒 Yellow Onions ☛ serving size: 1 cup chopped = 87 g; Calories = 107

🥒 Yellow Snap Beans ☛ serving size: 1 cup 1/2 inch pieces = 100 g; Calories = 31

Yellow Sweet Corn ☞ serving size: 1 cup = 145 g; Calories = 125

Yellow Tomatoes ☞ serving size: 1 cup, chopped = 139 g; Calories = 21

Yuca Fries ☞ serving size: 1 cup = 140 g; Calories = 374

Zucchini ☞ serving size: 1 cup, chopped = 124 g; Calories = 21

HEALTH AND NUTRITION WEBSITES

American Diabetes Association

(www.diabetes.org)

American Heart Association

(www.americanheart.org)

Centers for Disease Control and Prevention

(www.cdc.gov/healthyweight)

Cooking Light

(www.cookinglight.com)

Eating Well

(www.eatingwell.com)

eMedicine Health

(www.emedicinehealth.com)

Fruits and Vegetables Matter

(www.fruitsandveggiesmatter.gov)

Health

(www.health.com)

Hormone Foundation

(www.hormone.org)

National Heart, Lung, Blood Institute

(www.nhlbi.nih.gov)

National Institute on Aging

(www.nia.nih.gov)

National Institutes of Health

(http://health.nih.gov)

Nutrition.gov (www.nutrition.gov)

Prevention (www.prevention.com)

Printed in Great Britain
by Amazon

81535429R00322